Anthikad's
APPLIED PSYCHOLOGY
for Graduate Nurses

Anthikad's
APPLIED PSYCHOLOGY
for Graduate Nurses
(General and Educational Psychology)

As per the Revised Syllabus for BSc Nursing

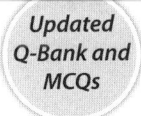

Sixth Edition

Revised and Edited by
Deepa Marina Rasquinha MA MPhil PhD
Assistant Professor
Department of Clinical Psychology
Manipal College of Health Professions
Manipal, Karnataka, India

Foreword
Kavyashree KB

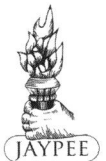

JAYPEE BROTHERS MEDICAL PUBLISHERS
The Health Sciences Publisher
New Delhi | London

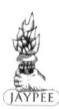 **Jaypee Brothers Medical Publishers (P) Ltd.**

Headquarters
Jaypee Brothers Medical Publishers (P) Ltd
EMCA House
23/23-B, Ansari Road, Daryaganj
New Delhi - 110 002, India
Landline: +91-11-23272143, +91-11-23272703
+91-11-23282021, +91-11-23245672
Email: jaypee@jaypeebrothers.com

Corporate Office
Jaypee Brothers Medical Publishers (P) Ltd
4838/24, Ansari Road, Daryaganj
New Delhi 110 002, India
Phone: +91-11-43574357
Fax: +91-11-43574314
Email: jaypee@jaypeebrothers.com

Overseas Office
J.P. Medical Ltd
83 Victoria Street, London
SW1H 0HW (UK)
Phone: +44 20 3170 8910
Fax: +44 (0)20 3008 6180
Email: info@jpmedpub.com

Website: www.jaypeebrothers.com

Website: www.jaypeedigital.com

© 2023, Jaypee Brothers Medical Publishers

The views and opinions expressed in this book are solely those of the original contributor(s)/author(s) and do not necessarily represent those of editor(s) and publisher of the book.

All rights reserved. No part of this publication may be reproduced, stored or transmitted in any form or by any means, electronic, mechanical, photocopying, recording or otherwise, without the prior permission in writing of the publishers.

All brand names and product names used in this book are trade names, service marks, trademarks or registered trademarks of their respective owners. The publisher is not associated with any product or vendor mentioned in this book.

Medical knowledge and practice change constantly. This book is designed to provide accurate, authoritative information about the subject matter in question. However, readers are advised to check the most current information available on procedures included and check information from the manufacturer of each product to be administered, to verify the recommended dose, formula, method and duration of administration, adverse effects and contraindications. It is the responsibility of the practitioner to take all appropriate safety precautions. Neither the publisher nor the author(s)/editor(s) assume any liability for any injury and/or damage to persons or property arising from or related to use of material in this book.

This book is sold on the understanding that the publisher is not engaged in providing professional medical services. If such advice or services are required, the services of a competent medical professional should be sought.

Every effort has been made where necessary to contact holders of copyright to obtain permission to reproduce copyright material. If any have been inadvertently overlooked, the publisher will be pleased to make the necessary arrangements at the first opportunity.

Inquiries for bulk sales may be solicited at: jaypee@jaypeebrothers.com

Anthikad's Applied Psychology for Graduate Nurses

First Edition	:	1998
Second Edition	:	2001
Third Edition	:	2004
Reprint	:	2005
Fourth Edition	:	2007
Reprint	:	2008, 2009, 2011
Fifth Edition	:	2014
Sixth Edition	:	**2023**

ISBN: 978-93-5465-680-4

Printed at: Sterling Graphics Pvt. Ltd., Manesar

Dedicated to

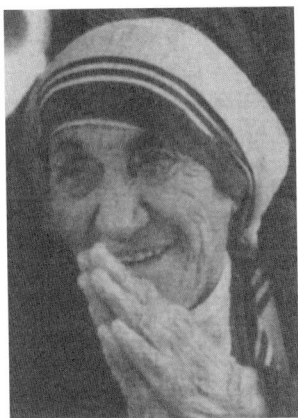

Blessed Mother Teresa
who has given a new meaning to the word compassion in reaching out to the destitutes and the lonely. Generations of student nurses will be inspired by her noble work among the poorest of the poor.

And
My beloved uncle Late Joy Moras,
My mother AE Moras,
My husband Peter Frank and
My daughter Kiara Frank

FOREWORD

I am delighted to pen down this foreword not because I know **Dr Deepa Marina Rasquinha,** Assistant Professor, Department of Clinical Psychology, Manipal College of Health Professions-Manipal Academy of Higher Education (MCHP-MAHE), Manipal, Karnataka, India, but also because she is my teacher and mentor, and I believe deeply in the hard work she puts into the task assigned to her to make it best.

The book *"Anthikad's Applied Psychology for Graduate Nurses"* authored by Dr Deepa provides a simple and clear explanation of the concepts in Psychology that can be easily related to the nursing field. The book covers contemporary aspects of psychology in nursing and the application of psychology concepts with examples and theories which have enriched the content of the book.

I am sure that the meticulous work and dedication put forward to write this book meets and covers the entire curriculum for various nursing courses as prescribed by different universities and also the Nursing Council of India. It is my hope that this book will provide an effective learning experience as a textbook and referenced resource for all nursing professionals leading to optimal client care. May all derive benefit from it.

Kavyashree KB MSc PhD (Psychology)
Assistant Professor
Department of Clinical Psychology
Manipal College of Health Professions-
Manipal Academy of Higher Education
Manipal, Karnataka, India

PREFACE TO THE SIXTH EDITION

Psychology is a science that provides better understanding of behavior. The sixth edition of *Anthikad's Applied Psychology for Graduate Nurses* integrates a variety of topics from the field that foster students' understanding of psychology and its impact on their everyday lives. I feel much relieved after years of effort put forth have been fruitful. Among the variety of changes incorporated, I am happy that edition includes details of important concepts depicted in table and the concepts are also explained with relevant examples and research evidences which helps students to get quick review of the topics included in the chapter. The modules/chapters are thoroughly revised including chapter outline, learning objectives in the beginning of each module. Key points and study questions have been appended at the end of each chapter as suggested that include essay questions, short answers and multiple choice questions (MCQs). As the book has been recommended for MSc (N) also, the following theories of personality development find brief mention in Developmental Psychology (Chapter 18) for the benefit of postgraduate students:

- Havighurst's Development Tasks Model
- Kohlberg's Moral Development
- Mahler's Theory of Object Relationships
- Hildegard E Peplau's Theory of Interpersonal Relations

In this edition as per the INC guidelines a special chapter on Soft Skills and Nursing Empowerment is being included.

Deepa Marina Rasquinha

PREFACE TO THE FIRST EDITION

My teaching experience of the last four decades has convinced me that a nursing student will be relieved of her anxiety to take down notes, if she has a concise textbook covering the subject matter, thereby she can concentrate more on the classroom lecture.

The absence of such a textbook covering general psychology and educational psychology is a serious handicap felt by students and teachers alike, and here is a sincere attempt to fill the gap. This book can be used as a textbook for physiotherapy students as well.

The author has consulted most of the books available on psychology and most gratefully acknowledges the help of the many sources used in the preparation of this text.

Although great care has been taken in writing the subject matter, it is likely that the author might have committed some errors and misconceptions of which he is not aware. Comments and criticism from teachers and students will, therefore, be appreciated and incorporated in subsequent editions.

I am particularly grateful to Shri Jitendar P Vij (Chairman and Managing Director) and other staff of M/s Jaypee Brothers Medical Publishers (P) Ltd., New Delhi, India, without whose efforts this book would not have come out in time and in such an elegant form.

Jacob Anthikad

ACKNOWLEDGMENTS

Working on this book has been an overwhelming experience, exploring more areas and incorporating more ideas. On completion of this book I would like to thank each and everyone who were a part of this journey and helped me through it successfully.

Firstly, I thank God Almighty for granting boundless blessings, knowledge and opportunity to accomplish this goal.

I am extraordinarily grateful to my colleagues and students at Manipal Academy of Higher Education for their support and encouragement.

My sincere thanks to my Psychology teachers, Dr YT Balakrishna Acharya, Professor Kareem Mukhdham, Professor Ganesh Rao, Professor Gopal Patwardhan and Dr MY Manjula for being amazing subject experts and training me to apply the knowledge of Psychology throughout my life.

I remain completely indebted to my family. My parents, AE Moras and *Late* Frank Rasquinha, for their love and support. I am grateful to my husband Peter Frank, who is a constant source of inspiration beyond my expectations. With immense love I take this opportunity to thank my daughter Kiara Frank. My extended family also plays a central role in my life and I remain ever grateful to all of them.

I also offer great thanks to the whole team of M/s Jaypee Brothers Medical Publishers (P) Ltd., New Delhi, India, for all their support to work in this project and make it a success. I extend my thanks to Shri Jitendar P Vij (Group Chairman), Mr Ankit Vij (Managing Director), Mr MS Mani (Group President), Dr Madhu Choudhary (Director-Educational Publishing), Ms Pooja Bhandari (Production Head), Ms Sunita Katla (Executive Assistant to Group Chairman and Publishing Manager), Ms Samina Khan (Executive Assistant to Director-Educational Publishing), Jitika Royal (Development Editor), Mr Rajesh Sharma (Production Coordinator), Ms Seema Dogra (Cover Visualizer), Mr Kapil Dev Sharma (DTP Operator), Mr Rahul Jadli (Proofreader), and Mr Ankush Sharma (Graphic Designer) of M/s Jaypee Brothers Medical Publishers (P) Ltd., New Delhi, India for this opportunity.

Last but not the least, I would like to thank Mr Santhosh Kumar (Senior Executive Key Accounts) of Bengaluru Branch for his support in completing this project.

CONTENTS

1. **Psychology and its Relation to Nursing** — 1
   Definition of Psychology   2
   Importance of Psychology   11
   Psychology and Nursing   12

2. **Body-Mind Relationship** — 18
   Integrated Responses   18
   The Behaving Organism   20
   Levels of Functioning or Levels of Consciousness   20

3. **Biology of Behavior** — 24
   Nervous System   24
   Sense Organs: Psychology of Sensations   29
   Muscular Control of Behavior   29

4. **Nature and Nurture: Individual Differences** — 34
   Nature—Heredity   34
   Nurture—Environment   35
   The Nature-Nurture Controversy   41

5. **Observation: Attention, Sensation, and Perception** — 44
   Attention   45
   Observation   49
   Parapsychology   57

6. **The Learning Process** — 61
   Domains or Types of Learning   62
   Modes of Learning   63
   Steps in Learning Process   76
   Factors Influencing Learning   76
   Transfer of Learning   78
   Learning and the Nurse   79

7. **Memory: Remembering and Forgetting** — 83
   Three Stages of Memory   84
   Factors Influencing Memory   87
   Remembering and Forgetting   90
   Process of Memory and Recall   91
   Forgetting   92

Methods to Improve Memory 98
Studying to Remember 99

8. **Thinking and Reasoning: Concept and Language** 103
   Kinds of Thinking 104
   Errors in Thinking 109

9. **Intelligence and its Measurement** 117
   Definitions of Intelligence 117
   Types of Intelligence 118
   Theories of Intelligence 118
   Assessment of Intelligence 127
   Types of Intelligence Tests 130
   Limitations of the Concept of IQ 131
   Individual Differences 132
   Practical Experiment 137

10. **Aptitudes (Capacity or Innate Potential)** 141
    Aptitude 141
    Practical Experiment 142

11. **Motivation** 146
    Types of Motivation 147
    Motive 147
    Theories of Motivation 151
    Motivation and the Nurse 155

12. **Frustration and Conflicts** 159
    Sources of Frustration 160
    Reactions to Frustration 165

13. **Stress and its Management** 170
    Symptoms of Stress 171
    Sources of Stress 172
    Types of Stress 172
    Emotional Reactions to Hospitalization 175
    Adaptation Theory (Dr Hans Selye) (1945) 175

14. **Defense Mechanisms** 181
    Anxiety and Fear 181
    Adjustment Mechanism or Defense Mechanism 182

15. **Emotions in Health and Disease** 194
    Importance of Emotions 200
    Emotions and Disease 200
    Development of Emotions 201

An Emotion Acts as a Motive   201
Theories of Emotions   202
States of Emotion   205
The Nurse and Control of Emotions   206

16. Attitude: The Way We See Things   210
Positive and Negative Attitudes   215

17. Personality (Is What the Man is)   220
Classifications of Personality   221
Theories of Personality Development   224
The Five Factor Model or the Five Traits Theory   233
Methods/Techniques of Personality Assessment   233
Assessment of Personality   234
Personality Development   237

18. Developmental Psychology   244
Nature–Nurture Debate   245
Development: Continuous or in Stages   245
Stability or Change Issue   245
Emotional Development in Children   246
Development in the Life Cycle   248
Eight Psychosocial Stages of Erikson   250

19. Mental Health and Mental Illness   265
Mental Hygiene Movement   266
Medical Classification of Mental Illness (World Health Organization)   267
Mental Health—its Meaning and Nature   267
Foundations of Mental Health   269
Role of Nurses in Psychotherapy   271
Shared Responsibility   274
Counseling   274

20. Psychological Tests: Measurement of Individual Differences   279
Kinds of Psychological Tests   279
Prerequisites of a Test: Reliability and Validity   282

21. Attributions: Our Explanations of Behavior   285
Pan Posthema's Case   286
Attributional Biases: Different Attribution for Ourselves and Others   286
Changing Attributions   287
Results and Conclusion   288
Factors Influencing Attributions   288

Modifying our Attributes 289
Attributions and the Nurse 289

22. Educational Psychology: Scope and Methods — 292
Education 292
Psychology 293
Educational Psychology 294

23. Effective Teaching — 300
Education as a Process of Communication 300
Transmission 304
Training Aids: Value and Characteristic 307
Curriculum Appraisal 308
Lesson Plan 309
For Effective Health Teaching 314

24. Role and Functions of a Teacher — 316
Instructional Role 316
Faculty Role 317
Individual Role 317
Qualities of a Good Teacher 317
Characteristics of Effective Teaching 318

25. Evaluation — 321
General Functions of Evaluation 321
Principles of Evaluation 322
Methods of Evaluation 323
Evaluation of Instruction 323
Benefits of Evaluation 324
Qualities of a Good Test 324
Types of Tests 325

26. Our Social World — 328
Scope of Social Psychology 328
Group—the Unit of Study 329
Antisocial Behavior 329
Staff Groups in Hospitals 330
Leadership 332

27. Soft Skills and Nursing Empowerment — 336
Soft Skills 336
Nursing Empowerment 338

Answer Keys 341

Index 343

INC SYLLABUS

APPLIED PSYCHOLOGY

PLACEMENT: I SEMESTER

THEORY: 3 Credits (60 Hours)

DESCRIPTION: This course is designed to enable the students to develop understanding about basic concepts of psychology and its application in personal and community life, health, illness and nursing. It further provides students opportunity to recognize the significance and application of soft skills and self-empowerment in the practice of nursing.

COMPETENCIES: On completion of the course, the students will be able to:

1. Identify the importance of psychology in individual and professional life.
2. Develop understanding of the biological and psychological basis of human behavior.
3. Identify the role of nurse in promoting mental health and dealing with altered personality.
4. Perform the role of nurses applicable to the psychology of different age groups.
5. Identify the cognitive and affective needs of clients.
6. Integrate the principles of motivation and emotion in performing the role of nurse in caring for emotionally sick client.
7. Demonstrate basic understanding of psychological assessment and nurse's role.
8. Apply the knowledge of soft skills in workplace and society.
9. Apply the knowledge of self-empowerment in workplace, society and personal life.

COURSE OUTLINE
T – Theory

Unit	Time (Hrs)	Learning outcomes	Content	Teaching/learning activities	Assessment methods
I	2 (T)	Describe scope, branches and significance of psychology in nursing	**Introduction** • Meaning of psychology • Development of psychology: Scope, branches and methods of psychology • Relationship with other subjects • Significance of psychology in nursing • Applied psychology to solve everyday issues	Lecture-cum-discussion	• Essay • Short answer
II	4 (T)	Describe biology of human behavior	**Biological basis of behavior—Introduction** • Body-mind relationship • Genetics and behavior • Inheritance of behavior • Brain and behavior. • Psychology and sensation—sensory process—normal and abnormal	• Lecture • Discussion	• Essay • Short answer
III	5 (T)	Describe mentally healthy person and defense mechanisms	**Mental health and mental hygiene** • Concept of mental health and mental hygiene • Characteristic of mentally healthy person • Warning signs of poor mental health • Promotive and preventive mental health strategies and services • Defense mechanism and its implication • Frustration and conflict—types of conflicts and measurements to overcome	• Lecture • Case discussion • Role play	• Essay • Short answer • Objective type

Unit	Time (Hrs)	Learning outcomes	Content	Teaching/learning activities	Assessment methods
IV	7 (T)	Describe psychology of people in different age groups and role of nurse	• Role of nurse in reducing frustration and conflict and enhancing coping • Dealing with ego **Developmental psychology** • Physical, psychosocial and cognitive development across life span—prenatal through early childhood, middle to late childhood through adolescence, early and mid-adulthood, late adulthood, death and dying • Role of nurse in supporting normal growth and development across the life span • Psychological needs of various groups in health and sickness: Infancy, childhood, adolescence, adulthood and older adult • Introduction to child psychology and role of nurse in meeting the psychological needs of children • Psychology of vulnerable individuals —challenged, women, sick, etc. • Role of nurse with vulnerable groups	• Lecture • Group discussion	• Essay • Short answer
V	4 (T)	Explain personality and role of nurse in identification and improvement in altered personality	**Personality** • Meaning, definition of personality • Classification of personality • Measurement and evaluation of personality—Introduction	• Lecture • Discussion • Demonstration	• Essay and short answer • Objective type

Unit	Time (Hrs)	Learning outcomes	Content	Teaching/learning activities	Assessment methods
			• Alteration in personality • Role of nurse in identification of individual personality and improvement in altered personality		
VI	16 (T)	Explain cognitive process and their applications	**Cognitive process** • **Attention**—definition, types, determinants, duration, degree and alteration in attention • **Perception**—meaning of Perception, principles, factor affecting perception, • **Intelligence**—meaning of intelligence: Effect of heredity and environment in intelligence, classification, introduction to measurement of intelligence tests—mental deficiencies • **Learning**—definition of learning, types of learning, factors influencing learning—learning process, habit formation • **Memory**—meaning and nature of memory, factors influencing memory, methods to improve memory, forgetting • **Thinking**—types, level, reasoning and problem solving • **Aptitude**—concept, types, individual differences and variability • Psychometric assessment of cognitive processes—Introduction • Alteration in cognitive processes	• Lecture • Discussion	• Essay and short answer • Objective type

INC Syllabus

Unit	Time (Hrs)	Learning outcomes	Content	Teaching/learning activities	Assessment methods
VII	6 (T)	Describe motivation, emotion, attitude and role of nurse in emotionally sick client	**Motivation and emotional processes** • **Motivation**—meaning, concept, types, theories of motivation, motivation cycle, biological and special motives • **Emotions**—meaning of emotions, development of emotions, alteration of emotion, emotions in sickness—handling emotions in self and other • **Stress and adaptation**—stress, stressor, cycle, effect, adaptation and coping • **Attitudes**—meaning of attitudes, nature, factor affecting attitude, attitudinal change, role of attitude in health and sickness • **Psychometric assessment of emotions and attitude—Introduction** • Role of nurse in caring for emotionally sick client	• Lecture • Group discussion	• Essay and short answer • Objective type
VIII	4 (T)	Explain psychological assessment and tests and role of nurse	**Psychological assessment and tests—introduction** • Types, development, characteristics, principles, uses, interpretation • Role of nurse in psychological assessment	• Lecture • Discussion • Demonstration	• Short answer • Assessment of practice
IX	10 (T)	Explain concept of soft skill and its application in work place and society	**Application of soft skill** • Concept of soft skill • **Types of soft skill**—visual, aural and communication skill • The way of communication	• Lecture • Group discussion • Role play • Refer/complete soft skills module	• Essay and short answer

Unit	Time (Hrs)	Learning outcomes	Content	Teaching/learning activities	Assessment methods
			• Building relationship with client and society • **Interpersonal relationships (IPR):** Definition, types, and purposes, interpersonal skills, barriers, strategies to overcome barriers • **Survival strategies**—managing time, coping stress, resilience, work—life balance • Applying soft skill to workplace and society—presentation skills, social etiquette, telephone etiquette, motivational skills, teamwork, etc. • Use of soft skill in nursing		
X	2 (T)	Explain self-empowerment	**Self-empowerment** • Dimensions of self-empowerment • Self-empowerment development • Importance of women's empowerment in society • Professional etiquette and personal grooming • Role of nurse in empowering others	• Lecture • Discussion	• Short answer • Objective type

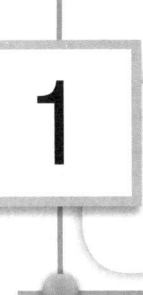

Psychology and its Relation to Nursing

"Mental disorders arise from physical ones and likewise physical disorders arise from mental ones".
—***Mahabharata***

Chapter Outline

- Psychology
- Introspection
- SQ4R
- Clinical Method
- Experimental Method
- Survey Method
- Structuralism
- Functionalism
- Psychoanalysis
- Gestalt
- Humanism
- Pure/Applied Fields of Psychology

Learning Objectives

♦ Students will be introduced to definition, schools/perspectives, scope, and methods in psychology.
♦ Orients nursing students to the relevance of psychology.

INTRODUCTION

The beginnings of psychology are to be found in the curiosity of primitive man about himself and his companions. The development of psychology as a science has followed a long and somewhat uncertain course through the centuries.

Psychology was considered to be a branch of philosophy until 1870s. The Greeks were the first to study mental illness scientifically and separate the study of the mind from religion. Aristotle (384–322 BC) described mind as a function of bodily processes. He emphasized the release of repressed emotions for effective treatment of mental diseases. Hippocrates (460–370 BC), father of medicine ruled out the possibilities of deities as the cause of mental diseases. They are due to brain pathology. With the fall of Roman Empire, superstitions came to dominate human thinking for many centuries. During the middle ages, the mentally ill were not considered as outcasts but as people to be helped. St. Augustin believed that although God acted directly in human affairs, people were responsible for their own actions.

In 1547, the monastery of St. Mary of Bethlehem in London was officially converted into a mental asylum. Rene Descartes introduced the idea of **dualism**, which asserted that the mind and body were two things that interact to form the human experience. The 17th Century British Philosopher John Locke believed that children are born into the world with minds like "blank slates" (*tabula rasa* in Latin) and experiences determined what kind of adults they would become.

In 1773, the first mental hospital in the US was built in Williamsburg, Virginia. In 1793, Philippe Pinel (1745-1826) removed the chains from mentally ill patients confined in BICETRE, a hospital outside Paris, thus bringing about the first revolution in psychiatry. In 1908, Clifford Beers, wrote the book, "the Mind that found itself" based on his bitter experiences in the mental hospital. He founded the American Mental Health Association, which made a major contribution to improve the condition of mental hospitals.

DEFINITION OF PSYCHOLOGY

It was in the year 1590 that Rudolf Goeckle used the word Psychology. It is derived from two Greek words "Psyche" and "logos". "Psyche" means soul or spirit. "Logos" means knowledge or study of. Psychology thus was the study of the soul. The word soul was used vaguely and attained religious significance with the rise of Christianity. Therefore, William James (1842-1910) used the term "mind" in place of soul in 1890. But this definition also became unsatisfactory because mind was abstract and could not be seen or understood, unless what the mind did was seen. Behavior is what the mind does. Therefore, psychology was defined by Watson as the scientific study of behavior and mental processes. Behavior includes all our outward or covert actions and reactions, such as talking, facial expressions, and movement. Mental processes, refer to all internal covert activity of our mind, such as thinking, feeling, remembering, etc. Clifford T Morgan says "Psychology is the science of human and animal behavior and it includes the application of this science to solve human problems".

Behavior is classified as described in **Table 1**.

Table 1: Classifications of behavior.

Types	Meaning	Activity (Examples)	Nature
Cognitive	Mental	Thinking, perception	Cannot be observed
Conative	Motor	Swimming, walking	Observable
Affective	Emotional	Feeling happy, sad	Observable

NL Munn defines "Psychology is the science of human behavior".

Defining psychology as the scientific study of behavior does not exclude mind and other internal processes from the field of psychology; what a person does—his or her behavior—is the outcome of the internal mental processes.

Psychology is a Positive Science

A science is a body of systematized knowledge that is gathered carefully observing and measuring events. Psychologists do experiments and make observations, which others can repeat and verify. It is this method of science that distinguishes psychology from art and philosophy.

Objectivity, reliability, validity, and predictability are characteristics of science.

Behavioral sciences are concerned with the observation and explanation of human behavior either in single individuals or in groups.

Behavior includes all human activities—motor activities like walking and speaking, cognitive activities, such as perceiving, remembering, thinking, or reasoning and emotional activities like feeling happy, angry, or sad. Behavior includes all our reactions and responses to the environmental stimuli. Behavior is anything that can be observed.

Psychology is related to many other behavioral sciences like anthropology (study of man in different cultures), sociology (study of human behavior in a group) geography, history and economics, which study various aspects of human behavior.

Psychology is a very young science having separated from philosophy in 1879 when Wilhelm Wundt (1832–1920) established the first psychological laboratory in the University of Leipzig, Germany. Wundt was the first to measure human behavior accurately and is called the "Father of Psychology". Titchner, James, Pavlov, Watson, Skinner, Freud, Rogers, and Maslow were all important in the different areas of development of psychology as a science.

Systems of Psychology or Schools of Psychology

Structuralism

Like complex chemical compounds are made of elements, psychologists made a similar approach and started looking for mental elements of which complex phenomena were composed of. As water was analyzed into elements hydrogen and oxygen by chemists, the taste of lemonade (a perception) was considered to be composed of psychological elements (sensations), such as sweet, sour, salt, and bitter. These elements were arrived at by the method of careful, trained introspection (i.e., looking within oneself). Use of introspection as the sole procedure for understanding mental elements was mainly due to the work of EB Titchner (1867–1927), an American Student of Wundt. This system is called structuralism, because it proposes to describe the mental structure. The school mainly focused on "what happens" when we engage in mental activity. Presently, this system has only historical importance.

Functionalism

Psychologists like William James of Harvard University did experiments on ways in which learning, memory, problem solving, and motivation helped people and animals adapt to their environment. The school was interested in knowing the functions of mind and behavior. Functions mean one of two things:
1. How the mind operates, that is, how the elements of the mind work together?
2. How mental processes promote adaptation?

Functionalists were more concerned with "how it happens" and "why".

Psychoanalysis

Psychoanalysis was founded by Sigmund Freud (1856–1939). It is different from structuralism, functionalism, behaviorism, and Gestalt psychology. In the course of his practice with neurotic patients in Vienna, Freud developed a theory based on unconscious motivation. The socially forbidden, personally unacceptable and painful desires, impulses, urges, and wishes of the individual are being pushed away into the depths of the unconscious portions of the mind from the conscious layers. This process is known as repression. However, these repressed impulses are active and try to occupy the conscious mind at least in a disguised manner, i.e., dreams, slips of pen and tongue, and unconscious mannerisms. Sometimes, they find socially acceptable expressions like the artistic, literary, and scientific pursuits. According to Freudian theory, these repressed unconscious impulses are sexual in nature. Actually, this attribution of sexuality to all motives bought unpopularity to Freud and his thinking.

According to psychoanalysis, the nature of the unconscious materials may be made conscious and the patient helped to remember them, which would help the individual to recover. This is done by the methods of free association and dream interpretation.

Freud gave us ideas like libido the motivating force in human life, regression, transference, sublimation, Id, ego, superego, conscious, preconscious, and unconscious oedipus complex and psychopathology of dreams. According to Freud, most of the humans activated from the unconscious.

Behaviorism

Although both structuralism and functionalism had considered the method of introspection as a valid one, behaviorism, under the leadership of John B Watson (1878-1958) rejected it as being something of a private experience and not available for testing, observation, and checking. The whole idea of consciousness is absurd.

Behaviorism emphasized that conditioned reflexes were the elements and not sensation that constitute the behavior. Conditioned reflexes are simple learned responses to stimuli. According to Watson, human behavior was made up of sets of conditioned reflexes. He stated that he could make anything out of an infant—a beggar, a lawyer, or a criminal. Behaviorism does not admit of instincts or inborn tendencies. It emphasized the need for objective study forming the basis of understanding of human and animal behavior. Behaviorist is not interested in feeling of fear because it is not measurable but he pays attention to changes in heart rate and blood pressure which are the effects of fear and can be objectively measured. The theory is based on Pavlov's classical conditioning. Pavlov had concluded that all behavior is response to some stimulus (S–R) in the environment.

Gestalt Psychology

This school of psychology was founded in Germany in 1912 by Max Wertheimer (1883-1943) and his colleagues Kurt Koffka (1886-1941) and Wolfgang Kohler (1887-1967). They felt that the structuralists were wrong in thinking the mind as made up of elements. They maintained the mind was not made up of a combination of simple elements. The German word "Gestalt" means "form" or "configuration" (an organized whole in contrast to the collection of parts). Perception is always related to the total situation. The Gestalt psychologists maintained that the mind

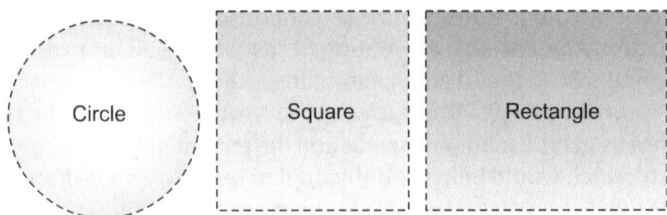

Fig. 1: Perception of patterns.

should be thought of as resulting from the whole pattern of sensory activity and the relationships and organizations within their patterns. For example, we recognize a tune in music, when it is transposed to another key; the elements have changed but the pattern of relationship has remained the same. Or to take another example, when you look at the dots in **Figure 1**, your mental experience is not just the dots or elements, but a circle, rectangle, and a square. It is the organization of the dots and their relationships that give the patterns, which you perceived.

The whole is more important than the parts; the parts themselves do not have much meaning except for their contextual position. Thus, behavior is more than the sum of conditioned reflexes. Experience and behavior are patterns or organizations somewhat similar to a magnetic field where changes in one part of a field are affected by changes in another part. One should look at a tree as a whole and not see only a few flowers, leaves, or fruits.

Humanism

When personality development focuses upon the development of self, it is called humanism.

This was developed in the United States by Abraham Maslow (1908-1970), and Carl Rogers (1902–1994). It focuses on the person's subjective experiences, freedom of choice, and motivation toward self-actualization. Humanists believe that behavior is controlled by our own free will and not by the unconscious or by the environment. They are interested more in solving human problems than in the laboratory experiments. They want each person to reach his full potential, i.e., self-actualization.

Methods of Psychology

Introspection or Self-observation Method

To introspect means to look within. It is internal perception or self-observation. The individual himself observes his internal activities and processes whenever and wherever he likes to do so. It is indispensable for the study of internal behavior. For example, a patient after an operation may be asked to report how he feels. The patient will try to look within and recall what happened and how he is feeling now.

Introspection does not involve any expenditure as it does not need any laboratory or apparatus. We get a direct knowledge of the mental experience of the individual. But the method cannot be used by children or mental defectives. It is a purely private affair and cannot be verified by other observers. In many cases, the patients may not have the insight to know about their conditions or language to describe them accurately. It can be used as a supportive method. The psychoanalysts have widely utilized this method but the behaviorists are vehemently opposed to it.

Observation Method or Systematic Observation

It consists of collection of data by means of observing behavior by somebody other than that person. For example, when a nurse is asked to make an observational report on a patient with an undiagnosed illness, she reports her observations, such as the patient's temperature, pulse, color, facial expression, restlessness, etc. Observation of the patient is very important in clinical medicine. The method is widely used also in studying the behavior of children and animals.

Experimental Method or Experimentation or Laboratory Method

In this method, made popular by Wundt, the psychologist studies under carefully controlled conditions, the effects of a dependent variable of changes in an independent variable. Many experiments are being conducted on people and animals dealing with learning, forgetting and many other mental activities. The tremendous progress of psychology during the 20th Century is mainly due to this method. The experimental method controls all variables.

The following are the steps in an experiment:
1. Identifying a problem, e.g., effect of noise on learning.
2. Formulation of the hypothesis.
3. Distinction between independent and dependent variables.
4. Arranging the environment and collecting data.
5. Analysis of the result (experimental data).
6. Testing of the hypothesis by the result of the experiment.

If the experimenter wants to know the influence of high temperature and pulse rate, temperature is considered as independent variable.

The advantage of this method is that experiments are objective and can be repeated and results confirmed. Limitations are that it cannot always be used, especially if the experiment might be dangerous to the subjects and are obtained in artificial situations of laboratory, e.g., crowd, riot, propaganda. Besides limited field, it has difficulty in securing the cooperation of subjects. As spontaneous behavior may be qualitatively different from artificial behavior of the laboratory, results may not be equally true in actual social situations. The method is expensive. Also the subject may suffer from anxiety or shyness.

Survey Method or Inventory Method

This method uses questionnaires, checklists, rating scales, ranking, and inventories to assess different aspects of behavior, emotional experiences, and aptitudes. It is also used for problems that cannot be directly observed. Surveys are used to gather information about political opinion, customer preferences, health needs, and sexual behavior. Data is collected by questionnaire method or interview method. The results of a survey of a large number of people have to be carefully analyzed before conclusions are made.

Questionnaire consists of a series of written questions or general statements. Method is simple to collect responses of a large sample. They can be even mailed, if subjects are at different places. However, the application is limited to literate classes.

Advantages
a. Flexibility
b. Can be applied to many populations
c. Broadness of scope
d. Can be used for many topics.

Disadvantages
a. Relatively superficial
b. Rarely probes deeply into complexities of behavior.

Test Method

Abilities, interests, attitudes, and intelligence are measured by this method by making use of carefully devised and standardized tests.

The test can be administered to a large number of personnel at the same time saving a lot of time, energy, and dislocation of routine work, e.g., Group IQ test to test.

Case History or Clinical Method

It involves an in-depth analysis of an individual, group institution, or other social units. It is used regularly in the medical and nursing setting. It aims at studying the causes and basis of people's anxieties, fears, and personal maladjustments. It makes use of case histories, interviews, home visits, and psychological tests for that purpose. It gathers information from what the subject can recall.

Case histories are scientific biographies. It consists of collecting all the information about an individual's past. This can be done by interviewing the individual himself and/or his family members, friends, classmates, teachers, and others who knew him and who can provide relevant information about his past. Documents like cumulative records, personal diaries and articles can throw light on his past and reveal some impressions about him directly or indirectly. Thus, case histories are done on the basis of remembered events and recorded data, using methods like observation, interview, and tests.

The method is also known as clinical as the method is conveniently used in hospitals by Doctors and Nurses since they often meet relatives of patients who may furnish reliable information about the incidents before the development of the present complaints. This information helps the doctor to detect the causes of the disorder and the nurse in assisting the patients to regain the sense of security and capability they have lost. Data should be valid, scientific, complete, and confidential.

Genetic or Developmental Method

Psychologists study not only the behavior of a particular time, but also its development from birth to death, the influence of heredity and environment in the development of the person and conditions favorable and unfavorable for normal development and abnormality.

It studies the growth of behavior. For example, to understand the learning behavior of an adult, the study will start from the childhood and adolescence.

Subfields of Psychology or Scope of Psychology

1. **Clinical psychology** is the largest subfield of psychology (55%). It is the study of techniques, which are employed in the diagnosis and treatment of mentally and emotionally abnormal personalities. A clinical psychologist has an MA or PhD in psychology and is trained to apply psychotherapeutic techniques, to diagnose psychological disorders and to conduct tests and do research. However, being not a doctor he cannot prescribe medicines. Psychiatrists are doctors holding an MD degree and specialized in behavioral problems. Being a physician, he uses drugs and other medical methods for treating the mentally ill. Psychoanalysis is different from clinical psychology and psychiatry. A psychoanalyst uses the special psychotherapeutic techniques developed by Sigmund Freud.

2. **Counseling psychology** is similar to clinical psychology but deals with people with relatively mild personal or emotional problems.
3. **Educational psychology** deals with the learning problems and their remedies. The main focus is designing curriculum, assessment methods, and various teaching methodologies.
4. **Industrial and organizational psychology** applies psychological principles to industry. They are also referred as personnel psychologists. They mainly deal with employee-employer relationship, absenteeism in workplace, increasing productivity, etc.
5. **Social psychology** deals with the behavior of an individual as it is influenced by others and how an individual influences others' behavior. It studies various types of group phenomena like public opinion, propaganda, attitudes, beliefs, and crowd behavior.
6. **Experimental psychology** involves basic research into the fundamental causes of human behavior by studying such basic processes as learning and memory, sensation and perception, and motivation. Physiological psychology concerns the structure and functions of sense organs, nervous systems, muscles and glands underlying all behavior. It lays emphasis on the influence of bodily factors on human behavior.
7. **Development psychology** studies the behavior as it develops from birth, through childhood, adolescence, and maturity to old age. It studies the factors that influence the growth or development of human behavior. Child psychology studies the behavior of children from birth to about the age of 12 years.
8. **Abnormal psychology** deals with the behavior of individuals who are unusual. It studies mental disorders, their causes, and treatment.
9. **Community psychology** is a broad field where social problems and the attempts of people to adapt to their work and community living are studied in the light of the principles of general psychology **(Table 2)**.

Table 2: Branches of pure and applied psychology.

Branches of pure psychology	Branches of applied psychology
General psychology	Educational psychology
Abnormal psychology	Clinical psychology
Experimental psychology	Industrial psychology
Physiological psychology	Legal psychology
Parapsychology	Military psychology
Developmental psychology	Political psychology

In pure psychology, we generate theories and discuss principles, which find their applications in applied psychology.

In the USA during 2005, 55% of psychologists worked as clinical psychologists in either private practice or therapy setting, 27% in academic settings of universities and colleges, 8% in other jobs, 6% in industry (business, corporation and consulting firms), and 4% in secondary schools conducting academic and career testing, and counseling for minor psychological problems.

IMPORTANCE OF PSYCHOLOGY

Psychology—the science concerned with behavior—both humans and animals—is only 125 years old. Despite its youth, it is a broad discipline, essentially spanning subject matter from biology to sociology. Biology studies the structures and functions of living organisms. Sociology examines how groups function in society. Psychologists study two critical relationships—1. between brain function and behavior, and 2. between environment and behavior.

1. **In the field of education:** Psychology has contributed a great deal towards the improvement of the processes and products of education. The application of psychology in the field of education has helped learners to learn, teachers to teach, administrators to administer and educational trainers to plan efficiently and effectively. It has helped in the assessment of natural abilities and acquired characteristics. Theories of learning, motivation, and personality are responsible for shaping and designing educational systems, according to the needs of the students.
2. **In the field of medicine:** Behavior counts much more than medicines and behavior can be learned only through psychology. It has removed many superstitions in the diagnosis and cure of mental and physical diseases. Psychology has contributed many valuable therapeutic measures like behavior therapy, group therapy, shock therapy, and psychoanalysis. A doctor, nurse, or any other person who attends the patient needs to know the science of behavior to achieve good results.
3. **In the field of guidance and counseling:** Knowledge of psychology helps to provide guidance and counseling to persons with problems of adjustment, in the field of education, employment and private life.
4. **In the field of industry and business management:** In the field of manufacturing, sales, or advertising—one has to apply the principles of psychology, such as needs, motives, interests,

and individual differences for good returns. Psychology has helped in selection, training, and placement of staff in industry. It has increased working capacity and efficiency of both men and machine and helped in the establishment of harmonious relationship between the employer and employee, manufacturer and consumer resulting in maximum economy and output.
5. **In the field of law:** Psychology has changed our outlook on criminology. The criminals are no longer treated as degenerated beasts. Efforts are accordingly made for their rehabilitation as useful members of the society. Background knowledge of psychology is very useful for our lawmakers to know the formal and informal laws of the country.
6. **Psychology as a teaching subject:** Psychology has a large scope as a teaching subject in colleges and universities. Background knowledge of human behavior is essential for various professions including senior administrators (e.g., IAS cadre) psychology can be taken up also as a fulltime profession.
7. **In the field of self-development:** Psychology helps the individual to know his assets and limitations, abilities and short comings, habits, and temperament. This knowledge may lead one to set realistic levels of aspirations, change his habits, and seek self-control, adequate adjustment, development, and progress. It may help him control his emotions, building of proper sentiments and character. It will enhance his decision making and problem solving abilities and self-actualization leading to a well-balanced and integrated personality.

Other important uses of psychology are in the fields of politics, military science, mental health, human relations, and world peace.

The move toward preventing illness, rather than merely diagnosing and treating it, requires people to learn how to make healthy behavior a routine part of living. Indeed many of the problems facing family today are problems about behavior, for example, drug addiction, poor interpersonal relationships, violence at home and in the street and the harm we do to our environment. Psychologists contribute solutions to problems through careful collection of data, analysis of data, and development of intervention strategies.

PSYCHOLOGY AND NURSING

Psychology has very vast scope with its numerous sub-branches as enumerated above. Medical psychology is a new area and deals with patients suffering from disorders of the mind. Mental health nursing is an important aspect of community health nursing. Health psychology explains the relationship between psychological stress and physical ailments. It promotes healthy ways of behavior and physical health. It promotes assertive skills, adjustment techniques and better coping skills, so that people are able to meet everyday stress, strain, and tension effectively.

A nurse, doctor, or any person who has to deal with patients, should know the science of behavior for better results. Behavior counts much more than medicines, and behavior is the subject matter of psychology. Physical and mental sickness may be caused by psychological factors and require psychological remedies as well.

Psychology has removed a lot of superstitions in the diagnosis and treatment of mental and physical sicknesses. Psychology has also contributed many therapeutic measures including behavior therapy, play therapy, group therapy, shock therapy, and psychoanalysis for the diagnosis and treatment of patients suffering from psychosomatic diseases.

Relevance of Studying Psychology by Nurses

The nurse occupies a central position in a system of human relationships, namely the health care system. Not only does she want to understand herself, she also wants to understand others as well. In the hospital, there are patients. At home, there are people who need her care. In the community health nursing field, there are people of all ages who need to be educated and also other members of the health team. Every one of these people can be better understood, if the nurse knows something of human behavior by studying psychology.

The physical and mental well-being of a patient depends largely on the nurse. In her professional capacity, the nurse has her share of anxiety, sorrow, anger, fear, and even hostility. These are raw edges of human emotions.

Today's nurse is living in a fast changing world with all its technological achievements. With the mechanization and urbanization of society, her working conditions are rapidly changing. The family, which is one of the basic institutions of society, is undergoing rapid changes in both form and function. Old and comfortable securities will soon be a thing of the past. The nurse has to deal with different people having different problems both physically and mentally. To serve them satisfactorily, knowledge of human psychology is essential.

Nursing care: After a detailed study of the basic principles of psychology, the nurse can apply the same principles in her dealing with her patients. A patient is an individual even though suffering from an ailment. He has his own likes and dislikes, fears and anxieties, prides and prejudices. For example, when a patient is posted for an operation, he should not only be prepared physically and clinically but also mentally and emotionally for the event. In this connection, nurses should remember:

1. Illness is painful and discomforting. It causes patients feel insecure and uncertain about their future.
2. Illness lowers self-esteem. Many patients show infantile regression during illness.
3. Nurse's approach should be human and individualized to each patient. The patient should be received as an honored guest, with utmost courtesy and genuine warmth. Calling patients by names and children by their nick names will instill confidence in them.
4. A patient is very tense on his arrival at the ward. He should be allowed to relax and all his fears and anxieties gently removed.
5. A patient should be introduced to the ward and well-oriented with the facilities available and to the people he is likely to meet in the ward.
6. Be a patient listener. Let the patient narrate his case in his own words and style.
7. The overmodest patient should be helped to lose his self-consciousness.

Psychology and the Student Nurse

Psychology has become an integral part of every profession including nursing. The study of human behavior is of great value to a student nurse in a number of ways:

1. **It will help her to understand herself:** She will get an insight into her motives, desires, emotions, and ambitions. She will realize how her personality is highly individualistic and complex, how she arrives at decisions in her life and how she solves her problems. By knowing her strengths and weaknesses, she can best use her own personality characteristics. This will let her direct her own life more productively and relate more easily with others, enabling her to control situations and attain self-discipline.
2. **It will help her to understand other people:** Leading to personal and professional adjustment. She will become sympathetic, alert, hardworking, and love humanity. She will become emotionally mature and cultivate an active mind and habits and enjoy teamwork. The student nurse has to study, work, and live with

other nurses, doctors, patients and their families. With her scientific knowledge of human nature, she will understand them better and thus achieve greater success in interpersonal relationships.

3. **It will help her to improve situations by helping others solve problems:** Illness and physical handicaps often bring about the need for major adjustments. Many diseases, such as heart disease and cancer are not cured by medical treatment, but are instead controlled. These diseases are for life and require special coping skills and health care. A nurse trained in educational psychology can be an effective health educator and can help in this kind of adjustments.

   In the health care setting, the patient's role in treatment is a major factor. A good understanding of the patient by the nurse can be the best social support to patients who are hospitalized and also while coping with chronic mental illness.

4. **Psychology helps to provide effective health teaching to clients:** An understanding of psychology can be of great help to a nurse to become a good health teacher to explain to the patient and relatives:
   a. The nature and diagnostic examination, findings, and treatment
   b. Principles of health and prevention of diseases
   c. After care programs and rehabilitation.

5. **She will appreciate the necessity of changing the environment and guide her how to do it:** The change in the environment is often necessary for adjustment and happiness. For example, eye glasses and hearing aids have been developed and introduced into the environment of those with sensory deficiencies to assist them in their attempts to achieve a more harmonious relationship with their surroundings.

   A child who is denied completely the affectionate care of parents may do better when given the care of foster parents. Irresponsible or highly dependent children may do better when placed in a residential school.

6. **She will understand the close interdependence of body, mind, and spirit:** She will recognize how her emotions affect her body and she will recognize the same in her patients. This will help her to control her life and recognize the similar needs in her patients.

7. **Psychology will help the nursing student in the following areas as well:**
   - Planning study by
     – Organizing the daily program
     – Arranging the study environment

- Developing basic abilities with
  - Motivation
  - Prompt warming up by checking reading ability and eye sight
  - Preparing for examination
    » Developing a positive attitude
    » Studying with examination in view.

For nursing student and emotions refer Chapter 15.

Key Points ● ● ●

- Psychology is the science of human behavior.
- Wundt was the first to measure human behavior accurately and is called the "Father of Psychology".
- Structuralism, functionalism, psychoanalysis, gestalt psychology, and humanism are some of the major schools contributed to the field of psychology.
- Branches of psychology are divided into pure and applied fields.
- Various methods are used in psychology to gather information.

EXERCISE

Make an introspection report on your joining for the BSc (nursing) course.

STUDY QUESTIONS

Long Essays

1. Define psychology. How does psychology help in good nurse-patient relationship?
2. Describe the scope of psychology. Explain its relevance to nursing.
3. Explain the various methods in psychology. What are the implications of psychology to students of nursing?
4. Discuss the various methods used to study behavior.

Short Essays

1. Discuss the scope of psychology.
2. Advantages and limitations of introspection method.
3. Explain the experimental method in psychology.
4. Bring out the similarities and differences between observation and introspection.

Chapter 1: Psychology and its Relation to Nursing

Short Answers

1. What is behavior?
2. Difference between a Psychologist and a Psychiatrist.
3. What are the methods used in psychology?
4. Explain nursing and psychology.
5. What is the experimental method?
6. What is introspection?

Write Short Notes on

1. Behaviorism.
2. Gestalt psychology.
3. Survey method.
4. Clinical method.
5. Definition of psychology.

Multiple Choice Questions

1. Who established the first laboratory in psychology?
   - a. Freud
   - b. Wundt
   - c. Maslow
   - d. Kohler
2. Structuralism: Titchener: Functionalism:_____
   - a. James
   - b. Miller
   - c. Skinner
   - d. Beck
3. _____ method involves in depth analysis of individual/group.
   - a. Case history method
   - b. Introspection
   - c. Observation
   - d. Survey
4. _____psychologists are also called personnel psychologists.
   - a. Industrial
   - b. Forensic
   - c. Counseling
   - d. Developmental
5. BF Skinner was a _____psychologist.
   - a. Gestalt
   - b. Humanistic
   - c. Psychoanalytic
   - d. Behaviorist

2

Body-Mind Relationship

Chapter Outline

- Behavior
- Mind-Body Relationship
- Self-sufficiency
- Altered State of Consciousness
- Hypnosis
- Meditation
- Empathy
- Psychoactive Drugs

Learning Objectives

♦ Students will be familiarized with mind-body relationship.
♦ Orients students to altered states of consciousness.

Behavior that is elicited by a stimulus is known as response. Behavior has cognitive, affective, and conative components. The process or result of the unification of these components into a whole is called integrated response.

INTEGRATED RESPONSES

Psychology studies the relationship between mind and body. Mind and body affect each other. The mind operates at the levels of thinking, emotion, and action. Mind and body cannot act independently on parallel lines. This is an integrated response, inseparable from each other.

When angry thoughts cross your brain, they stimulate both the halves of the autonomic nervous system—the sympathetic, which energizes you and the parasympathetic which calms you down. You may consider the former as a car's accelerator and the latter as its brake. You would be having a bumping ride, if you apply brake while accelerating. This is what would happen to your heart when you are constantly being resentful. The conflicting messages trigger jerky, ragged heart rhythms.

To arrest potential for physical damage, researchers in the field of heart-brain communication have found that you need to shift into a positive state of mind. As emotions, such as empathy and mercy, overpower negative feelings and thoughts, the symptoms of heart disease disappear. When you are treated unjustly by others, resent is the natural response. If those resentful feelings are not resolved, a grudge will form. Victims may want to hold a grudge, because it gives them a regained sense of control and superiority. However, when nursing a grudge, you are continuing as a victim and inviting anger to become a companion in your everyday life—and a toxin to your body.

Emotions depend on a complex combination of bodily responses and mental processes. Body provides energy to fight, flee, cope, hug, sing, or dance. Mind contributes to the understanding to offer an explanation for one's own actions or the actions of others. Just as the body produces epinephrine to fight out danger, the mind helps to decide whether the raised fist is a sign of rage, playfulness, or a threat.

Our emotions including moods, such as depression and complex feelings, such as hatred and love—are greatly affected by our interpretation, memories, and expectations. These emotions lead to think more positively about ourselves and the world around us feel better.

Action of Mind upon Body

1. All physical and motor activities begin by the motivation in the mind.
2. Negative emotions like fear, anger, and jealousy produce illness. They make us depressed. Emotional conflicts lie at the root of peptic ulcers, coronary heart diseases, blood pressure, and neurosis.
3. Deep thinking and concentration can cause physical fatigue.
4. Soldiers put in superhuman effort and win the war when their morale is high.

Action of Body upon Mind

1. Rise in blood pressure leads to mental excitement.
2. Fatigue retards intellectual activity.
3. Sudden emotion causes mental imbalance.
4. Constipation makes people irritable.
5. Dyspepsia (indigestion) makes people gloomy.

6. Hyperthyroidism leads to excitement and hypothyroidism causes lethargy.
7. Bad throat and septic tonsils can reduce concentration.

An understanding of the above facts is useful for the nurse to learn the etiology of diseases.

THE BEHAVING ORGANISM

The human being is capable of behavior and, therefore, is a living organism. The individual is in active relation with the environment and his environment influences and changes him. His behavior consists of his dealings with the environment. All behavior is a function of the individual and his environment, both of which undergo changes because of their interaction with one another.

Characteristics of Behaving Organism

a. **Unity:** The living organism behaves as one unit.
b. **Self-sufficiency:** Unlike machines, the living organism is autonomous. It is self-maintaining, self-changing, self-regulating, and self-reproducing. It moves from within as per its own laws.
c. Every living organism is unique. No two human beings are exactly alike.
d. A living organism changes and grows not only from within but also because of what happens from outside. An organism does not grow in an isolated vacuum.

LEVELS OF FUNCTIONING OR LEVELS OF CONSCIOUSNESS

1. Conscious,
2. Unconscious, and
3. Preconscious.

For details, see personality dynamics described in Freud's psychosexual theory of personality development (Chapter 17).

Altered State of Consciousness (ASC)

Besides conscious, unconscious, and preconscious, there are altered states of consciousness or ASC, which influence our lives. They include sleep, dreaming, drugs, hypnosis, and meditation.

Hypnosis is an ASC during which a person becomes very relaxed and open to suggestion. Hypnosis can be used to reduce pain, improve attention, become more relaxed and change harmful habits.

Meditation is an ASC brought about by focusing one's thoughts on a particular sound or idea. It can be used for relaxation or religious purposes. Meditation has been found to promote health by reducing the harmful effects of stress in life.

Six Steps in Meditation
1. Sit quietly in a comfortable position.
2. Close your eyes.
3. Deeply relax all your muscles beginning with your feet and progressing to your face. Keep them deeply relaxed.
4. Breathe through your nose and as you breathe out, say the word "one" silently to yourself.
5. Do not worry about whether you are successful or not in becoming relaxed. If distracting thoughts come to your mind, and you can expect them, ignore them; keep repeating the word "one".
6. Practice this once or twice a day.

Psychoactive drugs: Drugs, which alter consciousness are called psychoactive drugs and they act directly upon the brain. They can be stimulants, depressants, or hallucinogens. Stimulants include caffeine, nicotine, cocaine, and amphetamines. Alcohol, barbiturates, and marijuana are depressants. Lysergic acid diethylamide (LSD), *hashish, ganja,* and *bhang* are hallucinogens. Drug dependence or substance abuse is a major health problem. Drug is a journey to the unknown. It is difficult to stop but not impossible.

Nurse and Levels of Consciousness
The interrelationship of the body, mind, and everything happening to the person is extremely important in nursing care. A patient who had a surgery may have a very slow recovery, if he has serious problems at home or in his relationship with others. It is necessary to study a person's entire physical and psychological situation to provide him the most helpful nursing care.

The nurse must be aware of the power of the unconscious in her as well as her patient's behavior. She may feel uneasy when she is in the operation theater or in pediatrics ward. Patients may have unexplained fear of hospitalization or laboratory procedures.

Sleep is an essential need of all people. Often, hospital routines interrupt sleep of patients. Sometimes, this may be unavoidable, but whenever possible, more flexible routines should be used. Sometimes, health personnel including nurses have to keep awake and sleep at unusual hours or short periods. Loss of sleep should be made up at the earliest by sleep and good rest. Use of drugs to avoid sleep must be strictly avoided.

Health personnel and patients may wish to meditate for relaxation and religious reasons. A quiet place must be earmarked for this purpose in the hospital.

Key Points

- Behavior is a function of individual and their environment.
- Freud speaks of three levels of consciousness.
- Sleep, dreaming, drugs, hypnosis, and meditation are altered state of consciousness.

STUDY QUESTIONS

Long Essay

1. What is the physiological basis of behavior? What are the levels of functioning? How are the responses integrated?

Short Answer

1. What are integrated responses? What are the levels of thinking?

Multiple Choice Questions

1. Who proposed the three levels of consciousness?
   a. Freud b. Rogers
   c. Bandhura d. Hook
2. Alcohol is a_____.
   a. Stimulant b. Opiate
   c. Depressant d. Hallucinogen
3. Thoughts that are not in our current awareness but can be recalled is_____.
   a. Subconscious b. Preconscious
   c. Ultraconscious d. Nonconscious
4. Which of the following is not considered an altered state of consciousness?
   a. Dreaming b. Divided attention
   c. Hypnosis d. Meditation

5. The_____nervous system energies our body and the _____nervous system calms our body.
   a. Sympathetic, parasympathetic
   b. Parasympathetic, sympathetic
   c. Somatic, sympathetic
   d. Somatic, parasympathetic

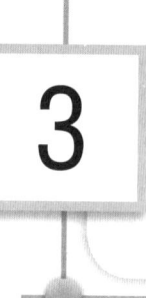

3

Biology of Behavior

Chapter Outline

- Brain-Behavior Relationship
- Sense Organs
- Endocrine System
- Neuron
- Neurotransmitters
- Central Nervous System
- Autonomic Nervous System
- Peripheral Nervous System

Learning Objectives

♦ Students will be familiarized with brain behavior relationship.
♦ Help students gain an insight into the various biological and physiological processes in human beings.

NERVOUS SYSTEM

Nerve is the most important part of our response mechanism. It joins the receptors and the effectors. The nervous system is divided into two parts (**Fig. 1**):
1. Central nervous system, and
2. Peripheral nervous system.

Neuron/Nerve Cell

A nerve cell with all its branches is called a neuron. Nerve cells or neurons are the information carriers of the nervous system. Neuron has a cell body that contains the machinery to keep the neurons alive and has two types of fibers: (a) Dendrites, and (b) Axon. The dendrites are relatively short and have many branches, which receive stimulation from other neurons. Axon is quite long and conducts nerve impulses to other neurons or to muscles and glands. Since, the dendrites and the cell body receive information that is then

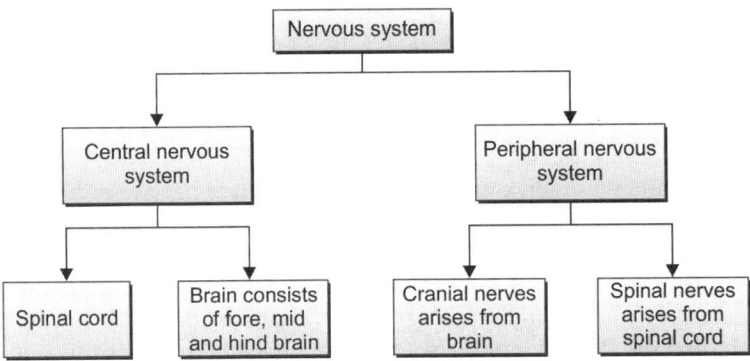

Fig. 1: Nervous system.

conducted along the axon; the direction of transmission is from dendrites to the fine axon tip.

In many cases, the axon has a white fatty covering called myelin sheath. This covering increases the speed with which nerve impulses are sent down the axon. However, it is the cell membrane, which immediately surrounds the cell body, the dendrites and the axon that is essential for the generation and conduction of nerve impulses down the axon.

Neurons form a vast, miniaturized informational network that allows us to receive sensory information, control muscle movements, regulates digestion, secrete hormones, and engage in complex mental processes, such as thinking, imagining, dreaming, and remembering.

A neuron is a brain cell with two specialized extensions. One extension is for receiving electrical signals and a second larger extension in for transmitting electrical signals.

How does a neuron impulse travel further from one neuron to another? Synapse is the connection for the flow of the current between the axon of the neuron and the receiving dendrite of the next. Synapses are the areas of functional contact between neurons. Enlargements of axon endings of transmitting neurons called boutons contain neurotransmitter chemicals, which are stored in small vesicles. A nerve impulse reaching these boutons causes neurotransmitters to be released into the synaptic cleft and then to excite or inhibit the receiving neurons. Some of the major neurotransmitters are acetylcholine, dopamine, epinephrine, norepinephrine, serotonin, glycine, and glutamic acid.

Central Nervous System

Mainly consists of spinal cord and the brain.

Spinal Cord

Roughly cylindrical structure containing a bulge in the lower middle region and gradually tapering to a point in lower back region. It is a segmented structure with each segment having both a sensory nerve and motor nerve on its left and right sides. Spinal cord runs through a hole, which is called spinal foramens. Spinal called is as mini brain, because it helps in maintaining posture, organization of gait, reaction to noxious stimuli, controls a portion of sexual behavior in both genders, and controls locomotion of the body.

Brain

Brain weighs 1.2–1.4 kg. CSF reduces 80 g of weight of the brain. Brain floats in the CSF. It is classified into hind, mid, and forebrain.

Hindbrain: Hindbrain is around the brain stem. It coordinates the movement of head. Medulla controls a number of reflexes breathing, heart rate, vomiting, salivation, coughing, and sneezing. Reticular formation is a complex loosely defined network of about 100 tiny nuclei and their interconnections that occupy the central core of the brain stem from the caudal boundary of the myelencephalon to the rostral boundary of the midbrain. ARAS plays an important role in arousal, sleep, attention, movement, muscle tone, and various cardiac, circulatory and respiratory reflexes. Pons plays a role in generating dreams. Cerebellum takes care of the muscle timing so there are no jerky movements. Damage leads to jerky movements and if damage is too much the person cannot stand.

Midbrain: It forms the top of brainstem. Two main parts are: (a) Tectum, and (b) Tegmentum.. The parts of the tectum include the superior, and inferior colliculi. The superior colliculi is involved in eye movements, and visual attention. It is connected to visual cortex thus controls movement of eyes, head, trunk, and limbs in response to visual impulses. The inferior colliculi has the auditory function. It plays a role in localization of sound. Tegmentum has dopamine secreting neurons, degeneration of which leads to Parkinson's disease.

Forebrain: Forebrain is mainly classified into diencephalon and telencephalon. Thalamus is considered the relay station of the brain. The different nuclei in thalamus are involved in various functions. Hypothalamus is one by tenth the size of thalamus. It has an important role in regulation of several motivated behaviors. Mamillary bodies play important role in memory. Telencephalon is the largest division of human brain. It mainly involves the limbic system, cerebral cortex, lobes, and major fissures.

Cerebral cortex: To consider the functions of the cerebral cortex (the gray matter), in behaviors and mental processes, it is convenient to divide it into sensory areas: motor areas, and associate areas. The primary sensory areas receive input, which originates in the sensory receptors. Visual sensations are represented in the occipital lobe; hearing and taste in the temporal lobe, and touch, pain, and pressure inputs reach the parietal lobe. The principal motor or movement areas of the cortex are in the central lobe. This area is organized, so that various parts of it are concerned with the movement of particular bodily structures.

The associative areas receive inputs from various regions of cerebral cortex and from lower portions of the central neurons system; they are involved in such complex functions as perception and the production and understanding of language.

The associative areas are those parts of the cortex, which would be included in the motor area. The associative area is divided into two parts: 1. Associative area is situated in the occipital, temporal, and parietal lobe between several motor areas. 2. Associative area is situated in the motor area and cerebrum in the front part. The associative areas are separated by association of fibers. If these fibers are damaged, some sensitive part of the brain is also damaged, e.g., with the destruction of association fibers of the cortex, everything learned is forgotten. With the destruction of the areas near the motor cortex, the capacity of speaking and writing is destroyed with the destruction of the visual area, it becomes impossible to understand language and man cannot understand words even while seeing them. Some severe damage to the areas of the front part of the brain results in forgetting of something immediately learned though one can remember something of childhood.

The cerebral hemispheres are specialized to perform different functions. The left is specialized for the processing of language. The right has only rudimentary language capabilities but has advantage over the left in pattern recognition and spatial abilities. In most people, the right hemisphere is specialized for recognition and memory of visual, auditory, tactile, and spatial patterns of stimulation.

Man acts with whole of his organism. There is an integration of mind and body. Human behavior reveals the influence of both mental and physical factors. When we analyze the bodily factors of human behavior, we find that the important elements involved in bodily functions are:
1. Receptors or the sense organs,
2. Effectors or the muscle and endocrine glands, and
3. Integrating mechanism or the nervous system.

The anatomy and physiology of the above systems are taught in anatomy and physiology classes. Here, we are concerned with their psychological roles.

Limbic system: Limbus means border or ring. It forms a border around brain stem. It is called ring, because it rings around thalamus. It also plays a role in emotions, motivation, circadian rhythm, and memory.

Basal ganglia: Plays role in muscle tone, motor control, controlling gross motor activities, and posture.

Amygdala: Amygdala means almond size is involved in feelings and expression of emotions, emotional memories, and recognition of signs of emotions in other people.

Major fissure/sulci: Large furrows in a convoluted cortex are called fissures. The largest fissure is the **longitudinal fissure** that divides brain into two equal parts the left and right hemisphere. It transfers motor, sensory, and cognitive information between the brain hemispheres. Only area where hemisphere meets is called **Corpus Callosum**—a set of neurons forming a fibrous structure. **Central fissure** divides frontal lobe from parietal lobe. **Lateral fissure,** which divides temporal lobe from parietal lobe and frontal lobe. **Calcarine fissure** is found in the occipital lobe.

Peripheral Nervous System

Peripheral nervous system is the nervous system outside the skull and spine. Sensory fibers carry excitation from receptors to CNS. They are afferent nerves. Motor fibers carry excitation from CNS to the glands or muscles. PNS is not protected by bone of spine and skull or blood brain barrier. PNS has two divisions (a) somatic, and (b) autonomic nervous system.

Somatic Nervous System

The somatic nervous system (SNS) is the part of the PNS that interacts with the external environment. It is also referred as thoracolumbar system. The SNS is the portion of the nervous system responsible for voluntary body movement and for sensing external stimuli. All five senses are controlled by the SNS.

Somatic nervous system consist 31 pairs of spinal nerves and 12 pairs of cranial nerves.

Autonomic Nervous System

The autonomic nervous system (ANS) is the part of PNS that regulates inner environment. Afferent nerves of the ANS carry signals from the organs of the body to the CNS and efferent nerves carry information from CNS back to the organs. Motor component of the ANS controls heart rate and blood pressure. The sensory component of the ANS includes sensations of satiety and illness. It is further classified as sympathetic and parasympathetic nervous system.

Sympathetic nervous system: Sympathetic neurons arise in the lateral part of the ventral horn of the spinal cord in the thoracic and lumbar region and are thus controlled by spinal cord. It stimulates, organizes, and mobilizes energy resources to deal with threatening situations. It also secretes epinephrine to increase heart rate, blood sugar, and dilates the pupil of the eye.

Parasympathetic nervous system (PSNS): It is called the rest and digests system. Originates in cranial and sacral regions and is controlled by brain and spinal cord. It is also referred as craniosacral system. Growth and repair functions are served by parasympathetic system. Functions of PSNS are opposite to sympathetic nervous system. Though they function in opposite directions both are usually active at the same time in varying degrees. Parasympathetic neurons arise from the ventral horns of the caudal spinal cord and also from ventral side of the brain. PSNS makes the mouth salivate, activates digestive system, slows down heart rate, pupillary constriction, and goose flash reaction is controlled **(Fig. 2)**.

SENSE ORGANS: PSYCHOLOGY OF SENSATIONS

Sense organs are gateways of knowledge. Without the vision, touch, hearing, smell, and taste we shall know nothing of external world. We will have no ideas, no concept; we will not be able to communicate with each other nor recognize the faces. Our sense organs are affected by these changes in the world around us and our bodily conditions. These changes are called stimuli and the sense organs response to stimuli.

Our sense organs consist of the receptors, specialized sensitive cells associated with the endings of sensory nerve fibers and various accessory apparatus and tissues, which contribute to the effectiveness with which sense organs functions. Each sense organ has distinctive and specific functions to perform. There is no duplication or overlapping of any functions.

MUSCULAR CONTROL OF BEHAVIOR

Our behavior involves action of different parts of our body. We move our limbs when we take bath, eat, dress, run, or walk. Besides outward movements of our limbs, there are movements of our internal organs.

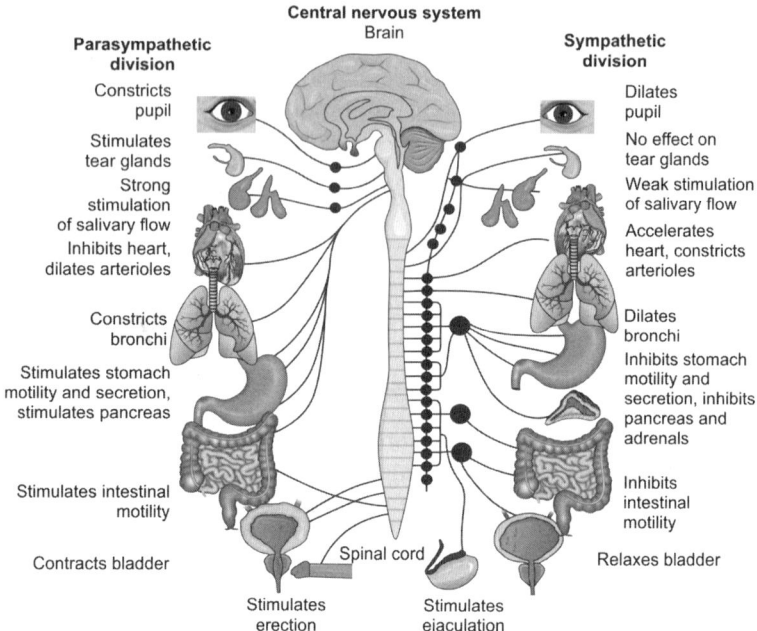

Fig. 2: Central nervous system.

In digestion, breathing, and blood circulation, there are movements of internal organs and tissues. Our muscles are responsible for the bodily movements, internal, and external.

The skeletal muscles enable the individuals to make movements by contracting and relaxing. These movements may be outwardly visible as in walking, running, gesticulating, and eating. The speed, strength, and precisions of movements involved in these activities depend on the coordination and control of the muscles.

The muscle control is lost when the nerve centers or fibers are injured or diseased. With exercises the muscles become fatigued. In fatigue, the muscles loose contractibility. By rest their strength and capacity are restored. Muscle tone means, the readiness of the muscles to contract. It ensures smooth and ready responses. It is the tone of muscles of legs, trunk, and neck, which enables us to perform such activities as solving a problem, listening to a lecture or aiming at a target.

General muscular tension causes irritability and excitement. Patients are likely to have defective muscle bone, which cause difficulties in digestion of food, elimination of waste, resting, and relaxation. This should be appreciated by nurses.

Glandular Control of Behavior

Endocrine System

There are two major systems for sending signals to the body's muscles, glands and organs. One is the nervous system, and the other is the endocrine system. The endocrine system is made up of numerous glands that are located throughout the body. These glands secrete various chemicals called hormones, which affect organs, muscles, and other glands in the body. The hypothalamus, which is located in the lower middle part of the brain, controls much of the endocrine system by regulating the pituitary gland, which is located directly below and outside the brain.

Major Endocrine Glands in the Human Body

The major endocrine glands in human body are described in **Table 1**.

Table 1: Major endocrine glands in the human body.

Gland	Functions	Dysfunctions
Posterior pituitary	The rear portion of the pituitary regulate the water and salt balance	Lack of the hormone causes a less common forms of diabetes
Anterior pituitary	The front part of the pituitary regulates growth through secretion of growth hormone and produces hormones that control the adrenal cortex, pancreas, thyroid and gonads	Too little growth hormone produces dwarfism, too much cause gigantism. Other problems in the pituitary cause problems in the glands it controls
Pancreas	This organ regulates the level of sugar in the blood stream by secreting insulin	Lack of insulin results in the more common forms of diabetes while too much causes hypoglycemia (low blood sugar)
Thyroid	This gland which is located in the neck, regulates metabolism through secretion of hormones	Hormone deficiency during development leads to stunted growth and mental retardation under secretion during adulthood leads to reduction in motivation. Over secretion refers to high metabolism, weight loss, and nervousness

Contd...

Contd...

Gland	Functions	Dysfunctions
Adrenal glands	The adrenal cortex (outside part) secretes hormones that regulate sugar and salt balances and help the body resist stress, they are responsible for growth of pubic hair, secondary sexual characteristics. The medulla (inside part) secretes two hormones that arouse the body to deal with stress and emergencies: epinephrine (adrenaline) and norepinephrine (noradrenaline)	With a lack of cortical hormones, the body's responses are unable to cope with stress
Gonads	In the females, the ovaries produce hormones that regulate sexual development, ovulation, and growth of sex organs. In males, the testes produce hormones that regulate sexual development, production of sperm, and growth of sex organs	Lack of sex hormones during puberty results in lack of secondary characteristics (facial and bodily hair) muscles in males, breasts in female)

Key Points ● ● ●

- CNS consists of spine and brain.
- Neurons are classified based on structure, and functions.
- The two hemispheres meet at corpus callosum.
- Sensory fibers are called afferent and motor fibers are called efferent.
- Sympathetic and parasympathetic nervous system function in opposite directions both are usually active at the same time in varying degrees.
- Endocrine system is made of gland that secretes chemicals called hormones.

STUDY QUESTIONS

Long Essays

1. Discuss the components of nervous system and their functions.
2. What are the different types of glands in the human body? Explain their functions.

3. Describe the various types of muscles in the human body with their functions.
4. Explain the general pattern of growth and development.

Short Essays

1. What is the importance of glands in nursing?
2. Describe the structure and functions of neuron.

Multiple Choice Questions

1. Degeneration of dopamine secreting neurons leads to:
   a. Parkinson's disease   b. Alzheimer's disease
   c. Kluver-Bucy syndrome d. Neglect syndrome
2. _____ divides the frontal lobe from parietal lobe.
   a. Longitudinal   b. Calcarian
   c. Central   d. Lateral
3. _____ is the largest endocrine gland in the human body.
   a. Adrenal   b. Gonads
   c. Pancreas   d. Thyroid
4. How many pairs of cranial nerves are there?
   a. 8   b. 12
   c. 31   d. 14
5. The _____ nervous system energies our body and the _____ nervous system calms our body.
   a. Sympathetic, parasympathetic
   b. Parasympathetic, sympathetic
   c. Somatic, sympathetic
   d. Somatic, parasympathetic

4

Nature and Nurture: Individual Differences

Chapter Outline

- Heredity
- Genetic Endowment
- Individual Differences
- Chromosomal Abnormalities
- Nature-nurture Controversy
- Dominant Gene
- Recessive Gene

Learning Objectives

♦ Students will be oriented to the nature-nurture controversy.
♦ Familiarize students to different chromosomal abnormalities.

NATURE—HEREDITY

Heredity refers to the biological process of transmission of certain biological and psychological characteristics from parents to their children through genes.

Evidences in Support of Heredity

1. Unequal intelligence levels of different occupational groups.
2. Unequal intelligence levels of different racial groups.
3. The close relationship between a child's physical and moral qualities indicating that both these qualities should have been inherited from the same sources. If a person is tall, long armed, dark eyed, and handsome, certain moral qualities can be safely attributed to him.
4. Studies by Galton and others into the ancestral history of twins, scientists, judges, artists and kings clearly demonstrated that distinctive mental ability is the result of inheritance rather than education. For example, the study of famous families of Edwards

and degenerate families of Jukes. In the USA, toward the end of the 19th century, some 1391 descendants of Jonathan Edwards were identified, out of which, more than 295 were college graduates, among whom 13 became college Principals and one became Vice-President of USA. There were no convicted criminals among them. The depressive history of Juke's family also supports heredity. Of 1,667 members, 300 died in infancy, 310 spent 2,300 years in poor houses, 410 were destroyed by disease, 400 were wrecked by their own wickedness, 7 were murderers, 60 habitual thieves who spent 12 years on average in prison, 130 were convicted criminals, and only 20 learned a trade. Such studies show that education is all paint; it does not alter the nature of the wood below, only improves the appearance a little!

NURTURE—ENVIRONMENT

Environment is anything immediately surrounding an organism and exerts a direct influence on it. The role of environment is so great that it can affect our society and behavior.

Freud has expressed the opinion that personality of a person is fashioned in the first 6 years of life, the rest of life being an expression of tendencies already developed. The influence of family environment upon the character, nature, habits, mental tendencies, and behavior of the individual is truly great. This has been verified by comparison of children brought up in families and those bred in orphanages. In childhood, parental love affects the stability of the emotions of the child, excessive love and care spoil the children; lack of affection leaves their feelings underdeveloped, which are then unnaturally expressed. Alfred Adler maintained that even the birth order of the child in the family affects his personality.

Individual Differences

No two individuals are exactly the same. Individuals differ from one another not only in height, weight, color, appearance, and speed of reaction but also in behavior. Some grow fast, some grow slowly. Some like music but not others. Some are aggressive and assertive, others are submissive. These are differences in intelligence, interest's attitudes and aptitudes. Individual differences in personality temperament can be observed from the birth itself.

In educational set up, understanding of individual differences helps in planning course material and training programs. All students do not learn in the same way.

Individual Differences in Intelligence

Character of the foster home definitely affects the degree of intellectual ability attained by the children subjected to its influence. Intelligence is much more responsive to environmental changes. There exists wide difference among individuals regarding intelligence. Not even identical twins or individuals matured in similar environment have equal intelligence (mental energy).

Development psychologists study the changes that occur during the life span, in the process of perception, learning, thinking, social activity, and other aspects of human behavior.

The relationship between IQ and closeness of genetic relationship

The relationship between IQ and closeness of genetic relationship has been described in **Table 1**.

Heredity/Genetic Endowment

Many aspects of human behavior and development ranging from physical characteristics, such as height, weight, eye, and skin color, the complex patterns of social and intellectual behavior are influenced by a person's genetic endowment. They also include physical deficiencies and the nature of glandular functioning. Functional units of heredity are the genes. Heredity is a source of both similarities and differences among individuals. The same heredity mechanisms that lead to resemblance of parent and offspring produce differences among members of a family. Fire that melts butter hardens the egg.

Table 1: Relationship between IQ and closeness of genetic relationship.

Relationship	Rearing	Correlation
Identical twins	Together	0.86
Fraternal twins	Together	0.62
Siblings	Together	0.41
Siblings	Apart	0.24
Parent-Child	Together	0.35
Parent-Child	Apart	0.31
Adoptive parent-child	Together	0.16
Unrelated Children	Together	0.25

0.41 and 0.24: Difference between two correlation show impact of environment

0.25: The relatively low correlation for unrelated children raised together shows the importance of genetic factors

Chromosomes and Genes

Biological inheritance is determined by chromosomes and genes. Females have 23 pairs of XX chromosomes. Males have 22 pairs of XX plus two singles represented as X and Y. The X and Y are called sex chromosomes because sex depends upon XX or XY combinations. Sets of chromosomes from different persons of the same sex look alike but internally they are very different, especially in unrelated individuals.

The heredity factors hidden within the chromosomes are the genes. They are "packets of chemicals" strung along the chromosomes like small beads on a thread. Within each chromosome there are about 1,000 genes. These genes contain two chemical substances DNA and RNA, which are responsible for transmitting the genetic code message from parent to offspring.

Transference of the traits was studied scientifically by Gregor Mendel, an Austrian monk. His work led to the knowledge of dominant and recessive genes in explaining the hereditary transmission of traits and related facts about mutation inheritance.

Mendel's Laws of Inheritance

Mendel formulated certain laws to explain the inheritance of characters:

1. **Law of unit characters:** All characters are units by themselves and certain factors (now called genes) control the expression of these characters during the development of the organism.
2. **Law of dominance:** Factors or genes occur in pairs. One factor may mask the expression of the other. The character that expresses itself in the F1 generation (first generation) is said to be the dominant and the character that does not appear in F1 generation is said to be recessive.
3. **Law of segregation:** When germ cells are formed, Mendel supposed that the opposed factors are separated, or segregated, so that each germ cell carries one or the other of the two factors and not both, Mendel's work provided the basis of the study of inheritance.

An offspring is found to derive a gene pair in one of the following forms:
   a. A dominant gene from one parent and recessive gene from the other.
   b. Dominant genes from both the parents.
   c. Recessive genes from both the parents.

A dominant gene must exhibit its dominance over the recessive genes. *For example,* if one parent furnishes a gene for brown eyes (known to be dominant) and the other provides a gene for blue (a recessive one), the offspring will have brown eyes (characteristic of the dominant gene).

Sex is determined by the X and Y sex chromosomes. All female eggs have only one type of sex chromosome (i.e., X) but sperm cells of the male may contain both types of X and Y.

At the time of conception, therefore, the mother can contribute the same X chromosome, while the father can contribute either X or Y. If he is transmitting X chromosome, then it results in a girl or if he transmits Y chromosome, a boy is produced.

Action of the genes on the cytoplasm changes the shape and other characteristics of cells. The heredity basis of individual differences lies in the unlimited variety of possible gene combinations that can occur. No two siblings get an identical heredity, as they do not get the same genes from the parents. Fraternal twins or dizygotic are different from each other because of different pairs of gene cells. However, identical or monozygotic twins develop from the same sperm and ovum and hence have exactly the same set of genes and, therefore, resemble each other completely.

Chromosomal Abnormalities

Mutation leads to different abnormalities in humans.

Some mutagens in nature are: Industrial chemicals, pesticides, food adulterants, drugs UV rays, medical and dental X-rays, and radiation from nuclear power projects.

Some of the chromosomal disorders are as follows:

1. **Klinefelter's syndrome:** It is due to an inability to metabolize phenylalanine. The incomplete oxidation results in the accumulation of phenylpyuric acid in the brain causing severe mental retardation, 47 chromosomes instead of normal 46, XXY. Individuals with this syndrome usually are phenotypically male, have verbal deficits, and show excessive aggressive behavior.
2. **Turner's syndrome:** A genetic disorder with 45 chromosomes instead of 46. Some of the common features include poorly developed ovaries, webbed neck, low set ears, broad chest with under developed breasts, amenorrhea, reproductive sterility unusual-shaped mouth and ears, learning difficulties, renal and urinary tract abnormalities, and cardiac defects.
3. **Down's syndrome:** It is also called trisomy 21. Affected persons are mentally retarded, short stature, open mouth, protruding furrowed tongue, hands and feet with short fingers and toes, tongue is too

long and outside the mouth, fifth finger incurved. 47 chromosomes instead of 46

4. **Fragile X syndrome:** Fragile X syndrome (FXS) is a genetic syndrome that is the most widespread single-gene cause of autism and inherited cause of mental retardation among boys. It results in a spectrum of intellectual disabilities ranging from mild to severe as well as physical characteristics, such as an elongated face, large or protruding ears, and large testes and behavioral characteristics, such as stereotypic movements (e.g., hand-flapping), and social anxiety.

5. **Cat cry syndrome:** It is also called cat cry syndrome from the characteristic cry of affected infants, which is similar to that of a meowing kitten, due to problems with the larynx and nervous system. Some of the behavioral problems shown are hyperactivity, aggression, tantrums, and repetitive movements, excessive drooling, severe cognitive, speech and motor delays. Affected females reach puberty, develop secondary sex characteristics, and menstruate at the usual time. In males, testes are often small, but spermatogenesis is thought to be normal.

6. **Fetal alcohol syndrome:** Children with mental and physical disorder because of excessive intake of alcohol during pregnancy by the mother. Children have low-birth weight, malformed head and face, MR, short stature, hyperactivity, vomiting, tremors, impulsivity, cognitive deficits, behavior problems, and learning difficulties.

Environment

It has been found that the environment also plays its role in human behavior and development. The temperature of the environment can affect the development of skin color in certain rabbits and eye color in fruit flies even though these attributes are genetically controlled. When we treat patients in hospitals, we try to bring about change by influencing the environment.

The environmental influences are those which act upon the organism at the earlier stages of development within the mother's womb and later external environment after birth.

The nucleus, chromosomes and genes are surrounded by a jelly-like substance known as cytoplasm. The cytoplasm is an intracellular environment, because the genes surrounded by it are influenced by and in turn influence its characteristics. The outcome of the organism is determined by the cytoplasm as well as its heredity. A new internal environment comes into existence, after the interaction of genes and cytoplasm has produced several cells. The actual structure of a cell depends upon its relation to the other cells. Development in specific locations determines that part of the body.

The growing organism is surrounded by amniotic fluid and attached to the mother by the umbilical cord. Thus, growth of the embryo depends on the nourishment provided by the mother.

Individuals are different from each other even at birth, in physical appearance, mobility, and temperament. These differences become more pronounced and complex with age and maturity. They acquire more characteristics as a result of their interaction with their environment, which is different for each individual. Environmental factors refer to all outside conditions and factors, which affect an organism.

Later endocrine glands and hormones produce another intercellular influence. Many congenital deformities are the result of over-active or under-active endocrine functioning.

The endocrine glands produce hormones which have the power to raise and depress the activity of the various organs. They influence emotional behavior. They bring about changes in physical appearance, motor functioning, intelligence, and emotional stability. The physical conditions of the body caused by drugs, toxins, and diseases also affect our behavior. The social/psychological environment in which the child is born provides social heritage. The customs, socioeconomic status, family environment, interaction among family members, and later peers and the school environment cause a variety of conditions to determine individual differences.

The social aspects of an individual's environment affect the personality decisively. If the home provides peace, love, mutual understanding and harmony, the child will develop into a healthy and self-confident individual. An overprotected child, not given independence and initiative will develop into an under-confident and over dependent personality. Repressive discipline may produce rebelliousness. The only child, if given extra protection and care will become a self-centered individual.

In the school, most children start learning to adjust the larger groups of people. The personality of the teacher, methods of teaching, studies, play and co-curricular activities, and the type of discipline—all these will shape the child's personality.

When we speak of environment, we generally think of the external world and all the forces that affect the individual directly or indirectly. But we have to consider two other environments. They are the intercellular environment and the intrauterine environment. The intercellular environment relates to embryonic development. Intrauterine environment shelters the baby during prenatal life. It deals with substances, which by passing the placental barrier can adversely affect the unborn child. Viruses, bacteria, and drugs cause damage to the child. So, the nurse as a teacher can help pregnant women to understand their responsibility for maintaining the necessary hygiene for the growth of a healthy infant.

Children bought up in an impoverished kind of environment where intellectual stimulation is lacking, show lower IQ than children who were exposed to an enriched environment. Children of parents, who are in intellectually superior professions and those living in urban areas show higher intellectual capacity when compared to children of rural areas. Several studies have been conducted on twins and most of them have brought out results, in favor of the influence of environmental factors on human development and behavior. Experiments conducted on identical twins reared separately have proved that there exist a lot of differences between identical twins. These differences could be attributed only to the variation in the environmental factors received by them.

THE NATURE-NURTURE CONTROVERSY

The nature (heredity)-nurture (environment) debate really concerns the relative importance of heredity, and environment. Today no one believes that nature alone or nurture alone, completely determines the course of our development. Psychologists agree that development is shaped by the interaction of heredity and the environment. Within this interaction, our genetic endowment for many characteristics provides us with a reaction range of possible levels that we may ultimately reach, depending on the quality of our experience in the environment.

However, it is still not possible to say with certainty what type of behavior or trait is influenced by heredity and what by environment. Heredity factors are more prominent in the following characteristics: Reflex and instinctive behavior, blood type, finger prints, eye color, color, and texture of the skin and hair, chromosome abnormalities and defective genes, schizophrenia, hemophilia, tuberculosis, and some cancers.

Environmental factors influence human interests, attitudes, aptitudes, habits, temperaments, social and cultural norms as well as manners and etiquettes.

Heredity, and environment are interdependent forces. Heredity supplies the potential talent, which the favorable environment brings out. Heredity determines the possible limits of accomplishment for any individual in any given situation. The environment determines how close to these limits of performance any individual can achieve in a given situation.

Key Points ● ● ● ●

- Nature refers to heredity and nurture refers to environment.
- Gregor Mendel is the father of genetics.
- Human beings have 23 pairs of chromosomes.
- Mutation leads to different abnormalities in humans.

STUDY QUESTIONS

Long Essays

1. Describe the importance of biological inheritance as foundation of behavior.
2. Describe the general pattern of behavior.
3. Explain the interaction between heredity and environment in shaping behavior.

Short Essays

1. Explain the role of inheritance in psychological development.
2. Principles of heredity.
3. Identical and fraternal twins.
4. Chromosomes.
5. Heredity.
6. Environment.
7. Nature-nurture controversy.

Multiple Choice Questions

1. _____ is a genetic disorder with 45 chromosomes.
   a. Turner's syndrome   b. Down's syndrome
   c. Fragile X syndrome   d. Cat cry syndrome
2. The "nature" part of the nature/nurture controversy refers to:
   a. The behavioral we acquired throughout our lives
   b. The environment
   c. The biological dispositions we're born with
   d. The outside world

3. Exposure to radiation or certain chemicals can injure our genes. Such occurrences are referred to as:
   a. The genetic code
   b. Nucleotides
   c. Heritability
   d. Mutations
4. Phenotype refers to _____ of an individual.
   a. Genetic make up
   b. Actual physical appearance
   c. Recessive alleles
   d. Hidden characteristics
5. Who is known as the "Father of Genetics"?
   a. Morgan   b. Mendel
   c. Watson   d. Bateson

5

Observation: Attention, Sensation, and Perception

Chapter Outline

- Sense Organs
- Sensory Experiences
- Involuntary Attention
- Voluntary Attention
- Span of Attention
- Distraction of Attention
- Perception
- Gestalt Laws of Perception
- Perceptual Constancies
- Imagery
- Extrasensory Perceptions

Learning Objectives

♦ Students will learn the process and association between sensation, attention, and perception.
♦ Orients students to sensory experiences, types, and factors of attention and principles of perception.

INTRODUCTION

Sensations are the result of physical stimuli operating on our nervous system. The process of sensing, attending, and interpreting is called perception.

Various physical energies in the Environment Act on the sense organs. The receptors in them are stimulated from which nerve impulses are transmitted to the brain. Perception of objects and events are produced when these nerve impulses are processed.

There are eight basic sensations involving eight different sense organs and resulting in eight different types of sensory experiences **(Table 1)**.

Chapter 5: Observation: Attention, Sensation, and Perception

Table 1: Sense organs and sensory experiences.

Name of the sensation	Sense organs	Sensory experience
1. Vision	The human eye	Light, color, shape, form, etc.
2. Audition	The ear—the basilar membrane	Different sounds
3. Gustation (taste)	The tongue—the taste buds	Sweet, sour, bitter, spicy, salty, and umami
4. Olfaction (smell)	The nose—receptors in the nasal passage	Sweet, fragrant, pungent, etc.
5. Cutaneous	The skin	Heat, cold, pain, and pressure
6. Kinesthetic	The muscles—receptors in the muscles	Sense of pull, push and strain
7. Organic	Receptors and muscles of the internal organs	Bodily sensations like hunger, thirst, nausea, etc.
8. Static or posture sense	Ear, semicircular canal	Sense of equilibrium, dizziness, reclining, etc.

Sensory Process and the Ward Nurse

1. A patient reacts to colors. There are some colors, which are soothing. The patient who needs rest should use subdued light. For stimulation and encouragement, bright light can be used in the ward.
2. A sick person cannot tolerate loud noise and becomes irritable. The nurse should do her best in reducing the noise level in the ward.
3. Wards in a hospital often have disagreeable smells and odors. The nurse should see that the doors and windows are kept open to reduce the bad smell in the wards.
4. To help the patient relish their food, it should be warm, fresh, clean, and tasty.
5. Nurses must have highly developed kinesthetic sense and should move slowly but deliberately and gracefully in the ward. Jerky movements of the nurse in the ward will result in discomfort to the patients.

ATTENTION

Attention is the focusing of consciousness on a particular object or idea at a particular time, to the exclusion of other objects or ideas.

Types or Varieties of Attention

Our attention can be involuntary (non-volitional), voluntary (volitional), or habitual.

Non-volitional *or involuntary attention* does not require any conscious effort to attend to an object. We give involuntary attention to loud sounds, bright lights, and strong penetrating odors.

In *volitional or voluntary attention,* we have to make a deliberate effort, e.g., uninteresting lectures, difficult assignments.

In *habitual attention,* there is no conscious effort or sensation so striking to attract our involuntary attention. We attend to them because of our attitudes, habits, or interests, e.g., the attention that a nurse gives to her patients or books on nursing arts.

Span of attention: The maximum amount of material that can be attended to in one period of attention is called "span of attention". If you are able to note five digits or five letters in a single act of attention, your span of attention is five. The normal span of attention is seven, e.g., when a car runs fast, the traffic police will not ordinarily be able to take note of than four numbers. Hence, registration plates of a motor car contain usually only four figures.

Tables 2 and 3 describes the external and internal determinants of attention.

Table 2: Objective conditions or external factors which increase attention (present in the environment).

Conditions	Examples
1. Nature of stimulus	More attractive stimulus catches our attention. Pictures attract more than words. Human pictures catch our attention more than animal. Colored more than black and white.
2. Location of stimulus	A stimulus in the center attracts. A picture in the center of the page of a newspaper attracts more than others.
3. Intensity/Change in the intensity of the stimulus	Loud sounds, bright colors, intense odors. Ticking of a clock in our room may not attract our attention but when it stops, our attention is attracted. Early morning music may not awaken us if it is of constant soft volume. But we will awaken, if it suddenly becomes very loud or stops. Experienced speaker changes the volume of his voice while addressing an assembly.
4. Movement	A fast moving electric sign attracts our attention. Moving toys have greater appeal to children.

Contd...

Contd...

Conditions	Examples
5. Size	The bigger size attracts more attention, but a small advertisement on a very wide background also attracts attention. Thus, attention of an object does not depend on size alone, but also on the background. We notice unusually tall people or midgets.
6. Contrast	Any objects different from its surroundings will stand out and attract our attention, e.g., a single man among many women, a spot on a clean white dress, a smudge on a clean wall.
7. Novelty	New and unusual hospital equipment, a new fashion in dress.
8. Repetition	A repeated cry, repeated ringing of a call bell; certain important facts repeated by the teacher for the attention of the students; commodities repeatedly advertised in the television; many posters of a movie stuck on the walls for effective advertisement.

Table 3: Internal factors or subjective conditions of attention (present in the individual).

Conditions	Examples
1. Interest	A sportsman eagerly looks for the sports column of the newspapers; a nurse may see news regarding employment, hospitals and new medical equipment.
2. Motives	When a child is hungry, he cries and looks for the feeding bottle ignoring even his favorite toys.
3. Experience	A child when seeing an apple for the first time does not perceive it as something to be eaten. Different people perceive the same object differently as per their experience.
4. Mental set or expectancy	Mental set means the tendency or bent of the whole mind. A person will attend to those objects towards which his mind is set. We attend to objects with which we are familiar. An individual's mental set represents his feelings, attitudes, interests, habits, needs, and expectation, e.g., while expecting a friend, we perceive any knocking sound as that of the friend's footsteps. In a psychological experiment, hungry students reported edible items when shown ambiguous pictures in dim light. Students who had their meals, perceived the same as play items like the bat, and ball.
5. Emotional state	Emotional states distort the perceptual field. Under stressful conditions we fail to perceive our surroundings fully.

Division and Degree of Attention

We cannot attend to a certain stimulus for a long time. Our attention is affected by and distributed among the stimuli around us. Continuous focusing is possible only with many shifting.

Shifting/fluctuation of attention is from one stimulus to another and more often from one aspect of the stimulus to another aspect of the some stimulus. Shifting of attention is normal, but it varies from individual-to-individual depending on subject and situational factors. Students who are in the habit of listening to music while studying can notice the fluctuation of attention. A person forced to carry on a particular task would definitely experience fluctuation of attention leading to distraction.

Distraction of attention refers to the shifting of attention from one stimulus to another. Distraction refers to an interference with our attention. The source of distraction may be external, such as noise, bad lighting, and uncomfortable seating or internal, such as lack of motivation, emotional disturbances, headache, ill health, fatigue, or boredom. To achieve the useful ends, one should try to overcome all forms of distractions.

Distraction causes harm. While reading a book one may hear the playing of his favorite music. In one case, he may listen to the music and stop reading. In the second case, he may continue reading the book, ignoring the favorite music. In a third case, he may read and hear the music simultaneously. In the fourth case, there will be total confusion leading to no music and no reading.

A teacher uses some of the above determinants to improve the attention of the students in the classroom.

Some major means of overcoming distractions are as follows:
a. Becoming more active in the work,
b. Disregard the distraction, and
c. Making distraction a part of the work.

Distraction forms an obstruction only where it is distinct or opposed to the activity since attention can be focused only on one object at a time. Therefore, another method of making a distraction ineffective is to make it a part of the work. Some people work better while listening to music, because they make music as part of their work.

Division of attention refers to the process of dividing attention equally and simultaneously between two or more objects. For example, listening to a lecture and writing down notes. Division of attention leads to the deterioration of the quality of all the tasks attended simultaneously.

Perception (Sensation plus Interpretation)

Sensation is the first step in perception. Perception is the process by which organisms interpret and organize sensations to produce a meaningful experience of the world.

What one perceives depends on selection, organization, and interpretation of stimuli. An individual selectively attends to certain stimuli and not to others. Factors influencing perception are as follows:
1. Functioning of the sense organs,
2. Functioning of the brain,
3. Previous experience,
4. Frequency of exposure,
5. Psychological state,
6. Interest,
7. Motivation, and
8. Behavior of the organism.

OBSERVATION

Observation involves two mental activities—(a) Attention, and (b) Perception. Perception is the interpretation of sensory stimuli, which reach the sense organs and brain. Interpretation gives meaning to sensation and we become aware of objects.

Perception is the process, by which we discriminate among stimuli and interpret their meanings and appreciate their significance, e.g., when we hear a sound, we are able to identify it as being produced by an aeroplane or an automobile. Perception gives meaning to sensation.

Human beings have perceptions corresponding to each sense organ visual perception, auditory perception, etc.

Theories or Laws of Perceptual Organization: Form Perception

Early in the 20th century, the Gestalt psychologists in Germany tried to discover the principles through which we integrate sensory information. They believed that the brain not only creates a coherent perceptual experience that is more than simply the sum of available sensory information but also that it does so in regular predictable ways. When several objects are present in the visual field, we tend to perceive them as organized into patterns or groupings.

The sensory impulses will be organized into meaningful units during perceptions. These organizing tendencies follow certain principles, which are known as laws of perceptual organization.

The most fundamental laws of perceptual organization is our tendency to perceive stimuli as: (1) Figure-ground, and (2) Grouping.

Figure-Ground Relationship

The most fundamental process in form perception is the recognition of a figure standing out from a background. Contours are whenever a marked difference occurs in the brightness or color of the background. Contours give shape to the objects in our visual world, because they mark an object off from another or from the background. Color also helps, e.g., a black panther can be seen easily against a white ground of snow but not a polar bear. This is because the polar bear is white in color. Another example is a picture hung on a wall. The faces of two men in the picture is the figure and the ground is the wall in which it hangs. When we read these sentences the black letters are perceived against the white background.

In **Figure 1**, if you see the light portion as a figure, you will see a water glass or candle holder, if you see the dark portion as a figure, you will see two faces. Either one is a figure against a background.

Grouping of Stimuli in Perceptual Organization

In grouping, the stimuli are grouped into the smallest possible pattern that has meaning. Objects are grouped on the basis of gestalt rule of perception organization. Important principles of grouping are proximity, similarity, symmetry, closure, common fate, and continuation.

Proximity

When objects are close to each other, the tendency is to perceive them together rather than separately. In **Figure 2**, we see three sets of two lines each and not six separate lines.

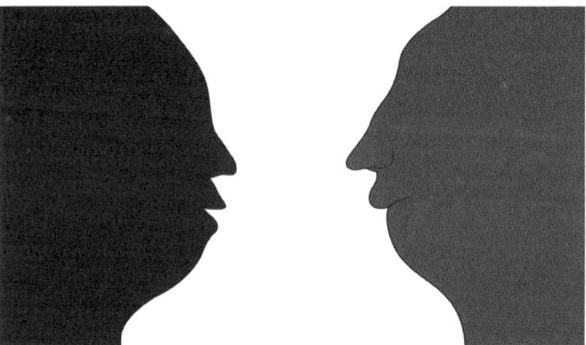

Fig. 1: Reversible figure and ground.

Chapter 5: Observation: Attention, Sensation, and Perception

Fig. 2: Proximity.

Similarity
Items that most closely resemble each other are perceived as units. In **Figure 3**, the circles and triangles are seen as two vertical rows of triangles and one row of circles and not as three horizontal rows of triangles and circles.

Symmetry
Items that form symmetrical units are grouped together. In **Figure 4**, we see three sets of brackets. We do not see six unconnected lines.

Closure
Items are perceived as complete units even though they may be interrupted by gaps.

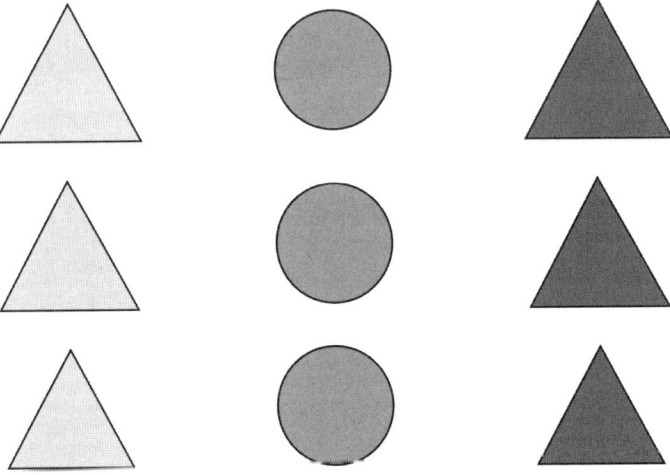

Fig. 3: Similarity.

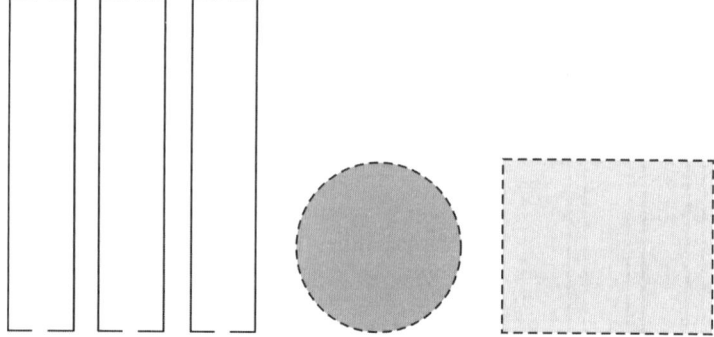

Fig. 4: Symmetry and closure.

Common fate

The law of common fate informs us that objects moving in the same direction appear to be grouped together. In **Figure 5**, in case these dots were mobile, those moving forward would be grouped apart from those moving downward.

Continuation

Anything which extends itself into space in the same shape, size, and color without a break is perceived as a whole figure. In **Figure 6**, we see a curved line and a straight line. We do not see a straight line with small semicircles above and below it.

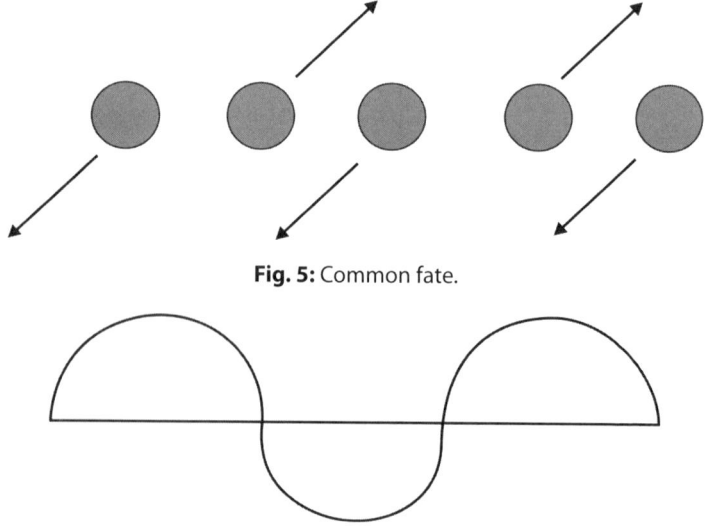

Fig. 5: Common fate.

Fig. 6: Continuation.

Perceptual Constancies

1. Shape constancy,
2. Size constancy,
3. Brightness and color constancy,
4. Perception of space binocular depth cues, and
5. Visual monocular cues.

Perceptual constancies refers to our tendency to perceive objects as relatively stable and unchanging despite changing information, e.g., the size of a man does not appear to change as he walks towards you even though his image on the retina of your eyes grows larger. Without this ability, we would find the world very confusing. Once we have formed a stable perception of an object (e.g., a white house) we can recognize it from almost any position, at any distance under almost any illumination—day or night. White paper is white despite varying illuminations.

Observer Characteristics

Our perceptual experiences depend largely on past experience and learning. Other factors, which affect perception are motivation, values, expectations, cognitive style, and factors related to growing up in a particular culture.

Depth Perception

Depth perception is the ability to perceive space and distances accurately. It is also known as the third dimension, without which we will perceive everything around us as flat. We need this ability to walk about, ride a cycle, thread a needle or do any meaningful movement with our body.

Cues are certain signs or clues, which help us to make judgments regarding distance and depth. There are two types of cues—(a) Binocular cues, and (b) Monocular cues.

Binocular cues: Cues which help in the perception of depth by integrating and synchronizing the images of both the eyes are called binocular cues. Two important binocular cues are: (a) Convergence of the eyes, and (b) Retinal disparity. These two cues help us perceive distance and depth. "Stereoscopic" vision (i.e., seeing with both eyes) obtained from merging of two retinal images makes perception of depth and distance more accurate.

Monocular cues: Cues which help in perception of depth and distance with the image of a single eye are called monocular cues. Interposition, linear perspective, aerial perspective, elevation, shadowing, texture gradient, and motion parallax are some of the monocular cues.

Errors or Abnormalities in Perception

Illusion is wrong perception (**Figs. 7A to F**) because of wrong interpretation of stimuli, e.g.:
a. A rope in the dark is perceived as a snake.
b. A moving dry leaf in the dark is perceived as a moving insect.
c. Illusion of motion picture on the screen (cinema).
d. Judging the taste of lemon juice as that of orange juice is gustatory illusion.
e. A stick in water appears bent.

Hallucination is an extreme form of inaccurate perception in which one sees something or hears some voice while nothing like that exists in the environment, e.g., perceiving a snake even in the absence of a rope, or seeing a ghost in the dark. Hallucination is felt by those who are mentally sick or emotionally maladjusted. Hallucination is due to subjective conditions. It is because of our inner fears and conflicts. We perceive things not as they are but as we are while illusion is wrong perception, hallucination is false perception.

Like illusion, hallucination sometimes depends on the mental state like fear, anxiety, and culture. The differences are given below:
a. In illusion, there is an external stimulus, which may not be present in hallucination (subjective perception).
b. While illusion often happens to ordinary people, hallucination is experienced by the mentally affected, tired, or intoxicated people.
c. In illusion, the stimulation is usually external while the stimulations in hallucination are in the person himself, who makes the later a kind of subjective perception, e.g., the vision of an Oasis at distance in a desert is hallucination. Another example, a woman in a white sari came at midnight and sat down on my bed and massaged my feet.

Abnormalities in Sensory Perception

- **Anesthesia** is a condition in which a person cannot respond to any sensory stimuli. It is caused by defective sense organs, drugs, or emotional stress. Some organs may be abnormal due to injury or illness. Drugs are used in the operating rooms to anesthetize a patient. We sometimes do not notice a pen or a bunch of keys lying before us and make a frantic search for it. We are either emotionally disturbed or preoccupied with some.
- **Hyperthesia** means excessive response to stimuli. Patients in the ward often show this behavior. They react violently to noises or bright

Chapter 5: Observation: Attention, Sensation, and Perception

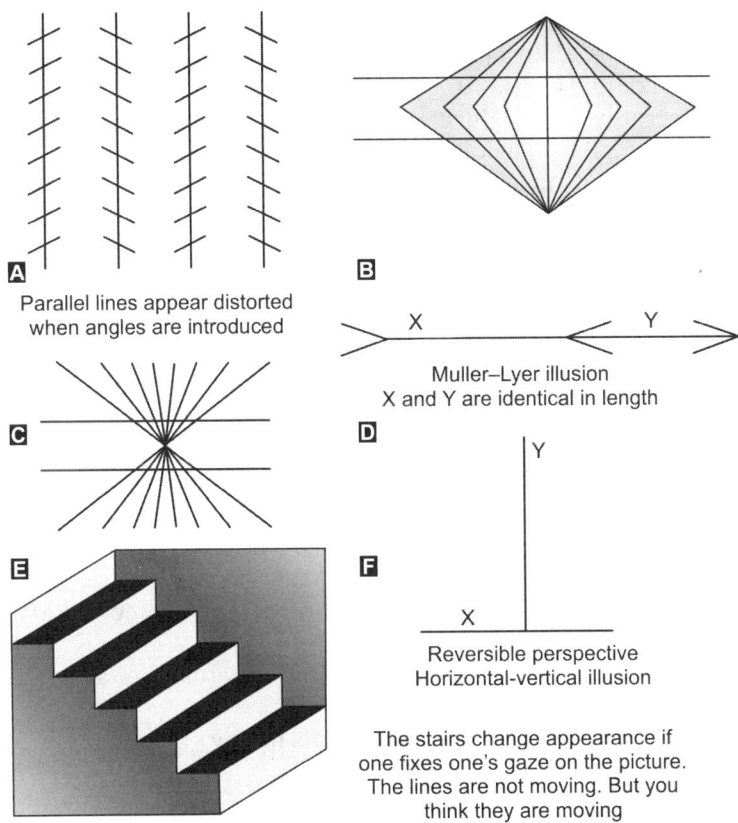

Figs. 7A to F: Some examples of perceptual illusions.

lights. When we are fatigued, we become hyperactive to lights, to sounds or to the weight of clothing.

* **Paresthesia** is grossly false sensation. A person of poor health or poor physiological balance may have sensations of offensive smells or bitter taste in the mouth when there is no reason for them.

Imagery

Imagery is the revival of past concept. It presupposes the perception of the object or situation in the past. The images recalled are at times equal to actual perceptions in all their details and sometimes they are vague and dim. It depends upon the images very often for thinking, reasoning, planning, painting, etc. It gradually reduces the habit of thinking in terms of imagery.

Depending upon the strength of voluntary imagery, Dalton classified people into imagery types, such as visible, audile, etc. Visual and auditory are usually stronger with the blind, auditory, and tactual imagings are stronger. With the deaf and dumb, tactual imagery is very strong. The strength of imagery also depends upon:
a. Pleasant and unpleasant feeling tone associated with the precept,
b. Habit of thinking in terms of images,
c. Law of recency and frequency, and
d. Age.

Imageful thinking is more prevalent among children than adults. Imagery is a very powerful aid to memory.

Observation (Attention and Perception) and the Nurse

The work of a nurse in the classrooms and clinics involve accurate observation. A nurse has to feel the pulse, read the thermometer, record readings on charts, note any changes in the patient's conditions follow instructions and administer doses of medicine to the patient. In all these activities, she has to be absolutely accurate.

Observation involves two mental activities—(a) Attention, and (b) Perception. To improve observation:
a. Give your full attention to each task. Undertake only one activity at a time. Avoid distractions.
b. Observe accurately and quickly but not hastily.
c. Keep your interest and motivation active.
d. Avoid personal bias or prejudice. It is possible to make only partial or inaccurate observations of those about whom you have negative feelings, e.g., the mentally retarded, the aged, the terminally ill, or those with socially unacceptable diseases, such as AIDS.
e. Cultivate the habit of observing accurately.

Observation and Perception by Nurse

Accurate perception and observation are advantageous for the nurse. Some positive results are accurate learning, adjusting more quickly, good judgment, better memory, more helpful and effective nursing care, improved recording and reporting, fewer accidents, and growing personal confidence.

Many patients find it difficult to distinguish between what they see and hear in the hospital. Particular attention must be given to a patient with any defect in vision or hearing, patients whose eyes are bandaged, those who are only partially aware of their environment because of sedation or those whose position in bed makes it difficult to observe

what is going on. Demonstrating and allowing the patient to touch, confirming the patient's perception when he is right, and correcting him when he is mistaken, are essential to good nursing. The nurse must:
1. Acquire sufficient knowledge of illusion and hallucination.
2. While making observation, the nurse must be conscious of the factors that must distort her observation.
3. She must be aware of her personal prejudices, tendencies and needs. She should not allow these to affect her observations.
4. Observations should be made with a broad and open mind and scientific spirit. Such habits can be acquired only after considerable practice.
5. Every part of human behavior should be observed with due care. Minor activities should not be ignored at the cost of major ones.
6. The nurse is to observe the patients in the ward, their facial expressions, physical and emotional changes and other activities. Her clinical observations are very important in the diagnosis and treatment of diseases.

PARAPSYCHOLOGY

There are certain types of behavior, which cannot be explained by normal theories of natural laws. Mysterious theories like precognition (predict events before happening), telepathy (ability to understand the thought processes of persons who are far away), psychokinesis (moving objects without physical force) and levitation (ability to float on water or walk on the surface of water) are some of the phenomena studied in parapsychology.

Extrasensory Perception

Extrasensory perception (ESP) involves the influencing of physical events by mental operations. They are areas of controversy in psychology and include the following:
a. Precognition
b. Telepathy
c. Clairvoyance or perception of objects or events not influencing senses, such as stating the number and suit of a playing card that is in a sealed envelope.
d. Psychokinesis (PK) whereby a mental operation affects a material body or an energy system. For example, wishing for a number affects what number comes up in the throw of dice.

Experimenters investigating these problems work in accordance with the usual rules of science and disallow any connection

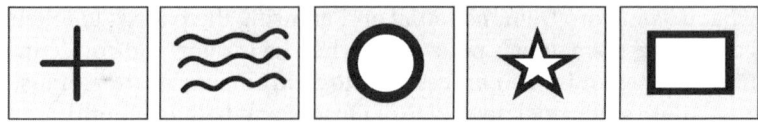

Fig. 8: Extrasensory perception.

between their work and occult doctrines like spiritualism and supernaturalism.

The case of ESP is based largely on experiments with cards, in which under various conditions, the subject attempts to guess the symbols on the cards randomly arranged in packs that he cannot see.

The usual ESP packs consist of 25 cards having five different symbols as shown in **Figure 8**.

The chance performance would be five hits for packet. Even very successful subjects seldom reach as high a level as 7 hits, but they may score above 5 often, to meet the acceptable standards of statistical significance. If the experimenter thinks of the symbol at the time the subject makes the response, the experiment is one on telepathy. If the experimenter does not see the card at all (it may be face down on the table before him or sealed in an envelope) then the experiment is one on the subject's clairvoyance.

Lack of Replicability

One of the chief reasons for the skepticism about ESP is that no method has been formed for reliably demonstrating the phenomenon. Procedures that produce results for one experimenter do not for another. Even the same experimenter testing the same individual for over a period of time may obtain significant results on one occasion and yet unable to repeat the same later.

Arguments against ESP

1. Many claims of ESP in the past turned out to be false on investigation (problem of dishonesty).
2. Improved investigation method did not provide improved results.
3. General lack of orderliness in the phenomena prevents theorizing to replace current vague speculation about what might be taking place.

However, these arrangements are not decisive and it is desirable to keep an open mind on ESP.

Chapter 5: Observation: Attention, Sensation, and Perception

Key Points ● ● ●

- Sensation is the first step in perception.
- Contours give shape to the objects in our visual world, because they mark an object off from another or from the background.
- Laws of perceptual organization were given by gestalt psychologists.
- Illusion is wrong and hallucination is false perception.
- ESP involves the influencing of physical events by mental operations.

STUDY QUESTIONS

Long Essays

1. Explain the attention process. What are the types of attention? How does the study of attention help a professional to carry on his duties?
2. How is perception organized? Explain perceptional disturbances with examples.
3. What are the determinants of attention?
4. Discuss the factors influencing perception.

Short Essays

1. Distinguish between sensation and perception.
2. Discuss the salient features of sensation and perception.
3. What is extrasensory perception?
4. What do you mean by sense perception?
5. What are the various factors that affect perception?
6. Differentiate between illusion and hallucination.

Short Answers

1. Explain the span of attention.
2. What is attention, types, and varieties of attention?
3. Define division of attention.
4. What is observation?
5. Write the factors influencing perception.
6. Write the factors influencing illusion.
7. Write the factors influencing hallucination.
8. Write the factors influencing errors of perception.
9. Define sources of distraction.

Multiple Choice Questions

1. What is the tendency to see an incomplete figure as complete called?
   a. Closure
   b. Proximity
   c. Continuity
   d. Good figure
2. Even though the retinal image of an object may change drastically, the object appears unchanged. This is the principle underlying_____.
   a. Perceptual closure
   b. Shape constancy
   c. Ambiguous stimuli
   d. Retinal disparity
3. Psychology that deals with ESPs is called_____.
   a. Physiological psychology
   b. Parapsychology
   c. Geopsychology
   d. Experimental psychology
4. _____is false sensation.
   a. Hypoesthesia
   b. Paresthesia
   c. Anesthesia
   d. Hyperesthesia
5. Which sense dominates our ability to taste foods and liquids?
   a. Olfactory
   b. Cutaneous
   c. Kinesthetic
   d. Gustatory

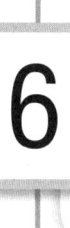

6. The Learning Process

Chapter Outline

- Aversion Therapy
- Reinforcement
- Classical Conditioning
- Schedules of Reinforcement
- Discrimination
- Shaping
- Extinction
- Sign Learning
- Flooding
- Social Learning
- Generalization
- Spontaneous Recovery
- Insight Learning
- Systematic Desensitization
- Laws of Learning
- Time Out
- Learning Curves
- Token Economy
- Learning Process
- Transfer of Learning
- Operant Conditioning
- Trial and Error Learning
- Punishment

Learning Objective

Familiarizes students to the learning process, types, and modes of learning.

INTRODUCTION

Cognition is the term given to those internal processes, such as thinking, learning, perceiving, remembering, and problem solving.

One of the most important characteristics of human being is their capacity to learn. Our personality, habits, skills, knowledge, attitudes, interests, and character is largely the result of learning. The main goal of learning is to increase individual and group experience.

Definition

Learning has been defined as a permanent change in behavior that occurs as a result of practice or experience and not due to maturation. A little girl, being indisposed is taken to a hospital. The nurse prepares the syringe, which the little girl looks on with interest. The nurse injects the medicine and the girl feels pain. When the little girl is taken to the nurse next time, she starts screaming when the nurse takes the syringe. She had learned by experience that injections are painful.

Learning caused changes in her behavior.

Learning is central to all our behavior as we learn to speak, write, think, and perceive. Our attitudes and emotional expressions are also learned behaviors. There are three important factors in the definition of learning:
1. Learning brings change in behavior (usually for the better).
2. Change takes place through practice or experience and not due to maturation.
3. The change in behavior should be relatively permanent lasting for years, months, or weeks.

DOMAINS OR TYPES OF LEARNING

1. **Verbal learning:** It helps in speaking language as use of communication devices like words, symbols, figures, sounds, and pictures.
2. **Motor learning:** It includes learning motor skills, such as walking, dancing, typing, cycling, and swimming.
3. **Affective learning:** It deals with emotional learning, such as learning of habits, interests, attitudes, appreciation, etc.
4. **Cognitive learning:** It includes learning of concepts, ideas, and problem solving. The learner acquires knowledge and information through which he forms concepts, sees relationships, and arrives at generalization.
5. **Serial learning:** It is when the learner is presented with types of learning that exhibits some sequential or serial order. For example, children learn to master lists of materials, such as alphabet, multiplication table, names of presidents and prime ministers.
6. **Skill learning:** A skill is a refined pattern of movement or performance based upon demands of the situation. The student nurse can learn by:
    a. Listening to directions and explanations,
    b. Reading a description,
    c. Seeing a demonstration, and
    d. Paying attention.

The practice depends on attitude and will of the learner and eradication of mistakes.

MODES OF LEARNING

1. Trial and error,
2. Learning by conditioning: Classical and Operant,
3. Imitation/Observation/Modeling,
4. Insight, and
5. Sign learning.

Trial and Error Method

Edward Lee Thorndike (1874–1947), the American psychologist, considered as the father of educational psychology conducted a series of experiments (1911) on trial and error method of learning by animals.

Experiment

A hungry rat was set free at the entrance of a wooden maze, which contained many pathways from the entrance to the center. But all the ways except one were blocked somewhere in the middle. A piece of bread was placed in the center of the maze. Seeing the bread, the hungry rat rushed to get it. It happened to enter the wrong path which was obstructed in the middle. Consequently, it had to return to the entrance but only to try other paths till it reached the bread. The next day, it made few errors. The experiment continued for several days till the rat was able to identify the right path at the very first glance without trying out other parts. Thorndike conducted similar experiments on a number of animals, e.g., monkeys, dogs, hens, and cats. The errors were reduced as the trials were repeated, i.e., SR connections were made.

From the rat's experiment and several other similar experiments, Thorndike formulated certain laws of learning. According to Thorndike, all learning is trial and error.

Laws of Effective Learning

1. **Law of effect:** Any response followed by a reward (food) will be strengthened. Any response, which is unsuccessful, will be weakened.
2. **Law of exercise:** The law of exercise states that there is a direct relationship between repetition and the strength of the stimulus-response bond. The law of exercise is based on the law of use and law of disuse. As per the law of use, any task that is repeated shows a tendency for the strengthening of the bond and as per the law of disuse, any task that is not repeated shows a tendency for the weakening of the bond. The learned activity (reading, writing,

typing, singing, drawing, dancing, etc.) is learned by constant practice over a long period.
3. **Law of readiness:** Learning takes place best when a person is ready to learn. If a person is ready to act, acting gives him satisfaction. A person cannot learn if he is not ready to learn. Readiness includes motivation, inclination, attitude, or mindset.

Thorndike ignored the role of intelligence and insight learning. Many scientific discoveries have taken place suddenly without any prior trial and error. Quite often individuals learn suddenly by insight rather than by trial and error, which is a very time-consuming process.

The method of trial and error is used when:
a. The learner is completely motivated and sees the goal clearly. The rat tries to enter the maze only, because it is hungry and knows that there is food inside the maze.
b. When perception or learned activities alone are not sufficient.
c. When the learner fails to find the solution to the problem through perception, understanding, intelligence, and language. Then he proceeds blindly, tries in various directions, commits errors; eliminates them and finally, arrives at the correct response.
d. Human beings learn most of the simple motor skills by trial and error.

Learning by Conditioning

Classical Conditioning

The study of classical conditioning began in the early years of the 20th century when Ivan Pavlov (1849–1936), a Russian Physiologist who had already won the Nobel Prize (1904) for research on digestion, turned his attention to learning. While studying digestion, Pavlov noticed that a dog began to salivate at the mere sight of the food dish. Pavlov decided to see whether a dog could be taught to associate food with other things, such as a light, or a tone. In classical conditioning, we learn to associate two stimuli and thus to anticipate events.

Pavlov's Experiment

In Pavlov's experiment, a researcher first attached a capsule to a dog's salivary gland to measure salivary flow. A bell was rung, every time, the dog Sam was given the meat powder. This was repeated several times. Later Pavlov observed that the dog salivated at the mere sound of the bell, without the meat powder being followed. Thus, the dog had been conditioned to respond to a new stimulus, which was previously an unconditioned response (UCR).

The meat powder is the unconditioned stimulus (UCS); salivation is the UCR sound of the bell is the conditioned stimulus (CS) and salivation at the sound of the bell is the conditioned response (CR).

Pavlov's theory is that CS (bell) simply as a result of pairing with the UCS (meat powder) acquires the capacity to substitute for the UCS in evoking the response. This means that an association is formed between the CS and the UCS, so that CS becomes the equivalent of the UCS in eliciting response.

Pavlov believed that this association took place in the brain. Two areas of the brain, one for the UCS and the other for the CS became activated during classical conditioning and the activation of UCS area resulted in a reflex or automatic response.

Pavlov showed us how a significant internal process, such as learning can be studied objectively.

Principles of Conditioning

Extinction and spontaneous recovery

When a CS is presented alone without the UCS for a number of trials, the strength of the CS gradually decreases. This process is called extinction. Thus, when the bell is presented alone without the meat powder for a number of trials, salivation gradually decreases. After a response has been extinguished, it recovers some of its strength with the passage of time. This is known as spontaneous recovery. This implies that the extinction procedure while decreasing the strength of a conditioned response does not entirely remove the tendency to respond to CS. Reconditioning is more rapid than original conditioning. Reconditioning occurs when CS and UCS are paired again.

Generalization

Stimulus generalization is the tendency to give conditioned response to stimuli that are similar in some way to the conditioned stimulus but have never been paired with the unconditioned stimulus. The greater the similarity of these stimuli to the original conditioned stimulus, the greater is the amount of generalization.

Stimulus generalizations are responsible for developing phobias in people. A child who is attacked by a dog can develop a fear for furred animals and even for Santa Claus who has a white beard. These irrational fears can be eliminated by the principle of extinction.

Discrimination

This is a process that is complimentary to generalization. It occurs when the individual learns to distinguish between similar stimuli and to respond differently to each. While generalization occurs due to similarities, discrimination results due to differences. Selective reinforcement and extinction cause discrimination. For example, in an experiment with animals, lights S_1 and S_2 on adjacent windows served as conditioned stimuli which lead to conditioned blinking to that light which was followed by an air puff to the eye as a conditioned stimulus. On the first day only S_1 was presented and reinforced. By generalization, it was developed for S_2 also.

When on the second day trials with S_1 and S_2 intermingled and presented when only S_1 was reinforced, conditioned blinking occurred only for S_1. This shows that the animal has discriminated between S_1 and S_2. Discrimination is the opposite of generalization.

The principles of classical conditioning can be used in the following areas of animal and human learning:

1. **Developing good habits:** Good habits, such as cleanliness, respect for elders, and punctuality, etc., can be brought about by using principles of classical conditioning.
2. **Breaking of bad habits and elimination of conditioned fears:** All learning is acquired in the social environment. Acquired learning may be deconditioned by using the principles of classical conditioning, e.g., for deconditioning anxiety and fear in maladjusted children.
3. **Training of animals:** Animals trainers have been using the principle of classical conditioning and operant conditioning for long without being aware of the underlying mechanism.
4. **Use in psychotherapy:** In deconditioning, emotional fears in mental patients.
5. Used to develop favorable or unfavorable attitude toward learning, teacher and the school.

Anxiety, which is a common symptom of emotional disorder, is a fear that is induced through classical conditioning. For example, a person develops fear of automobiles because of his painful experience of an accident.

JB Watson (1878–1958), father of the behaviorist school, showed that it is possible to condition children in the same way as dogs. He conditioned his nine-month-old child Albert to become afraid of furry animals by frightening him with a loud noise, every time he played with a previously beloved furry toy.

A number of activities we perform in our day-to-day life are merely conditioned reflexes learned through the process of conditioning. Some psychiatric symptoms may be the result of conditioning. Fear of open undefined spaces, sharp objects, blood, carrying out certain treatments may have occurred as a result of conditioning without the person's knowledge.

Applications of Classical Conditioning

Processes like extinction, spontaneous recovery, generalization, and discrimination are being successfully used in behavior therapy. Many of the unpleasant emotional responses that are the causative factors for much abnormal behavior can be eliminated by using the principles of classical conditioning. Some of the behavior therapies based on classical conditioning principles are given below:

a. **Systematic desensitization:** Mainly used to treat phobias and induce relaxation. Some of the most common fears treated with desensitization include fear of public speaking, fear of flying, stage fright, elevator phobias, driving phobias, and animal phobias. The number of sessions required depends on the severity of the phobia, usually 4-6 sessions up to 12 sessions for a severe phobia. The patient creates a fear hierarchy starting at stimuli that create the least anxiety (fear) and building up in stages to the most fear provoking images.

   The patient works on the fear hierarchy, starting at the least unpleasant stimuli and practicing their relaxation technique as they go. When they feel comfortable with this (they are no longer afraid) they move on to the next stage in the hierarchy. If the client becomes upset they can return to an earlier stage and regain their relaxed state. The client repeatedly imagines this situation until it fails to evoke any anxiety at all, indicating that the therapy has been successful. This process is repeated while working through all of the situations in the anxiety hierarchy until the most anxiety-provoking.

b. **Flooding:** Flooding aims to expose the sufferer to the phobic object or situation for an extended period of time in a safe and controlled environment. For example, a claustrophobic will be locked in a closet for 4 hours or an individual with a fear of flying will be sent up in a light aircraft. The experience can often be traumatic for a person, but may be necessary, if the phobia is causing them significant life disturbances. Flooding uses *in vivo* exposure, actual exposure to the feared stimulus. Flooding is rarely used and if therapists are not careful it can be dangerous. It is not an appropriate treatment for every phobia. It should be used with caution.

c. **Aversion therapy:** It is a form of psychological treatment in which the patient is exposed to a stimulus while simultaneously being subjected to some form of discomfort. This conditioning is intended to cause the patient to associate the stimulus with unpleasant sensations with the intention of controlling the targeted behavior. For example, placing unpleasant-tasting substances on the fingernails to discourage nail-chewing.

Operant Conditioning or Instrumental Conditioning (Table 1)

Instrumental conditioning is associated with the works of EL Thorndike (1874–1947) and BF Skinner (1904–1990). Thorndike was the first to conduct laboratory experiments (1898) on operant conditioning leading to the formulation of the law of effect which formed the basis of the principle of reinforcement. But it was Skinner who made operant conditioning popular with experiments on pigeons, rats, and human beings.

Table 1: Comparisons between classical and operant conditioning.

Classical conditioning	Operant conditioning
Response is emitted or not, the UCS will be presented	Response is elicited (the learner does not see the food (stimulus))
Time interval between CS and the UCS is rigidly fixed	Time interval depends on the organism's own behavior
The UCS occurs without regard to the subject's behavior	The reward is contingent upon the occurrence of response (reinforced by food)
Association between SR is on the basis of law of contiguity (things occurring closer in time and space get associated)	Association between SR) is on the basis of law of effect (effect of reward and punishment)
There is pairing of UCS and CS (response is emitted in the absence of stimulus)	No pairing of UCS and CS but pairing of a response and the reinforcing stimulus which follows
Reinforcement comes first as food is presented first to elicit the response	Reinforcement is provided after the response is made by the organism
UCS is presented regardless of whether the (CR) conditioned response occurs	Stimulus is presented only if the organism makes the desired response
Stimulus oriented (stimulus is conditioned)	Response oriented (response is conditioned)
Essence of learning is stimulus substitution	The essence of learning is response modification
Involuntary response (saliva flows automatically)	Voluntary response (knowledge-mind)
Involves autonomic nervous system organism is passive	Involves central nervous system organism is active

Skinner placed a rat inside a glass box (Skinner box) containing a lever and food tray. The animal was free to explore the box. Whenever the lever in the box was pressed, automatically a pellet of food was dropped on the tray. By a mechanical device, the number of times the rat pressed on the lever was recorded. Pressing of the lever was the response to be learned (the operant response) and the food was the stimulus consequence (reinforcement). The rate of presses increased notably with the rewarding of the rat with food each time he pressed the lever. By reinforcement, the rat learned the instrumental response. Reinforcement can be either positive or negative. Operants are actions, which animals and human beings do like walking, smiling, watching televisions, etc. The learner has to "operate" on his environment. The term "instrumental" points to the fact that the learner has some control over his circumstances. His action is instrumental to what happens to him.

Instrumental conditioning involves more activity on the part of the learner than classical conditioning. Generally, behavior directed towards gaining a reward or avoiding a punishment are examples of instrumental action. Intention and achievement are important in this kind of learning.

Basic Concepts in Operant Conditioning

Reinforcement

The process by which a stimulus increases the probability that a preceding behavior will be repeated. For example, bonuses, toys, praise, good grades, borrowing the family car from dad, or taking a break after an hour of study.

Types of reinforcers:

1. **Primary reinforcers:** Satisfies some biological need and works naturally, regardless of a person's prior experience.
   For example, food for a hungry person, warmth for a cold person, and relief for a person in pain.
2. **Secondary reinforcers/conditioned reinforcers:** It is a stimulus that becomes reinforcing because of its association with a primary reinforcer, e.g., money, token economies.
3. **Positive reinforcers:** Positive reinforces are that which strengthens the response by presenting a pleasurable stimulus after response. For example, the paychecks that workers get at the end of the week increase the likelihood that they will return to their jobs the following week.
4. **Negative reinforces:** Strengthens a response by reducing or removing something undesirable or unpleasant. For example,

student decides to clean up the mess in the room in order to avoid getting in a fight with the roommate.

Schedules of reinforcement
1. **Continuous reinforcement schedule:** Reinforcing of a behavior every time it occurs.
2. **Partial (or intermittent) reinforcement schedule:** Reinforcing of a behavior sometimes but not all of the time. It is classified into two types:
   a. Considering number of response: Ratio schedules
   b. Considering amount of time: Interval schedules

Skinner also developed variable schedules for both interval and ratio reinforcement where reinforcement appears after any time interval or number of responses.

1. **Fixed ratio:** Reinforcement depends on a definite number of responses. For example, reinforcing after every third time a child exhibits sharing behavior.
2. **Variable ratio:** The number of responses needed for reinforcement varies from one reinforcement to the next. For example, some teachers do not like giving marks to competed project but would like to see the project during various stages of progress and then mark it.
3. **Fixed interval:** A schedule in which a response results in reinforcement only after a definite length of time.
   Example: Reinforcement—20 seconds—reinforcement—20 seconds—reinforcement.
4. **Variable interval:** A schedule in which the time between reinforcements varies.
   Example: Reinforcement—20 seconds—reinforcement—30 seconds—reinforcement—35 seconds.

Punishment

The presentation of an aversive stimulus or removal of positive stimulus following a response that decreases the frequency of that response.

Two types of punishments are—(a) Positive, and (b) Negative.

a. **Positive punishment (Type I punishment):** This type of punishment is also known as "punishment by application". Positive punishment involves presenting an aversive stimulus after a behavior as occurred.
   Examples:
   • When a student talks out of turn in the middle of class, the teacher might scold the child for interrupting her.
   • Spending 10 years in jail for committing a crime.

Chapter 6: The Learning Process

Table 2: Pleasant and unpleasant stimulus.

	Rewarding (pleasant) stimulus	Aversive (unpleasant) stimulus
Adding/presenting	Positive reinforcement	Positive punishment
Removing/taking away	Negative punishment	Negative reinforcement

b. **Negative punishment (Type II punishment):** This type of punishment is also known as "punishment by removal". Negative punishment involves taking away a desirable stimulus after a behavior as occurred **(Table 2)**.

For example, a teenager comes home after curfew and the parents take away a privilege, such as cell phone usage. If the frequency of the child coming home late decreases, the privilege is gradually restored.

Applications of Operant Conditioning

Operant conditioning has practical importance in many area of behavior modification. Parents can reinforce their children's appropriate behaviors and punish inappropriate behaviors. One must analyze how complex the desired behavior is. Teachers reinforce good academic performance with small rewards of privileges. Behavior therapist uses it to treat adults and children with behavior problems or psychological disorders.

a. **Shaping:** An operant conditioning procedure in which reinforcers guide behavior toward closer and closer approximations of the desired behavior.

For example, a teacher is trying to teach a child to speak in front of the whole classroom. Child is a shy kid; he wouldn't be able to give a speech right away. So, instead of promising him some reward for giving a speech, rewards should be given to behaviors that come close.
* Giving him a reward when he stands in front of the class.
* Next, when he goes in front of the class and says hello.
* Then, when he can read a passage from a book.
* Finally, when he can give a speech.

b. **Time out:** A form of type II punishment in which a student loses something desirable for a period of time. Time-outs may be on a chair, step, corner, bedroom, or any other location where there are no distractions, and reduced access to fun items, activities, and people. Research has established that 15 minutes is the maximum time that a child should be kept in time out from reinforcers.

c. **Token economy:** A token economy is a form of behavior modification designed to increase desirable behavior and decrease undesirable behavior with the use of tokens. Individuals receive tokens immediately after displaying desirable behavior. The tokens are collected and later exchanged for a meaningful object or privilege. Mainly used in psychiatry set ups, special schools, anti-addiction centers, prisons. Individuals can also lose tokens (response cost) for displaying undesirable behavior. Initially, tokens are awarded frequently and in higher amounts, but as individuals learn the desirable behavior, opportunities to earn tokens decrease. By gradually decreasing the availability of tokens (fading), students should learn to display the desirable behavior independently, without the unnatural use of tokens.

Bandura's Social Cognitive Theory

Just as Tolman believed that rats gather information and form cognitive maps about their environments through exploring, Bandura believes that humans gather information about their environments and behavior of others through observation.

Social cognitive learning results from watching, imitating, and modeling and does not require the observer to perform any observable behavior or receive any observable reward.

Social cognitive theory emphasizes the importance of observation, imitation, and self-reward in the development and learning of social skills, personal interactions, and many other behaviors. Unlike, operant and classical conditioning, this theory says that it is not necessary to perform any observable behavior or receive any external rewards to learn.

Bandura believes that four processes—(a) Attention, (b) Memory, (c) Imitation, and (d) Motivation—operate during social cognitive learning.

Social Learning: Albert Bandura (Principle of Imitation)

There are many forms of learning which cannot be explained by conditioning, we also learn through observation. Albert Bandura and Richard Walters (1963) focused on the highly efficient from of learning known as observational learning or imitation. Imitation is defined as a response, that is, like the stimulus triggering the response; a person or animal watches or hears another do or say something; then responds in the same way. Bandura maintains that nearly all learning that can take place directly through instrument learning procedure can also take place through imitation. Many of the nursing skills like giving an injection, making bed or dressing of a wound are learned by observing the senior students perform the same. Even maladaptive behaviors like aggression are learned by observation. Television can have good as well as bad effects. It can enhance prosocial behavior through positive observational learning. Modeling is often the most efficient means of learning complex skills. It is also a valuable therapeutic too especially with phobias.

There are two ways that observational learning helps people acquire new behavior. Firstly, it provides information on the how of the behavior; the specific steps by which others are able to perform it. Secondly, it gives evidence of the "doableness" of the behavior; the fact that others can do it helps demystify the behavior, makes it less frightening, and encourages the belief that I too can do it.

Applications of Social Learning Theory to Nurse Education

The new nursing student must start her professional role and this can be developed by allowing the student to observe a prestigious staff nurse going about her daily work. The student will observe not only clinical skills but also interactions with patients and other members of the healthcare team, thus learning professional attitudes as well as techniques.

The nurse teacher must also act as a professional model when she is with the students, showing enthusiasm about nursing and the ability to do the job skillfully. It is a useful idea when working with student groups to pair the students, so that the weaker ones are working with the more able students and learning by observation.

Other uses of the social learning theory are as follows:
1. Both children and adults learn a great deal through observation and imitation. Young children learn language, social skills, habits, fears, and many other every day behaviors by observing their parents and other children.
2. Many people learn academic, athletic, and musical skills by observing and then imitating a teacher.
3. It has an important role in a child's personality development.
4. Fearful children become less fearful when they watch other children acting fearlessly in the same situation.
5. Demonstrating a fearless approach to a phobic situation may be useful to motivate a patient's approach to the feared object or situation.
6. Modeling is also used in weight reduction and smoking cessation programs.

Learning by Insight (Gestalt Psychology)

It was developed by a group of Gestalt psychologists, Kurt Koffka, Wolfgang Kohler, and Max Wertheimer who concluded that the individual learns by his ability known as insight and not by blind trial and error. According to them, a person can deduce the solution by insight, if he perceives the situation as a whole. The situation viewed as a whole will definitely look different from that viewed through its parts. The whole of an object or situation is not merely the sum total of its parts like water is quite different from its elements hydrogen and oxygen. Sum total of the parts may create a new entity, which is called as Gestalt. The emergence of a Gestalt produces in an individual an insight into the problem.

The most famous experiments conducted by Kohler (1887–1967) in relation to insight were those conducted with a chimpanzee called Sultan. Some bananas were placed inside the cage of hungry Sultan who was then given two sticks, so constructed that they could be fitted together.

The hungry Sultan tried to get the bananas by extending out his hands. Then he took up one of the sticks and tried to pull the bananas, an effort which he kept up for 1 hour. Then he got tired and started to play with the sticks. Meanwhile, one end of one stick got incidentally fastened into the ring fixed on the end of other stick with the result that both the sticks were joined together. Now Sultan used this joined stick to pull in the bananas and succeeded.

The Gestalt psychologists made a number of such experiments and concluded that individuals learn by insight which emerges suddenly as a result of perceiving the situation as a whole. Sultan's sudden learning was due to insight developed from his perception of the total situation consisting of the cage, sticks, and bananas as a whole.

The gestalists tried to interpret learning as a purposive, exploratory, and creative enterprise instead of trial and error or simple stimulus response mechanisms.

Characteristics of Learning by Insight

1. Insight is sudden.
2. Insight is due to understanding.
3. Insight alters perception.
4. Old objects appear in new patterns and organization due to insight.
5. Higher species of animals including man has more insight than members of lower species.
6. Insight develops usually after some trial and error.
7. Previous experience is of assistance to insight.
8. Maturity also helps insight as shown by the smoother working of insight in older age than in adolescents.

9. If pieces essential for the solution of the puzzle are presented together when perceived, insight comes about earlier.

While classical conditioning and operant conditioning (trial and error) belong to the stimulus-response (S-R) theories of learning, insight learning belongs to the cognitive learning stimulus-stimulus (S-S) theories.

Insight is often used in problem solving, puzzles and riddles. To emphasize the suddenness of the solution, it is also called as "Aha experience" or Archimedes "Ureka".

Insight learning is superior to trial and error in the following respects:
1. Trial and error emphasizes the acquisition of motor skill but insight learning emphasizes mental effort.
2. Trial and error depends upon perception but insight depends upon sensory motor-coordination.
3. In trial and error, the activity is goal directed but in insight, it is the unconscious mind that exerts the most, while the conscious activities are either very few and/or aimless.
4. Every new problem has to be tackled from the very beginning, if trial and error method is used. On the other hand, both generalization and differentiation are present in insight, which cause transfer of learning and the use of old insight for the solution of new problems.

Tolman's Theory of Sign Learning

According to Tolman (1930), learning is a total process. It takes place by cognition. Cognition includes concepts like knowledge, thinking, planning, inference, and purpose.

The learner through his experience recognizes some cues or signs and then relationships with goals. Learning consists in the recognition of signs and their meanings in relation to goals.

Tolman argued that the organism follows certain signs and clues to reach a goal. It learns its ways by following a sort of mental map and it does not learn only some movements but also their significance and meanings. Hence, this theory is called sign learning theory.

According to Tolman, during goal-directed behavior, cognitive maps are formed, which are used to reach the goal.

In a typical experiment by investigators in sign learning, a comparison was made between the two groups of hungry rats in a maze. In one group, each subject received food each time it ran the maze and steady improvement was noticed. In the other, each subject was given access to the maze without finding a food reward and little improvement occurred in time or error scores.

However, when food was introduced at the tenth trial, performance soon approximated that of the group which had been rewarded continually. Such sudden improvement suggests that the animals had acquired information about the maze, which they did not utilize until, after the 10th day, it became advantageous for them to do so. The rats had developed a cognitive map of the maze.

STEPS IN LEARNING PROCESS

1. Motivation within the learner.
2. Goal or goals become related to the motivation.
3. Barriers of difficulties are perceived and experienced and tension rises. Strong barriers may cause excessive tension, which may altogether discourage and confuse the learner.
4. The search for an appropriate solution to the problem or an appropriate line of action to reach his goal.
5. The most appropriate line of action is selected and practiced; inappropriate behaviors dropped.

FACTORS INFLUENCING LEARNING

Learning depends upon three main factors:
1. Nature of the learner,
2. Nature of the learning material or task to be learned, and
3. Nature of the learning situation or learning methods.

Nature of the Learner

a. **Perception:** Sense organs are the gateways of knowledge. The process of perception and the factors related to perception should be perfect.
b. **Organic defects:** Visual defects like hyperopia, myopia, astigmatism, and color blindness can affect learning adversely. Similar is the case with hearing impairment and infections.
c. **Fatigue:** Both mental and physiological. Compulsive learning, loneliness, strain, restlessness, and boredom can cause mental fatigue. Studying in a room lacking fresh air and sunlight and in places where waste materials and toxic substances are accumulated can cause physiological fatigue.
d. **Time of the day:** There is no variation in efficiency of learning throughout the day, provided other factors are present. Even adverse environmental conditions like heat and noise can be overcome with learner's willpower.

e. **Age and learning:** The capacity to learn improves up to 23 or 24 years. After 40 years, it declines.

Nature of Learning Materials

Lesser the number of learning elements in a material and less complexity, easier is the learning. Meaningful learning is easier than rote learning (learning a material without knowing the meaning). The better the individual elements of learning material are distinguished, the faster they are learned.

Nature of the Learning Method (Making Learning More Effective)

a. **Definite goal:** With a clear goal in mind, the student works toward a definite purpose. Clear aim enhances motivation. Intention to learn ensures better learning.
b. **Knowledge of results or psychological feedback:** Frequent and regular review of the amount of progress being made toward the goal, acts as a strong motive to promote continuing effort on the part of the learner.
c. **Distribution of practice periods:** Shorter practice periods are more effective than longer periods and when distributed over several days yield better result. This will reduce mental fatigue.
d. **Whole versus part method:** This is as per Gestalt theory. With easy units whole method should be adopted. If the material is difficult, smaller units can be learnt but they should still be as large wholes as a learner can manage efficiently. Try to learn in natural units. Rhyming helps to learn poems.
e. **Logical learning:** Instead of rote memorization, you should try to grasp the meaning of the text. Logical learning calls for an arrangement and also assimilation with ideas in mind.
f. **Rest:** Take rest in between your studies as mental fatigue prolongs the study process.
g. **Level of anxiety:** Mild degree of anxiety can be a useful aid to learning but undue worry, anxiety, and nervousness will have an inhibiting and interfering effect.
h. Overlearning/repetitions at regular intervals help to retain the material over a longer period of time.

Learning Curves

The rate of learning can be quantitatively measured by plotting it on graph. In some cases, we find that the increase in learning is small in the beginning but the rate increases with the progress of learning.

This is called positively accelerated curve (**Fig. 1**). In such a curve, an increasing rate is shown throughout. If the gains in the beginning are relatively more and decrease as learning progresses, we get a negatively accelerated curve. Negative acceleration is characterized by initial increase in gains followed by decrease with practice. These curves may be obtained for tasks, which are not able to sustain the motivation of a student. Positively accelerated curves are obtained when learning of simple things are involved.

A learning curve for tasks of uniform difficulty shows a slow start followed by increase in learning, then decrease followed by a period of almost no learning and then a period of learning or reaching the limit (S-shaped curve). The stages are referred to as initial lag, increasing gain, decreasing gain, plateau, and end spurt.

TRANSFER OF LEARNING

Transfer of learning or training occurs when learning of one set of material influences the learning of another set of material later, for example, driving a new car. The movements and responses in driving a new car will have similarities and differences when compared to movements and responses in driving the old car. The individual has to adapt his old habits and learn new ones.

To demonstrate the effects of transfer of learning, the following experiment is useful. Two groups of subjects are used. The first, experimental group learns task A and then task B. The second group (the control group) learns task (B) only without learning task (A). If

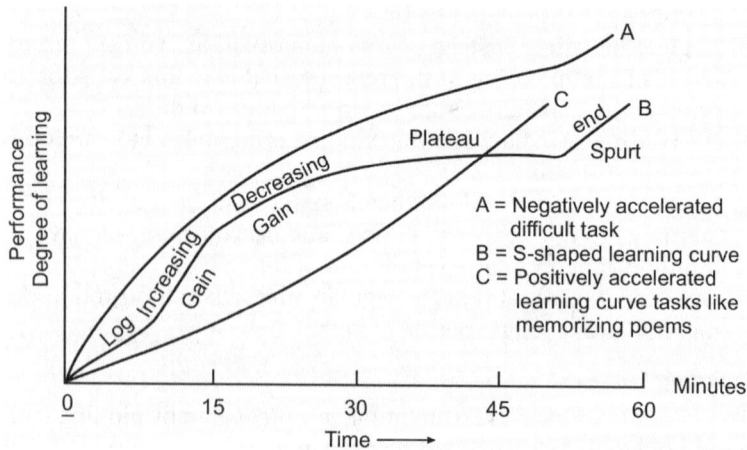

Fig. 1: Learning curves.

the experimental group learns task (B) more easily and effectively than the control group, we say that positive transfer has taken place. Positive transfer means the learning of the earlier task (A) has facilitated the learning of the later task (B). On the other hand, if the experimental group is found to be more difficult in learning task B, with poor performance, we may say that negative transfer has occurred. Negative transfer means that the learning of the earlier task (A) has interfered with or hindered the learning of the later task (B). If both the experimental and control groups learn the later task (B) in an equal manner, no transfer or neutral transfer has occurred.

For example, if learning to play the piano has facilitated the learning to play the violin, it is a case of positive transfer of learning. If learning Telugu has hindered the learning of Tamil, it is a case of negative transfer. If learning to play the piano has had no influence in learning geography, it is a case of neutral transfer.

In order to achieve maximum efficiency of learning, one has to reduce as much the negative transfer effects of learning

LEARNING AND THE NURSE

Modern nursing is a complicated and challenging profession. The student nurse must have clear goal interest to learn. She has to acquire a lot of information from books, lectures, and discussions. There are many complicated skills she has to learn with repeated practice.

Everyday newer techniques are being invented in medical science. The knowledge of learning process is helpful to the nurse not only while she is a student but throughout her career. The more she is prepared to receive new ideas, make new adjustments, and learn new techniques, the more she will be successful in her profession.

Every patient admitted in the hospital, has something unique about him. The nurse should have good understanding and learn more about each patient. This will lead to better adjustment and early cure.

Some diseases leave the patient crippled in one way or another. The nurse has to teach him new ways and techniques to substitute for the function of the crippled organ. This requires knowledge of the learning process by the patient and the nurse.

The following 25 suggestions listed by Crow, Crow and Skinner may be of practical value to the nurse in the development of the habits of effective study:
1. Study with a definite purpose in mind.
2. Evaluate immediate and remote goals.
3. Provide a definite place for study.

4. See that physical conditions are conducive to study.
5. Plan and follow a definite time schedule.
6. Look for the main ideas in the reading material.
7. Cultivate the habit of reading rapidly and carefully.
8. Outline the study material.
9. Make brief, well-organized notes in your own language.
10. Evaluate the difficulty of the material.
11. While reading, raise significant questions on the material to be learned; then answer them.
12. Study with intent to recall.
13. Attend carefully to all illustrative materials.
14. Complete all study assignments.
15. Let active study and rest period be interspersed with each other.
16. Try to learn the unit or the lesson as a "whole" when possible.
17. Concentrate on what you are studying at the time.
18. Shut out all emotional distractions.
19. Overlearn sufficiently so that delayed recall is possible.
20. Learn to summarize and review what you have learned or read.
21. Be alert to ideas emphasized by the teacher.
22. Think over the statements made by the author and try to challenge them.
23. Find out what the several authorities say about a topic or an idea.
24. Apply subject-matter learned in as many practical situations as possible.
25. Make intelligent use of the dictionary.

Key Points

- Learning is a process and it brings change in behavior.
- Thorndike conducted experiments on trial and error method of learning.
- Laws of learning where formulated by Thorndike.
- Pavlov is the proponent of classical conditioning.
- In classical conditioning, there is association between two stimuli.
- UCS is capable of eliciting a response (UCR).
- CS pairs with UCS and elicits a response (CR).
- Systematic desensitization used to treat phobias and induce relaxation.
- Flooding and aversion therapy based on classical conditioning principles.
- The proponent of operant conditioning is BF Skinner.
- Reinforcement and punishment can be positive or negative.
- Reinforcement based on no of response is ratio schedule and based on time is interval schedule.

Contd...

Chapter 6: The Learning Process

Contd...

- Operant conditioning has practical importance in many area of behavior modification.
- Bandura believes that observational learning has four processes—attention, memory, imitation, and motivation.
- Insight learning was put forth by Gestalt psychologists.
- Transfer of learning or training occurs when learning of one set of material influences the learning of another set of material later.
- Positive transfer means the learning of the earlier task has facilitated the learning of the later task.
- Negative transfer means that the learning of the earlier task has interfered with or hindered the learning of the later task.

STUDY QUESTIONS

Long Essays

1. Define learning. Discuss the various types and conditions of learning.
2. Explain Thorndike's trial and error theory of learning. What are its educational implications?
3. What do you mean by conditioning? Compare classical and instrument conditioning.
4. Learning and the nurse.

Short Essays

1. Laws of effective learning.
2. Insight learning.
3. Transfer of learning.
4. Social learning theory and its application to nursing.
5. Factors influencing learning.

Short Answers

1. Theories of transfer of learning.
2. Overlearning.
3. Extinction and spontaneous recovery.

Multiple Choice Questions

1. The random reappearance of a behavior after extinction:
    a. Spontaneous recovery   b. Acquisition
    c. Reconditioning   d. Start response

Chapter 6: The Learning Process

2. A child's toy is taken away after she hits her brother (to stop her from repeating it again) is an example of:
   a. Positive punishment
   b. Negative punishment
   c. Positive reinforcement
   d. Negative reinforcement
3. Observation learning is also known as_____.
   a. Modeling
   b. Manipulation
   c. Parallel conditioning
   d. Insight
4. A free pastry is given to customers after purchase of every seven pastries. This is an example of_____kind of reinforcement schedule.
   a. Fixed interval
   b. Fixed ratio
   c. Variable interval
   d. Variable ratio
5. Zero transfer is also known as_____.
   a. Neutral
   b. Negative
   c. Positive
   d. Bilateral
6. _____is the proponent of trial and error learning.
   a. Kohler
   b. Thorndike
   c. Tolman
   d. Ebbinghaus
7. _____is a behavioral therapy based on classical conditioning principles.
   a. Shaping
   b. Time out
   c. Flooding
   d. Token economy
8. The "aha" experience occurs in_____and it was put forward by_____.
   a. Insight learning; Bandura
   b. Insight learning; Kohler
   c. Latent learning; Kohler
   d. Sign learning; Tolman
9. _____is a type of punishment in which an individual loses something desirable for a period of time.
   a. Response cost
   b. Shaping
   c. Time out
   d. Aversion therapy
10. The theory of sign learning was introduced by_____.
    a. Kohler
    b. Tolman
    c. Ebbinghaus
    d. Bandura

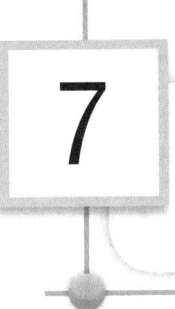

7. Memory: Remembering and Forgetting

Chapter Outline

- Memory
- Encoding
- Storage
- Retrieval
- Recall
- Retention
- Iconic Memory
- Echoic Memory
- Short-term Memory
- Mnemonic Techniques
- Episodic Memory
- Semantic Memory
- Forgetting
- Theories of Forgetting

Learning Objectives

♦ Students will be introduced to the process, types and various techniques to improve memory.
♦ The chapter orients students to forgetting and the theories of forgetting.

INTRODUCTION

Memory was the one of the first phenomena to be studied in a psychological laboratory (Ebbinghaus 1864). The power to store experiences and to bring them into the field of consciousness sometime, after the experience has occurred is called memory. The current trend in the study of memory emphasizes cognitive or mental processes. Cognition concerns the internal processing of information received from the senses. One aspect of this processing is memory. Memory is the encoding, storage, and retrieval of information. Memory is defined as the capacity to retain and retrieve information. Forgetting is the loss, permanent or temporary of the ability to recall or recognize something learned earlier.

Memory System = Information Processing

Ideas about memory that emphasize the processing of information in stages or steps are known as information processing theories. According to psychologist, John Kihlstrom, University of Arisona, this approach is modeled after the high speed computer (1987).

The memorizing process is organized in the form of memory traces, which functions like a computer.

Memory is said to consist of three cognitive processes mentioned in its definition–(a) Encoding, (b) Storage, and (c) Retrieval.

Three Memory Process

Encoding is the process of receiving sensory input and transforming it into a code that can be stored.
Storage is the process of actually putting the coded information into memory.
Retrieval is the process of gaining access to the encoded, stored information when it is to be used.

THREE STAGES OF MEMORY

Depending upon the differences in the rates of decay of the information, mainly three kinds of storage are described. They are as follows:
1. Sensory memory (SM) or immediate memory,
2. Short-term memory (STM), and
3. Long-term memory (LTM).

Sensory Memory or Immediate Memory

Sensory memory stores incoming information in a sensory register, which has large capacity. Information in sensory register lasts for a very short duration ranging from fraction of a second to a few seconds. Sensory image is like the flash of letters on a screen or the auditory image of a spoken word. The materials of SM may be processed into short-term or long-term memory or they may be discarded.

Types of Sensory Memory

Sensory memory is of two types:
1. **Iconic memory:** It is a form of SM that holds visual information for almost quarter of a second to 2 seconds. It makes things in your visual world appear smooth and continuous despite frequent blinks and eye movements. For example, iconic memory holds sparks in an electric sign as individual images as it travels in a circle, as a

result, you see a continuous circle of light rather than single dots of light.
2. **Echoic memory:** A momentary SM of auditory stimulus; if attention is elsewhere sounds and words can be still recalled within 3-4 seconds. It lets you to play back auditory information and gives you time to recognize sounds as words.

Functions of Sensory Memory

1. **Prevents from being overwhelmed:** SM keeps you from being overwhelmed by too many incoming stimuli. Anything you do not attend to, will vanish in seconds.
2. **Gives decision time:** SM gives you a few seconds to decide whether some incoming information is interesting or important. Information you pay attention to, will automatically be transferred to STM.
3. Provides stability, playback, and recognition.

Short-term Memory (STM) or Working Memory

Short-term memory holds a relatively small amount of information about seven items or chunks, for a short period of 15-30 seconds. The type of information stored consists of sounds, images, words, or sentences. Information is lost from STM by being displaced by new inputs. Information from STM may be transferred to LTM through either maintenance or elaborative rehearsal. If you pay attention, by rehearsing the information, such as humming the song you heard or taking the notes of a lecture, the information will be encoded for storage in LTM, that is, why it helps to take lecture notes. Whether or not recall the instructor's words for LTM depends partly on how it is encoded. Poor class notes result in poor encoding and poor recall on examination. Good encoding makes new association, which increases the chances of recall **(Fig. 1)**.

Long-term Memory (LTM)

Long-term memory has the unlimited capacity to store information for days, months, years, and even a lifetime. Information may be lost, or at least not retrieved, from LTM because of difficulties in the search process or because of interference by other LTMs.

It is by LTM that you always remember your name, your father's name, date of birth, and other personal data. LTM is of two types:
a. Episodic, and
b. Semantic.

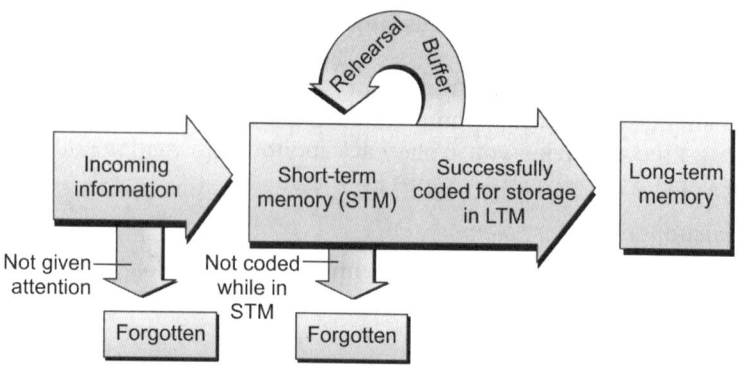

Fig. 1: Sensory memory, STM, and LTM.

Episodic Memory

Episodic memory is the memory related to our personal affairs like name, qualification, date of birth, and personal experiences. It is a record of what has happened to us, our remembrances of past things. It is less organized and hence will be forgotten faster.

Semantic Memory

It comprises of our knowledge and information related to the world. For example, 2 × 2 = 4 or Earth is round and goes round the sun. It also contains meanings of words and concepts; rules of using these in language. Semantic memory is not easily forgotten as the information is stored in a highly organized way, in logical hierarchies from general to specific ones. Such organizations enable us to make logical inference from information stored in semantic memory. Some people have very good episodic memory while some others have good SM **(Fig. 2)**.

The levels of processing theory of memory emphasize the depth of analysis and elaboration of incoming information. The most superficial depth on level is that of perception, the next deeper level is the structural level and the deepest level involves giving meaning to the input. Information reaching the meaning level and elaborated at this level has the best chance of being retained.

When we speak of memory, it is usually the LTM. Information in LTM is organized, categorized and classified like in a large library with a good cross-indexing system. The tip of tongue (TOT) phenomenon indicates that information is organized in LTM, e.g., a person is searching for the word "sampan" but cannot quite come up with it, but words with meanings similar to sampan are being retrieved indicating that items are stored in meaningful categories in LTM.

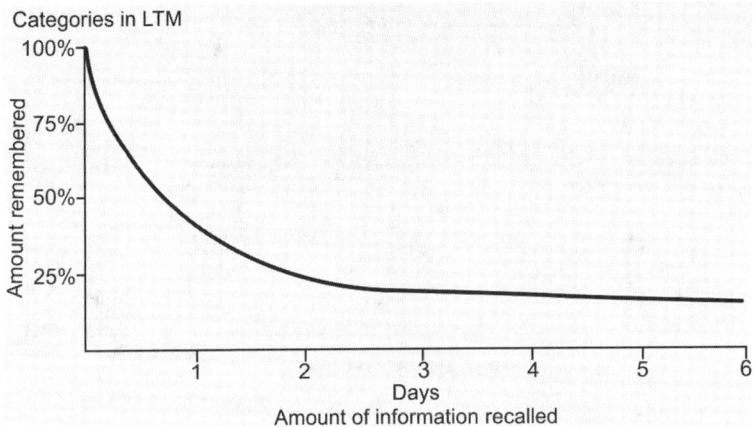

Fig. 2: Curve of forgetting (retention curve) notice the rapid falling within the first 24 hours.

FACTORS INFLUENCING MEMORY

Organization and Memory Network Theory

Memories are patterns of items, woven together by organization. When lists of words or other materials are studied; greater the degree of organization that the learner can develop on the material, the better the subsequent recall.

In an experiment to learn words, the experimental group was given the words organized in a hierarchical tree as shown in **Figure 3**.

The control group also studied the same words for the same length of time randomly without any organization chart **(Fig. 3)**. When tested later, the experimental subjects recalled 65% of the words while the control group could remember only 19%. Another example is the periodic table in chemistry.

Self-recitation During Practice

Recall during practice usually takes the form of reciting to oneself. Such self-recitation increases the retention of the material being studied. Suppose a student has 2 hours to study an assignment that can be read through in 30 minutes. Rereading the assignment four times is likely to be much less effective than reading it once and asking him questions about the material he has read. He can then reread to clear up the points that were unclear when he attempted to recall them.

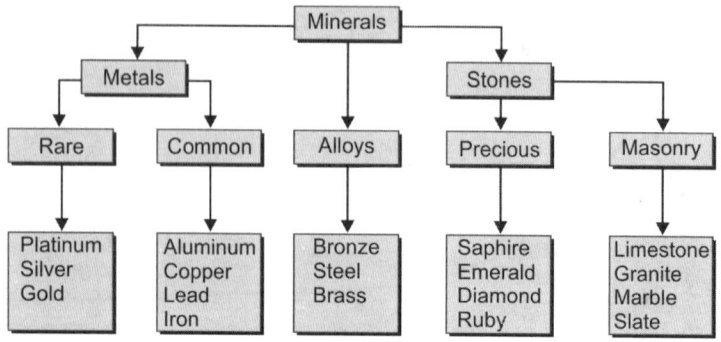

Fig. 3: Organization tree.

The percentage of study time that should be spent in self-recitation depends on the material and the type of test for which one is preparing. The percentage is usually higher. In a well-known laboratory experiment, the greatest efficiency in recall of historical materials occurred when as much as 80% of the study time was used for self-recitation.

The self-recitation in learning forces the learner to define and select what is to be remembered. In addition, recitation represents practice in the retrieval of information in the form likely to demand later on. Time spent in active recall with book closed, is time well spent!

Overlearning and Retention

Something to be long retained must be overlearned, that is learned beyond the point of bare recall. In an experiment, three groups of subjects were required to memorize a list of words by the serial anticipation method. Each group learned to a different degree of overlearning **(Fig. 4)**. For subjects in the group of 0% overlearning practice was terminated after one perfect recall. For the 50% overlearning group, member of trials were increased by half. For 100% overlearning group, the number of trials was doubled.

The results of the recall tests during 1–28 days is shown in **Figure 4**.

The curves indicate that the greater the degree of overlearning, greater the retention at all-time intervals. But the amount of retention cannot increase indefinitely with overlearning. A point of diminishing return is eventually reached. However, overlearning is always preferable to under learning.

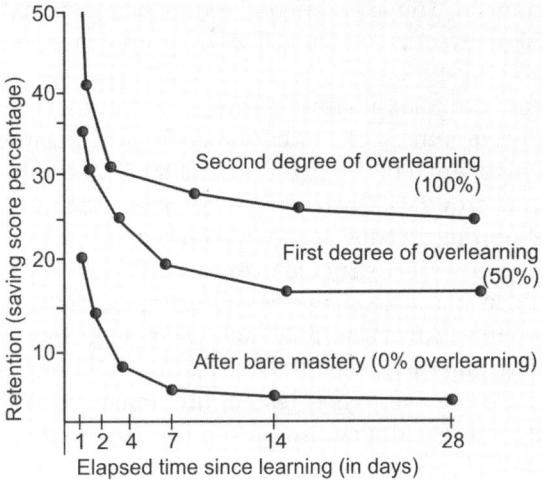

Fig. 4: Overlearning.

Method of Loci (Mental Stroll Method)

Try to visualize a walk through the apartment in which you live. You enter the front hall, move next to the living room, then to the dining room, the kitchen, and to the bedroom. If you were to use these loci to memorize a shopping list, e.g., bread, eggs, beer, milk, and bacon, then you would try to form a series of mental images. A loaf of bread hanging from a halfway light picture, an egg sitting as "Humpty Dumpty" on the pelmet in the living room, a spilled can of beer on the dining table, a cow in the kitchen, and a pig sleeping in the bedroom. When ready to recall the shopping list, you would take an imaginary walk trying to recall the image associated with each room.

Imagery as an Aid to Memory and Recall

Memory for pictures is often better than the memory for words. So use visual memory. Mental imagery is a powerful aid to memory. It has practical applications as an aid to learning. Recent experiments demonstrate that mental imagery may be applied with extraordinary effect to teaching foreign languages vocabulary.

Subjects who did not know Spanish studied a list of Spanish words for a fixed time period. They would hear each Spanish word pronounced and see its English translation on a screen. Later they took a test in which they gave the English translation as each word was pronounced. The experimental group, using mental imagery, averaged 88% correct as compared to 28% correct for the control group that used rote repetition.

In a laboratory experiment, the experimental group was presented with a deck of 100 cards; each card printed with an arbitrary pair of unrelated concrete nouns, such as dog-bicycle. The experimental group was instructed to associate the words on each card by imagining a visual scene in which they are interacting in some way. They were instructed to form bizarre or unusual images and include as many details as possible. For example, picturing a dog dressed in a Clown's outfit, pedaling an old fashioned bicycle. The control group was given the same learning task but simply told to study and rehearse. When tested, the imagery group showed 80% recall, whereas the control group remembered only 30% of the word pairs.

REMEMBERING AND FORGETTING

The act of remembering presupposes previous learning and involves three main steps:
1. Recognizing the request to recall and preparing to search the memory files,
2. Going to the correct file, receiving relevant memories, or association and selecting the particular items, and
3. Reproducing the memory through some medium of communication like speech, writing, or gestures. The pleasanter the original learning experience, the more readily it is remembered.

Certain extrinsic and intrinsic aspects of the material to be memorized affect the quality of learning:

Extrinsic Factors

a. Age,
b. Intelligence,
c. Motivation,
d. Physical factors, such as fatigue, cold, and
e. Stress.

Intrinsic Factors

a. Meaningful material,
b. Part versus whole learning,

c. Massed versus spaced learning,
d. Interference from previous learning, and
e. Sense modalities involved.

PROCESS OF MEMORY AND RECALL

Stage I: Perception of the Stimulus Material (Sensory Memory)

If anything is to be memorized, the stimulus must be recognized first. This is almost instantaneous and occupies only a very short period of time. The more unusual or complicated the material, the longer it takes for it to be recognized as a meaningful stimulus. Generally, the stimuli appear in series or chains against a background of sensory experiences. For example, when reading a passage in a book the reader may recognize individual words and his rate of reading is determined by the time taken to recognize each word in the chain. In order to achieve a faster reading rate, the background stimuli are ignored and selective attention given to some important words on the page. Patients listening to doctors reveal similar characteristics. Certain words or signals that have similar personal meaning for the patient may be attended to and an effort made to make sense of these particular bits of information.

Stage II: Short-term Memory

This stage in the storage of information normally requires the material to be turned into symbols for easy filing. Adults usually achieve this through language so that intense experiences may be retained directly from sensory store; for example, the recollection of strong odors or the recall of acute disturbances of autonomic functioning during a panic attack.

Young children are able to store detailed visual information as a kind of mental picture over a long period of time. This is referred to as eidetic imagery and this ability disappears with language symbols in adult life.

There is a limit to the amount of material that can be held in STM. Quite a lot of information is lost due to continuous presentation of more detail. This limit varies from person-to-person and also according to the type of material being held in the store. To overcome this problem, individuals employ various techniques like repetition, rehearsal, and deliberate attempts to cut out extraneous materials while retailing the gist or principle of what is necessary to be remembered.

When a doctor gives advice to the patient, the patient will store the information in the STM. The problem of encoding is assisted by providing repetition of instructions and in addition, by presenting the same in writing.

Stage III: Transfer to Long-term Store

The final step involves the use of symbols, usually language when the material to be retained is filed. The permanency of LTM is related to the number of associations attached to the information and the amount of learning that has gone into the memorizing process. New material can interfere with old material in the LTM.

FORGETTING

Munn (1967) defines forgetting as the loss, permanent, or temporary, of the ability to recall or recognize something learned earlier. Sometimes, what we think is forgotten in real sense is not forgotten, because it has never encoded and stored in the first place. Many students complain that they do not remember the contents after attending the class or forget after reading the text.

This is due to lack of attention. Some information does not reach STM from sensory register or due to inadequate encoding and rehearsal; the information may not have been transferred from STM to LTM.

Theories of Forgetting

There are four theories of forgetting:

1. **Consolidation theory**—*faulty memory process:* Many times, we forget as memory does not match events which had occurred. This happens due to the constructive processes, i.e., certain materials may be simplified or changed during encoding. We remember the gist or meaning of what we have read or heard, but not the actual words themselves.
2. **Memory trace decay theory:** We forget because of decay of memory traces with lapse of time. It is like rusting of iron. The decay theory supposes that when we learn something, a memory trace is formed because of neurological changes in the brain. This trace will gradually fade away, if the imprint is not occasionally reactivated. The way to remember is to rehearse and keep these traces active. As the individual ages, his memory stores begin to regenerate and a lot of material is lost, while at the same time, new knowledge is not retained because adequate capacity for

storage is no longer available and the material has to be packed into existing files where it gets lost. This is similar to a computer system in which the data storage tape gradually become degraded over time and new files are not opened. Clinicians have pointed out to the relationship between the degradation of the central nervous system and failing memory. Here, it is the new learning that is badly affected and there is poor recall of recent experiences. By contrast old learning, memories of long-past events may not be affected at all. The forgetting process in the elderly seems to progress backward such that a patient may have forgotten what happened last week, however important the event, but can well remember experiences of a decade earlier.

3. **Repression theory** is held better in explaining morbid forgetting of unpleasant events. We do not want to remember by processing them into our unconscious mind. Repression, according to Sigmund Freud, is a mental process that automatically hides, emotionally threatening, or anxiety producing information in the unconscious. Repressed memories cannot be recalled voluntarily.

4. **Interference (inhibition) theory:** Learning new things interfere with memory of what is learned earlier and prior learning interferes with memory of things learned later. STM has a limited capacity. Childhood experiences are well remembered, because the stores were large, empty, and available at that time. On usage, the stores fill up and material is retained only after competing with the existing information, some being lost and some retained.

   a. **Retroactive inhibition:** This is a technical name for new learning interfering with material previously learned. This is a backward effect. An experimental design for the retroactive inhibition is given in **Table 1**.

   For example, you may learn one chapter of anatomy in activity I, then learn one chapter of physiology in activity II, then try to recall what you have learned in physiology. The amount of information you forgot would be due to retroactive inhibition caused by learning physiology.

Table 1: Retroactive inhibition.

Groups	Activities		
	I	II	III
Experimental	Learn anatomy	Learn physiology	Test in anatomy
Control	Learn anatomy	Rest or unrelated activity	Test in anatomy

The control group learns the same chapter of physiology, rest for sometime, and afterward finds the recall much better as there is no retroactive inhibition.

b. **Proactive inhibition:** When prior learning interferes with the learning and recall of a new material, it is proactive inhibition. This is a forward process.

An experimental design for the proactive inhibition is given in **Table 2**.

Suppose you learn English (A), then French (B) you would find that the study of English interfering with your recall of French due to proactive inhibition, i.e., interference with subsequent memory.

In both types of interference, it has been found that the effect of interference is less with meaningful material and after attaining some mastery in the subject. Time tabling of lessons in various educational settings is designed to reduce forgetting due to interference. Very dissimilar subject follow each other. For example, in schools, a language might follow mathematics, in colleges of nursing, practical nursing then anatomy. At the beginning of your course, you should try to allot different study times to similar subjects to avoid interference.

Other Types of Interferences

Forgetting occurs owing to several other types of interference like items in the STM interfere with each other thus are continually forgotten. One tends to remember items at the start of a list (primary effect) and at the end of a list (recency effect) better than items in the middle (serial position effect).

Items in the LTM interact with each other; old items can be distorted or changed by the new inputs.

Some inputs are rejected by the lower centers of the brain because they are meaningless or unimportant while other inputs are deliberately repressed.

Table 2: Proactive inhibition.

Groups	Activities		
	I	II	III
Experimental	Learn A	Learn B	Recall B
Control	Rest or unrelated activity	Learn B	Recall B

Encoding, Organization, and Retrieval Problems

If the stored information is not encoded well or organized at the time of learning, it is forgotten. Retrieval cues are important in memory as we may not be able to recall information in one situation but may spontaneously remember in another situation. Retrieval is facilitated by organization of the stored material and the presence of retrieval cues that can guide our search through LTM for stored information. In the absence of proper retrieval cues, the desired items stored with LTM will not be found. Sometimes, you cannot recall something while actively searching for it but after giving up that search while doing something else, you recall that information. This is because your new activity has generated new retrieval cues.

Processes of Forgetting

Forgetting involves two processes:

a. **Cue dependent forgetting:** The inability to retrieve information stored in memory because of insufficient internally or externally generated cues.
State dependent memory: The tendency to remember something when one is in the same physiological or emotional state as during the original learning or experience. Without it, the person has difficulty in retrieval.

b. **Trace dependent forgetting:** Traces are conceived in the brain in the same psychological fashion. When these traces are not available at the time of recall it results in forgetting (may be due to lapse of time).

Motivated Forgetting

Many lapses of memory in daily life are due to motivated forgetting. We may forget the names of people whom we hate. We forget to buy a particular edible item, which the housewife had asked to buy, probably because it is not to our liking. Repression theory holds that we forget, because the retrieval of memories would be painful or unacceptable in some way.

Visitors to patients sometimes indulge in recollections of all the sad and unfortunate experiences, which they remember suddenly when the association with hospital. Sickness and death bring those memories to the fore. Patients do not find stories of other people's suffering, operations, treatments, and misfortunes at all comforting. Nurses may have to help visitors to remember positive, encouraging, and hopeful types of conversation by their own cheerful, optimistic attitude to visitors.

The patient may appear to forget his family and his work and may remember only the events which occur in the hospital. His conversation is about wards, nurses, other patients. He appears to have forgotten his family. Children in hospital show this to a very marked degree.

Emotional factors also play an important role in forgetting. If we encode while in one emotional state and try to recall it while in another, our recall suffers.

Anxiety or guilt-producing materials are more often forgotten than pleasant experiences. Suppose in a particular class, you were scolded by the instructor. You are likely to forget most of what was taught in the class that day. This is why punishment is not, in the long-run, effective in promoting learning.

Psychologists have also found that some persons cannot forget unpleasant experiences easily and this is related to personality.

Memory Disorders

Amnesia—Forgetting during Sickness

Amnesia refers to loss of memory due to disease. The person may forget his past experiences or may have impaired ability to encode, store, and retrieve making new memory difficult. Amnesia is a profound memory deficit due to either the loss of what has been stored or to the inability to form new memories. Amnesias are classified into two types: (a) Biological, and (b) Psychological.

a. **Biological amnesias:** These are caused by brain malfunctions. Examples are transient global amnesia, alcohol induced amnesia and the amnesia caused by certain diseases of the brain. Transient global amnesia is a short-lived amnesia attack due to change in the normal blood flow to the brain and characterized by retrograde and anterograde amnesia. High doses of alcohol result in amnesia for the events that occurred while drunk. In addition, heavy drinking over a period of years can produce brain damage and a pattern of systems known as the Korsakoff's syndrome. Anterograde amnesia and some loss of remote memory characterize the memory problems of this syndrome. Senile dementia and primary degenerative dementia, of which Alzheimer's disease is an example are instances of brain diseases that have amnesia as a major symptom. This is due to encode and store new information in the brain. Drug abuse also causes biological amnesia.

Chapter 7: Memory: Remembering and Forgetting

b. **Psychological amnesia**
   * *Childhood amnesia* is due to the differences in the ways young children and older people encode and store information. As adults, much of our memory is encoded verbally and tied into networks or schemata that are language based. But the young child without language encodes memories in a nonverbal form, perhaps storing information as images or feelings. Early childhood memories are thus said to be stored in forms no longer available to us as verbal adults. Our language dominated memories do not have retrieval cues appropriate for gaining access to the image and feeling memories of early childhood. Perhaps the memory machine is just not able to store LTMs until its maturation is essentially finished.
   Language ability and memory develop together because both depend on brain maturation. Repression is another explanation given for childhood and dream amnesias.
   * *Dream amnesia in dream amnesia,* the difference between the symbol system in dreams and in waking makes the waking retrieval of any information encoded during dreaming difficult. While usually considered to be psychological, childhood, and dream amnesia have a biological basis—the immaturity of the brain in childhood amnesia and the difference between the brain states in dreaming and in waking for dream amnesia. The forgetting of defensive amnesia protects the amnesiac from the guilt or anxiety that can accompany intense, intolerable life situations, and conflicts.

Memory and Brain Damage

When the brain is damaged by accident, operation, drugs or toxins, remembering is impaired. The amount of forgetting is related to the extent of brain damage. Because forgetting takes place most rapidly immediately after learning, before consolidation has taken place and much more slowly later on, the material most recently learnt is most completely forgotten after head injury. Old knowledge remains intact.

Patients who suffer from concussion may have forgotten what they were doing at the time of the accident. On recovery from electroconvulsive therapy, epileptic fits, or an anesthetic, the patient may forget where he placed his belongings, what was the last meal he ate or which part of the ward he is in.

METHODS TO IMPROVE MEMORY

Proper Learning Method

Proper learning method with training, practice, and motivation, memory can be improved. Learning by whole rather than by parts, improves learning. Similarly, recitation method helps to memorize better than continued rereading of the same material.

Our recall process can be improved by keeping ourselves away from harmful emotional factors, building self-confidence, and making the right associations. Learner's will, his interest, span of attention, and the right learning methods have vital roles to play in the process of remembering. Memory training aims to achieve a good memory.

Mnemonics or Memory Tricks

Mnemonics comes from the Greek word for memory and refers to the specific memory improvement techniques. Most mnemonics techniques rely on the linking or association of to be remembered material with a systematic and organized set of images or words with (oxidation), which we are very familiar, and therefore can provide reminder cues. Use mnemonic devices to remember a list of unfamiliar items, e.g., a sentence "Citric acid is Krebs' starting substrate for mitochondrial oxidation" to remember the names of acids in Krebs' cycle.

Memory Pegs

Memory pegs with the analogy of a clock room in mind, the reminder cues are called memory pegs to hang that to be remembered items, e.g., the letters of the word VIBGYOR can be used as "pegs" on which to hang the names of rainbow colors—violet, indigo, blue, green, yellow, orange, and red. Similarly, PVT TIM HALL to remember the essential amino acids.

Method of Loci

The word "loci" mean "places". The memory pegs of this system are parts of your image of a scene. The scene can be a street, a building with roads, the layout of a college campus, a kitchen or anything that can be visualized clearly and contains a number of discrete items in specific locations to serve as memory pegs. Suppose you want to remember for examination, classical conditioning. Then start by imagining a dog, experimental room, food, bell, and any person as an experimenter. Rehearse this image over and over until it is well-established in your mind. After you have formed your image, associate the events like stimulus substitution and extinction with this. The trick is to make association with as many concepts as needed.

Rhyming System

Think of the words that rhyme with numbers 1 is a bun, 2 is shoe, 3 is a tree, 4 is a door, 5 is knife, 6 is a disc, 7 is a pen, 8 is a light, 9 is fine, 10 is men, and so on. Now when you have a list to remember, you can associate the items on the list with your images of the numbers. If the first item on a grocery list is coffee imagine a steamed cup of coffee next to a plate of buns; if the second item is hamburger, you might see a giant shoe squashing hamburger into a patty, and so on.

Make a Story

If you have a list of unrelated items to remember a useful memory devise is to relate the items in a made-up story.

The story starts with the first item on the list and each succeeding item is included in that order. Doing this gives coherence and meaning to the otherwise unrelated items. It is a form of elaborative encoding.

Chunking

Suppose you want to remember your credit card number-20014609001, you can break the numbers into chunks, the first four digits could be remembered as the year you passed your school or associate with any significant thing that happened in that year—next four digits could also be taken as date, e.g., someone's birthday. The last three numbers form a chunk that is easy to remember by itself.

Overlearning

Retention is greater when subject matter is well-learned. Overlearning is the term used to describe practice that continues after a perfect recall has been scored.

STUDYING TO REMEMBER

Here are some tips to improve your memory:
a. Study is work and takes time, so plan a *study schedule* to cover the study content. Stick to this schedule firmly. If you study hard during your scheduled times, you will have plenty of time for your friends and television.
b. **Rehearsal** is crucial for transferring information from STM to LTM. Maintenance rehearsal consists of merely repeating information

while elaborative rehearsal consists of thinking about what is rehearsed in an effort to relate, it to other things that you know or you are learning. You should spend half of your study time in elaborative rehearsal. Make notes of important points as all the details of information cannot be remembered. Revise these notes often. You use imagery to visualize the material you are learning and give auditory stimulation by reading aloud. For example, while studying nervous system, visualize the structure of nervous system with minute detail and also read loudly. Multichannel stimulation will improve your memory.

c. Remember the importance of organization. Textbooks like this one are organized by headings, to provide a kind of outline. As you rehearse elaborately, give your own organization, under different topic headings and provide your own retrieval cues. For visual images of abstract ideas make a map of the contents in your mind.

d. Give a feedback to yourselves by testing your grasp. Do some additional work on any weak spot. Revise areas where you could not remember. By testing yourself, you will be practicing your retrieving skills.

e. Review before examination. Try to overlearn but do not get anxious as you have seen high anxiety level would interfere with your remembering.

f. Give some short rest pauses between your study times. It would help to consolidate the material you are learning.

g. Study repeatedly to boost long-term recall overlearn. To learn a name, say it to yourself after being introduced; wait a few seconds and say it again. To provide many separate study sessions, make use of life's little intervals—riding on the bus, walking across college campus, and waiting for the class to start.

h. Make the material personally meaningful. To build a network of retrieval cues make class notes in your own words. Mindlessly repeating information is relatively ineffective. Better to form images, understand and organize information, relate the material to what you already know or have experienced and put it in your own words without such cues, you may be stuck, when a question uses different phrasing than you memorized. To increase retrieval cues, use as many associations as possible.

i. Refresh your memory by activating retrieval cues. Mentally recreate the situation and the mood in which the original learning occurred. Return to the same location. Jog your memory by allowing one thought to cue the next.

j. Minimize interference. Study right before sleeping. Do not study topics in close proximity that are likely to interfere with each other, such as psychology and sociology or anatomy and physiology.

PRO: Planning, Rehearsal, Organization; FRO: Feedback, Review and Overlearning.

Key Points ● ● ● ●

+ Memory is the encoding, storage, and retrieval of information.
+ Sensory memory is of two types: Iconic memory and echoic memory.
+ Short-term memory is also referred as working memory.
+ LTM is of two types: Episodic and semantic.
+ Forgetting is the loss, permanent or temporary, of the ability to recall or recognize something learned earlier.
+ Mnemonic refers to memory improvement techniques.

STUDY QUESTIONS

Long Essays

1. Describe the different memory processes.
2. Illustrate the methods of improving memory.
3. Explain the factors affecting memory. Describe the various methods of memorizing.
4. What is forgetting? Explain the theories of forgetting.

Short Essays

1. Describe LTM. Differentiate it with STM.
2. Describe some salient factors affecting forgetting.

Short Answer

1. What are the causes of forgetting?

Multiple Choice Questions

1. Semantic and episodic memory are two kinds of:
    a. Short-term memory organization
    b. Retrieval process
    c. Long-term memory organization
    d. Rehearsal process

2. Learning, retention, recall, and recognition are said to constitute:
   a. Intelligence
   b. Memory
   c. Intuition
   d. Imagination
3. Memory for particular events is called_____.
   a. Semantic
   b. Sensory
   c. Episodic
   d. Procedural
4. _____ of forgetting explains forgetting of unpleasant events.
   a. Interference theory
   b. Repression theory
   c. Decay theory
   d. Consolidation theory
5. New learning interfering with previous learning is_____.
   a. Retroactive inhibition
   b. Proactive inhibition
   c. Amnesia
   d. Rehearsal

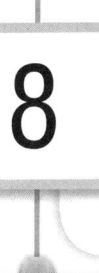

8. Thinking and Reasoning: Concept and Language

Chapter Outline

- Thinking
- Reasoning
- Images
- Symbols
- Concepts
- Creativity
- Problem Solving
- Concept Formation
- Language

Learning Objectives

♦ Students will be introduced to concepts of thinking, reasoning, and problem solving.

♦ Students will be oriented to the importance of language in communication.

INTRODUCTION

Man is differentiated from animals because of his ability to think and speak. More than 2000 years ago, Aristotle referred to man as a thinking animal. The term *homo sapiens* used by biologists to refer to human beings, means thinking or wise animal.

Thinking is a higher mental process, which involves verbal symbols, internal, visual, and auditory images, ideas, concepts, and mathematical symbols. It takes into account past experiences, future possibilities, and external realities as well. Thinking, usually, takes place when the individual is exposed to an unfamiliar situation in which habitual responses are inadequate for adjustment. Such a situation is known as problem situation. We conclude:

❖ Thinking is a cognitive activity.
❖ It is goal directed.

- It is a problem solving behavior.
- It is a process of mental exploration.
- The process of thinking involves use of symbols. A symbol represents some event or item in the world.
- Images, concepts, symbols, and languages are used as instruments of thinking.

KINDS OF THINKING

1. Perceptual or concrete thinking,
2. Conceptual or abstract thinking,
3. Creative thinking,
4. Reasoning or logical thinking, and
5. Problem solving.
   Directed thinking – Reasoning + Problem solving.

Perceptual or Concrete Thinking

It is based on perception. Perception is the process of interpretation of sensation according to one's experience. It is also called concrete thinking as it is carried over the perception of actual or concrete objects and events. Being the simplest form of thinking, small children are mostly benefited by this type of thinking. It is a one-dimensional and literal thinking.

Conceptual or Abstract Thinking

It does not require the perception of actual objects or events. It is abstract thinking and makes use of concepts or abstract ideas. It is superior to perceptual thinking as it economizes efforts in understanding and helps in discovery and invention. Language plays an important part in conceptual thinking.

Creative Thinking

The thinking of scientists or inventors is an example of creative thinking, e.g., Watson's discovery of DNA structure, Archimedes principle, etc. It refers to the ability for original thinking, to create or discover something new. It is not bound by any established rule. The person himself formulates the problem and he is free to gather evidences and to invent tools for its solution. Creative thinking is aimed at creating something new.

When an individual generates an original, unusual, and productive solution to a problem, the thinking involved in such a process is called creative thinking. Creative thinking is defined as personal, imaginative thinking, which produces a new, novel, and useful solution. Creative thinking uses divergent thought and not convergent thought. In divergent thinking, the individual attempts to generate a novel solution to a problem. Divergent thinking is not guided by rules or convention as in case of convergent thinking.

The processes involved in creative thinking are studied through the reports of great thinkers and inventors. Interviews, questionnaires, and introspective reports are used for this purpose. Creative thinking involves the following steps:
1. Preparation,
2. Incubation,
3. Illumination or inspiration,
4. Evaluation, and
5. Revision or verification.

Preparation involves formulation of the problem and collection of necessary and relevant data. Incubation occurs when the individual is unable to find a solution in spite of long and concentrated efforts. During this period, the ideas that interfered with the solution fade away. What he learns and experiences in the meantime may give clues to solution. During illumination, insight occurs—the sudden grasping of the solution to the problem. This is followed by evaluation when the correctness of the solution is verified; if found correct necessary modification to make it precise may be effected. If this apparent solution proves to be wrong on verification, he retraces the process of thinking. This is revision.

Characteristic Elements of Creativity

1. Creativity is a process and not a product.
2. The process is goal directed either for personal benefits or for the benefit of a social group.
3. It leads to the production of something new, different, and therefore, unique for the person whether to be verbal, nonverbal, concrete, or abstract.
4. Creativity comes from divergent thinking while conformity and everyday problem solving come from convergent thinking.
5. It is a way of thinking, it is not synonymous with intelligence, which includes mental abilities other than thinking.
6. The ability to create, depends on acquisition of accepted language.
7. Creativity is a form of controlled imagination that leads to some kind of achievement whether in painting, block building or day dreaming.

Creative Individuals

The following traits are, usually, present in creative thinkers:
1. Sensitivity to people, events and problems,
2. Broad range of knowledge and interests,
3. Ability to combine a wide variety of ideas easily,
4. Verbal fluency,
5. High energy level,
6. Impatience with routine tasks,
7. Like to take risk,
8. Persistence in tasks they enjoy,
9. Good sense of humor,
10. Independent, willing to be different, courageous,
11. Uninhibited in thinking and feeling,
12. Choose truth and beauty before recognition and success, and
13. Spontaneous and brilliant imagination.

Factors Affecting Creativity (for Developing Creativity in Children)

1. Rich environment, which stimulates creative thinking.
2. Allow free expression in arts and science.
3. Recognition to creative child and reinforcing his creativity.
4. Helping children to see relationships, contexts, and sequences.
5. Encouraging group contributions to individual creativity.
6. Recognition of readiness for creativity.
7. Recognition of the role of self-discovery in creativity.
8. Assisting children to develop a sense of self, through creative play, dramatics, drawing, painting, music, dance, and other fine arts.
9. Realizing importance of whole community as a stimulus to creative efforts.

■ Reasoning (Reflective Thinking or Logical Thinking)

Reasoning is one of the best forms of controlled thinking in which the thought process is directed consciously toward the solutions of a problem. It is guided by some logical principles.

Reasoning is the highest form of thinking to find out causes and predict effects. By this process, an individual tries to solve a problem by incorporating two or more aspects of his past experience. Reasoning enables to figure out the implication of certain facts or hypotheses and to derive certain generalization. It is a stepwise thinking and it is highly purposeful, controlled, and selective.

Reasoning may be broadly classified into two types— (a) Inductive reasoning, and (b) Deductive reasoning. Inductive logic (reasoning) arrives at a general principle based on particular instances. For example, having seen a number of crows to be black, one comes to the conclusion that all crows are black. Deductive logic (reasoning) deals with scales for drawing valid conclusions from assumptions. For example, we assume that all men are mortal. Then we talk about a particular man say, Socrates and derive the conclusion that Socrates is mortal. Causes for making errors in reasoning are faulty fact gathering, prejudice, emotional problems, cultural barriers, and fixation.

Problem Solving

Problem solving is an important kind of thinking. Problem solving behavior occurs in novel or difficult situations in which a solution is not obtainable by the habitual method of applying concepts and principles derived from the past experience in similar situations.

Problem situation occurs when there is an obstacle to reach the goal. The obstacle may be physical, social, or financial, which may hinder progress of the individual toward the goal.

Problem solving can be done by trial and error or mechanical means. But these methods are time-consuming and hence ineffective. Problem solving can also be done through insight, which is a sudden understanding that comes after studying the problem.

Problem Solving in Hospital Situations

Many problems arise in hospital situations. At the outset collect as much information on as many aspects as possible about the particular problem. The different components of the problem should be perceived and thoroughly understood. All the personnel concerned with that problem should be contacted for detailed discussion and their opinions and suggestions recorded. Examine if the past or present emotional or physical health status of any member has anything to do with the problem on hand. Solution to the problem has to be found subject to the existing rules, regulations, and policies of the hospital.

After collecting all the available data and studying the different dimensions of the problem, the concerned authority has to arrive at the correct conclusions and careful decisions which have to be intimated to all the personnel concerned. As a matter of routine, all these facts and probable alternatives involved in the problem and its solution should be recorded in writing for future reference.

Scientific Method of Problem Solving Involves Seven Steps (John Dewey)

1. **Recognizing the problem:** It is quite possible to have a problem and not be aware of it especially in its early stages.
2. **Defining the problem:** Identify and name the problem, so that you can find an appropriate solution. To state exactly what this problem is, i.e., identifying the problem in definite terms.
3. **Collecting relevant information data** from all possible sources that have bearing on the problem. Appropriate tools are gathered, books, and magazines collected.
4. **Formulation of hypothesis or possible solutions:** One tries to think of the various possibilities for the solution of one's own problem in the light of the information and his own experiences. Intelligence and other cognitive abilities also help in the formulation of an appropriate hypothesis.
5. **Evaluation of the hypothesis for possible solutions:** We put into practice the course of action we have chosen as the most appropriate and verify its rightness by the results or conclusions. All tentative solutions should be closely analyzed and evaluated.
6. **Verification:** The validity of the derived conclusion is tested by employing them in solution of various similar problems, if they are found suitable in solving these problems, they are accepted for the current situation also.
7. **Choosing another action, if unsuccessful:** If another action is necessary you will have to return to your list of possible solutions and choose again. Then you can begin the seven steps again and the cycle goes on. If your problem is, not getting good grades in the examination, it may be due to a serious health problem and you may need more extensive health care. If you have emotional problems, you may need counseling. If you have no funds for your education, you may have to apply for a scholarship. You could analyze any one of the problems listed above and find a number of reasonable solutions. The important thing is to evaluate the results, accept them as good or unsuccessful and then choose further or different action, if necessary.

Another example of problem solving is that of going from one place (x) to another place (y). If one recognizes this problem he might use a route map, refer to sign posts, and choose one of the many possible routes depending upon what he wants. If he wants to reach the destination soon, he will select the shortest route. If he wants a comfortable and safe journey, he will select a national highway and so on, bus or train, etc.

ERRORS IN THINKING

1. Specific abstraction,
2. Magnification,
3. Minimization,
4. Irrational conjunction, and
5. Errors caused by emotions like fear, anxiety, stress, pain, and discomfort.

Errors in inductive thinking often occur, because we do not look for disconfirming evidence. Errors in deductive reasoning are commonly due to distortion of premises. Both inductive and deductive reasoning are involved in problem solving, which require flexibility in thinking.

Thinking and the Nurse

Nursing practice is improved by an ability to think creatively and use reliable problem solving methods. The nurse can practice good habits of thinking and systematic problem solving in the profession and all areas of her life like planning her career, problems in family life, and difficulties in professional and personal relationships.

Daily problem solving is a major challenge for the nurse. It is important to have accurate data upon which to base reasoning or problem solving. Much of the data used by you will be gathered through your own observation and perception. Other data may be supplied through monitors, laboratory tests and from other members of the health team. Develop the following habits:

1. Collect as much factual information as possible.
2. Beware of your own prejudices as well as those of your patients.
3. Separate facts from opinion, important from minor details.
4. Search carefully for underlying physical and emotional problems.
5. Define the problem clearly.
6. Look for relationships between cause and effect.
7. Do not jump to hasty conclusions.
8. Think about all possible solutions.
9. Listen to all solutions suggested by others.

10. Choose one solution and test to see if you have chosen the correct solution.
11. Keep an open mind by constant questioning of self and others.

Elements of Thought (Tools of Thinking)
1. Images,
2. Concepts,
3. Symbols and signs,
4. Language, and
5. Decision making and judgment.

Concepts
Much of our thinking is in the form of concepts. A concept is a word or idea with a generalized meaning which represents entire class of objects, ideas, and events, e.g., sari, hospital, green, animal, or car. The word "sari" represents all kinds of saris: saris of 6 yards or 8 yards lengths; saris made of cotton, silk, nylon, saris with or without border. Similarly, the concept "hospital" can represent different kinds of hospitals, small, large, city, rural, general, and specialized hospitals.

Concepts save your time, which can be utilized for more abstract thinking. Concepts can also be transferred from something we are very familiar to something new. For example, if you have learned the concept of sterile technique in the operation theater, it will be easy for you to learn new sterile procedures at the bedside.

Concepts are formed
1. By first hand examples: A demonstration by the teacher helps you to learn a concept easily. If you only read a new procedure thoroughly and had no visual demonstration, it would be more difficult and slower to learn than if you could see the procedure demonstrated first. The same is true of learning various diagnoses, e.g., edema can be understood much better, if you could see a patient with edema.
2. By learning rules: These rules give the common characteristics of all things in a particular class. When these rules are learned the person can immediately classify any new thing with some thing he already knows. Usually, scientists adopt this method, e.g., animals are classified—as "insects", "reptiles", "rodents", and "mammals" based upon some of common qualities characteristics or rules.

Piaget's and Bruner's contribution to concept formation
Jean Piaget (Theory of cognitive development) holds the view that every child passes through a series of four stages in concept formation.

At every stage, children become biologically equipped to carry out certain mental processes, which result in their ability to form concepts. These processes determine the type of intellectual tasks that a child can accomplish at a particular age. In the first stage, it is called sensorimotor, the child develops the concept of object permanence. In the next preoperational stage, the child gets the conservation concept. In the next stage, the ideas are all "concrete" and in the last stage of development, the operations are all formal and the child becomes capable of abstract ideas/concepts.

Jerome Bruner (1957 and 1973) contrary to Piaget's biological approach theory, Bruner emphasized that intellectual development does not follow any set pattern of stages and the stages are necessarily age related. Different children follow different pattern of concept formation as per their experiences in thought development. There is a distinction between concept and precision, even though the distinction is not precise. It is quantitative rather than qualitative. One of the major differences is in the process involved. The perceptual act of categorizing is immediate. We feel that "A rose in a rose is a rose" without further analyzing what a rose is.

Language

Language is a highly developed system of symbols in which words within a grammar can be written or spoken in different combinations. Mankind's ability to communicate in language, distinguishes him from animals. Language is extremely important for thinking, because it allows new learning to be communicated to others and stored for future generations.

Words representing, objects and ideas are the symbols forming the basis of language. Words are made up of speech sounds called phonemes and meaningful combinations of these speech words are called morphemes. The letter C as it is pronounced in cat is a phoneme. The same letter C is another phoneme when pronounced in city. This is why, there will be more phonemes in a language than the number of alphabets. There are 26 letters in English alphabet and 40 phonemes. All the syllables need not be morphemes, since all syllables do not have meaning when they stand alone. For example, the word "ring" is a single syllable word. It is also morpheme. On the other hand, the word like taking has two syllables, but the "ing" syllable is not a morpheme since, it possesses no meaning by itself. In addition to symbols, a language must have grammar. A grammar is a set of rules for combining sounds into words and words into sentences. Language can help us to produce new ideas.

Language development in children

The reason for language development in a child is viewed in two different ways. One is what is known as behavioristic approach. This view holds that the child learns language in the same manner in which he learns other skills. Classical conditioning, instrumental conditioning, and modeling are the methods by which the child acquires language. Reinforcement of language pattern is thought to be very important, according to this view.

Another way in which language development is viewed is known as "cognitive" approach. According to this view, the child is born with the capacity to develop language skills. Exposure of the child to some language is all that is needed for the language to be learned.

Though there are supporting evidences for both view points, occurrences of spontaneous new word combinations by children favor the cognitive approach.

The cognitive development in an individual passes through a well set pattern (See Piaget's cognitive theory of development). The process seems to combine learning via rewords with active construction of rules by children themselves. By the age of 4 years, most children use adult-like grammar. Language expert Noam Chomsky (1968) proposed that there are universal grammatical rules used by all children everywhere and that this universal grammar is stimulated by an inborn language acquisition device. Chomsky did not give importance to environmental influences (hearing and practicing sounds) in language development.

Language and communication

Communication is the process by which one person conveys thoughts, feelings, and ideas to another. It is the foundation of interaction among human beings. It allows people to establish, maintain, and improve contracts with other. Caring relationships are the heart of nurse's work. An individual who comes to a health agency is there because he needs help in relation to his health. The nurse and other health professionals are there to help him. To develop a relationship whereby she can help the patient, she must develop skills in communication, since without communication, no relationship is possible. Communication is part

Chapter 8: Thinking and Reasoning: Concept and Language

of the art of nursing. A critical component of nursing practice is the ability to communicate effectively.

Basic elements of communication are the following:

Sender	Receiver
Message	Environment
Channel	Feedback

Message

A message refers to information or opinion that is directed to the target. Nurses can send effective messages by expressing themselves clearly, directly, and in the manner familiar to the receiver. Communication can be difficult when participants have different levels of education and experience. The nurse must be sure that her clients can read, before sending messages in writing.

Transmitting the right message to the right people at the right time is a crucial factor in successful communication. A good message must be:
a. Inline with the objective,
b. Simple,
c. Meaningful,
d. Based on felt need,
e. Clear and understandable,
f. Interesting,
g. Specific and accurate,
h. Timely and adequate,
i. Fitting the audience, and
j. Culturally and socially appropriate.

People express themselves through language, movement, gestures, voice inflections, facial expressions, and use of space. Many forms of communications merge to create meaning to sender's message.

Language: Verbal communication

Verbal communications involve the spoken or written word. Verbal language is a code that conveys specific meaning as words are combined. The most important aspects of verbal communication are given below:
1. **Vocabulary:** Communication is unsuccessful, if the receiver cannot translate the sender's words and phrases. A nurse works with persons of various cultures who speak different languages. Those who speak the same language may use subcultural variations of words, e.g., dinner may mean a midday meal or the last meal of the

day. Medical jargon may sound like a foreign language. Children may use special words to describe bodily functions or a favorite dress or toy. Adolescents often use words in unique ways that are unfamiliar to adults.
2. **Clarity and brevity:** Effective communication is simple, short, to the point to minimize confusion. Avoid verbal mannerisms. Avoid phrases, such as "I mean", "you know", or "OK?" in every sentence. Give examples to clarify messages for the receiver. Use short sentences and words that express an idea simply and directly.
3. **Denotative and connotative meaning:** A single word can have several meanings. The denotative meaning is shared by individuals who use a common language. The word baseball has the same meaning for all individuals who speak English, but the word "code" denotes cardiac arrest to health care staff. The connotative meaning is the interpretation of a word's meaning by the thoughts, feeling, or ideas people have about that word. Families who are told a loved one is in serious condition may believe that death is near but to nurses the term "serious" simply describe the nature of the illness.
4. **Intonation:** Tone of voice affects the meaning of a message and emotions directly influence tone of voice. A simple question or statement can express enthusiasm, anger, or concern. Talking rapidly, using awkward pauses can convey an unintended message. Long pauses and rapid shift to another subject may give the impression that one is trying to hide the truth. Speak slowly to enunciate clearly and use pauses to stress a particular point.
5. **Timing is critical in communication:** The best time for interaction is when a client expresses an interest in communicating. When a client is facing emergency surgery, discussing the risk of smoking is less relevant than explaining preoperative procedures.

Key Points ● ● ●

+ Thinking is a higher mental process.
+ Inductive logic (reasoning) arrives at a general principle based on particular instances.
+ Deductive logic (reasoning) deals with scales for drawing valid conclusions from assumptions.
+ Problem solving is an important kind of thinking.
+ Creative thinking uses divergent thought and not convergent thought.
+ Language is a highly developed system of symbols in which words within a grammar can be written or spoken in different combinations.

Chapter 8: Thinking and Reasoning: Concept and Language

STUDY QUESTIONS

Long Essay
1. Discuss the different kinds of thinking.

Short Essays
1. Elements of creativity and characteristics of creative individuals.
2. Problem solving.
3. Thinking and the nurse.

Short Answers
1. Concept.
2. Language development in children.

Multiple Choice Questions

1. The correct order of stages in creative thinking is_____.
   a. Preparation, Incubation, Illumination, Evaluation, Revision
   b. Preparation, Illumination, Incubation, Evaluation, Revision
   c. Preparation, Incubation, Evaluation, Illumination, Revision
   d. Preparation, Evaluation, Illumination, Incubation, Revision

2. People who are creative tend to use_____.
   a. Convergent thinking
   b. Divergent thinking
   c. Subordinate thinking
   d. Little or no thinking

3. When we just start completely agreeing with some deduced results or principles and try to apply to particular cases, it is known as:
   a. Deductive reasoning
   b. Inductive reasoning
   c. Divergent thinking
   d. Convergent thinking

4. Words are made of speech sound called_____.
   a. Morpheme
   b. Phoneme
   c. Syntax
   d. Grammar

5. The seven stages of problem solving are given by_____.
   a. John Dewey
   b. James Stuart
   c. Nicholas
   d. Bruner

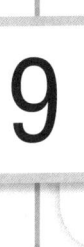

9. Intelligence and its Measurement

Chapter Outline

- Intelligence
- Two Factor Theory
- Fluid and Crystallized Intelligence
- Cubical Model of Intelligence
- Bruner's Theory of Concept Formation
- Cognitive Development
- Mental Retardation
- Intelligence Assessment
- Stanford–Binet Scale
- Wechsler's Intelligence Scale
- Raven's Progressive Matrices
- Intelligence Quotient

Learning Objectives

♦ Students will be familiarized to different types and theories of intelligence.
♦ Students will be oriented to causes and management of mental retardation.
♦ Orients students to the role of heredity and environment on intelligence and various ways to assess intelligence.

DEFINITIONS OF INTELLIGENCE

❖ *"Intelligence is the ability to give responses that are true"*—**Thorndike**
❖ *"Intelligence is the ability to carry on abstract thinking"*—**Terman**
❖ *"Intelligence is a biological adaptation consisting of process of assimilation and accommodation"*—**Piaget**
❖ *"Intelligence is a goal-directed behavior"*—**Binet**
❖ *"Intelligence is creativity"*—**Guilford**.

Intelligence is an individual personality characteristic. David Wechsler suggests that intelligence of a person is his ability to adjust to the world. Wechsler has defined intelligence as the aggregate or global capacity of the individual to think rationally, to act purposefully, and to deal effectively with the environment (1958). It includes the power of adaptation of an individual to his milieu and his ability to learn and do abstract thinking.

TYPES OF INTELLIGENCE

Intelligence can be divided into three kinds:
1. Mechanical intelligence,
2. Social intelligence, and
3. Abstract (or general) intelligence.

Mechanical Intelligence

It is the skill to "manipulate tools and gadgets" and in managing the working of machines. Mechanical engineers and trained industrial workers have an abundance of mechanical intelligence.

Social Intelligence

It means understanding of people and the ability to act wisely in human relationships. Salesmen, diplomats, and politicians are to be socially intelligent.

Abstract Intelligence

It is the ability to handle words, numbers, formulae, and scientific principles. A person with abstract intelligence is able to discover relations among symbols to solve problems, e.g., professionals like doctors, lawyers, and literary men.

In selecting personnel for various jobs, it is useful to know the type of intelligence of the applicants.

There are differences between intelligence and aptitude. Intelligence test is the assessment of the capacity or the potentiality that a person has, whereas the aptitude tests measure capacity that predicts what one can accomplish with training. An aptitude is a combination of characteristics indicative of an individual's capacity to acquire some specific knowledge or skill. It reveals an individual's ability in a given area.

THEORIES OF INTELLIGENCE

Factor Theories (Structural Theories)

Factor theories focus on factors, which constitute intelligence as an organization (of intelligence).

Chapter 9: Intelligence and its Measurement

Spearman's Two Factor Theory or G Factor Theory

According to the British Psychologist, Charles Spearman (1927) intelligence consists of a general ability that works in conjunction with special abilities. Fundamental to all intellectual functioning is the influence of "G" or general factor, but the presence of various special "S" abilities is responsible for the relationships that exist between specifically demonstrated abilities, such as musical, or athletic skill. Spearman thought that every test is composed of the G factor, which is universal plus a specific S factor that is found in each test alone. For example, an arithmetic test might tap both "G" and "S", a specific mathematical ability. The idea that intelligence can be largely summed up with one score (e.g., IQ) is closely related to Spearman's idea that intelligence consists of one general ability factor.

Spearman's two factor theory is the first attempt in the application of factor analysis to intelligence. Factor analysis is the correlation technique used by researchers to discover what the elements of intelligence really are.

Multifactor Theories (Thurston and Guilford)

a. **LL Thurston (1936)** found that general intelligence could be broken down into seven primary abilities **(Table 1)**.
   Thurston assembled a battery of tests to measure abilities. His primary mental abilities (PMA) test is still widely used.

b. **JP Guilford (1967)** expanded the concept of multiple components in intelligence. Guilford's is an alternative to Spearman's two factor theory and rejects the notion of a general intelligence factor. He described human activities in terms of three basic categories of mental abilities: (a) Operations (acts of thinking), (b) Contents (terms of words, symbols, etc.), and (c) Products (the ideas we develop, along these categories).

Table 1: Primary abilities and their descriptions.

Abilities	Descriptions
Verbal comprehension	Ability of grasp meaning of words
Word fluency	Speed in use of words
Number	Perform calculations accurately
Spatial ability	Ability to perceive distances and recognize shapes
Memory	Recall a list of words, numbers, and other materials
Perceptual speed	Grasp of visual details
Reasoning	Ability to logical thinking

Guilford has proposed a three dimensional theory of intelligence represented by a cubical model. The model provides for 120 factors of intelligence or primary abilities, which is a combination yield of four contents, five operations, and six products. According to Guilford, there are three types of thinking abilities **(Fig. 1)**:

1. *Cognition*— It deals with discovering and recognizing information.
2. *Production*—It reflects the use of known information. Productive ability may be either convergent, i.e., leading toward a single correct answer or divergent, i.e., taking a number of directions (answers), any one or more may be right.
3. *Evaluation*—The ability used in determining the adequacy and correctness of cognition and production.

To measure memory, there are numerous rote memory tests, such as learning tests of nonsense syllables, paired associates, etc. Tests of cognition may include such tasks as rearranging scrambled letters to form a word, e.g., CEIV, NERTE, to the familiar words VICE, ENTER. The content is "symbolic", since the test involves a set of letter symbols; the operation is "cognition" as it requires recognition of information and the product unit is a word.

Guilford's three dimensional model of intelligence has helped us to bring out tests that include items in which more than one answer could be correct **(Fig. 2)**. It has also given demonstration of creative thinking.

c. **Howard Gardner (1997):** Instead of one kind of general intelligence, there are eight kinds they are as follows:
1. *Linguistic intelligence:* Ability to understand, acquire and use language effectively. People with linguistic intelligence like reading, playing word games, making up poetry, or stories.

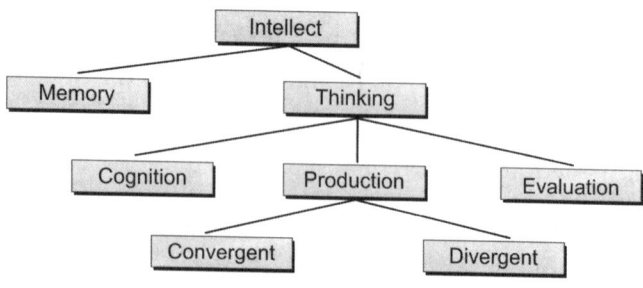

Fig. 1: Guilford's plan of intellect.

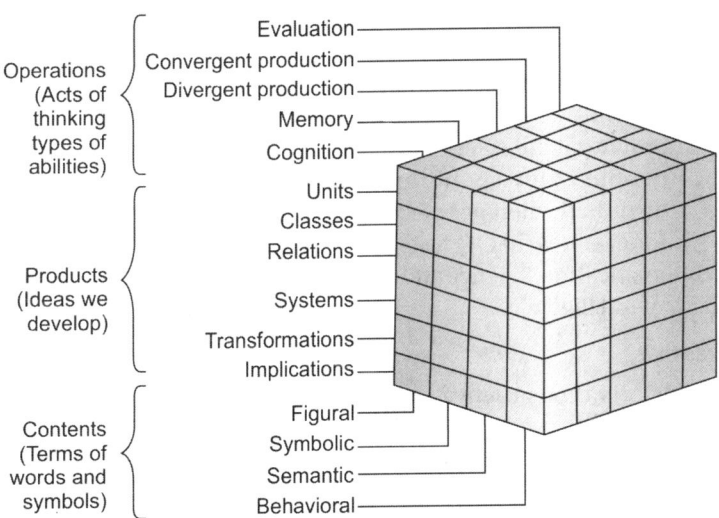

Fig. 2: Guilford's model of the intellect. The cubical model of intelligence. Each of the 120 small cubes represents a primary ability that is some combination of operations, products, and contents. Guilford defines information as that which the organism discriminates and disseminates along the two dimensions—(a) Contents, and (b) Products.

2. *Musical intelligence:* Ability to accurately perceive and/or produce acts of sound, rhythm, tone, and melody. People with this intelligence study better with music in the background. They can be taught by turning lessons into lyrics and speaking rhythmically.
3. *Logical/mathematical intelligence:* Ability to think analytically, in an orderly or practical manner and/or perform mathematical-related tasks. People like to experiment, solve puzzles, and investigate issues scientifically.
4. *Spatial intelligence:* Ability to manipulate objects within space and move objects around with precision. People like to do jigsaw puzzles, read maps, and daydream.
5. *Body movement (kinesthetic) intelligence:* Ability to be aware of the functioning of ones own body and others bodies as well as to demonstrate strong physical coordination.
6. *Interpersonal intelligence:* Ability to understand, interact with others. They are good listeners, and advisors. These students learn through interaction. They have many friends and empathy for others.

7. *Intrapersonal intelligence:* Ability to access one's own feelings, fears ability to draw on one's emotions to guide and understand one's behavior, recognition of personal strengths and weaknesses
8. *Natural intelligence:* Ability to tune into nature, (plants, animals) or natural life sciences (biological, chemical, physical). These people enjoy spending time with mother nature and are disturbed when people pollute environment.

Gardner states that IQ tests primarily measure verbal and logical/mathematical intelligence and neglect the other five equally important kinds of intelligence.

Creativity

Creativity is a constructive process which results in the production of essentially new products. The term creativity has become popular in educational circles. It is used in connection with Guilford's divergent thinking.

There is a consistent difference in the thinking process of high IQ youngsters and creative ones. The youngsters of high intelligence (but not high creativity) is conforming and restricted in his view point, whereas one of high creativity (but not high intelligence) rejects conformity and express himself in a free manner, not always acceptable to social institutions. He may produce a small number of ideas, but each idea may be quite original or unusual and of high quality. He may be able to take a simple idea and do an outstanding job of elaborating and expanding it or he may produce ideas which show a great deal of flexibility of thinking.

Process Oriented Theories of Intelligence

All the above mentioned theories are structural theories, which try to find the component parts of intelligence and describe "how" these parts fit together. But the process oriented theories focus on intellectual processes—the patterns of thinking that people use when they reason and solve problems. They prefer to use the term cognitive process in place of intelligence. They hold that intelligence is a process. Also they are more interested in how people go about solving problems and figuring out answers, than in how many right answers people get. They focus on the development of cognitive abilities.

Jean Piaget (1970) (Stage Theory of Cognitive Development)

The Swiss Psychologist Jean Piaget (1896–1980) proposed four main stages of intellectual development **(Table 2)** each of which builds on the previous one.

Chapter 9: Intelligence and its Measurement

Table 2: Stages in cognitive development (Development of mental or cognitive processes that enable a clued to know about the world).

Stages and age	Characterization
1. Sensorimotor Birth–2 years	The infant becomes aware of the relationship between what he can sense and what he can do with his muscles. He becomes aware of the relationship between his actions and their effects on the environment so that he can act intentionally and make interesting even lasts longer (If he shakes a rattle it will make a noise) learns that objects continue to exist, even though no longer visible (object permanence)
2. Preoperational 2–6 years	Uses language and can represent objects by images and words, is still egocentric (the world revolves around him) and he has difficulty in taking the view point of others; classify objects by single salient features; if A is like B in one respect A must be like B in other respects. Toward the end of the stage, begins to use numbers and develop conservation concepts
3. Concretely operational 6–12 years	Becomes capable of logical thought, achieve conservation concepts in this order: number (age 6) mass (age 7), weight (age 9). Can classify objects, order them in series along a dimension (such as size) and understand rational term (A is longer than B) loses egocentricity
4. Formal operations (adolescence)	Logical abstract thinking appears. Ability to reason realistically about future. Adolescents are now comfortable with verbal statements. And adolescent egocentrism exists

He focused on the development of knowledge through assimilation (modifying the environment to fit one's pattern of thinking and accommodation (modifying oneself to fit the environment).

The quality of one's problem solving abilities and one's ability to be creative in meeting life's challenges depend upon one's ability to think. By operation is meant mental activities like classifying, correcting, adding, subtracting, etc.

Intelligence is an adaptive process that involves interplay of biological maturation and interaction with environment. He viewed intellectual development as an evolution of cognitive processes, such as understanding the laws of nature, mathematical rules, and principles of grammar.

Four Stages of Development of Thinking (Piaget's Theory of Cognitive Development)

1. **Sensorimotor stage:** In Piaget's system, infancy birth to 2 years corresponds to *sensorimotor stage*. This stage involves sensory and

motor activity, e.g., sucking. The child begins simply acting on and experiencing the environment apparently without any significant thought. An important development is that of object permanence, the awareness that objects continue to exist even when they cannot be seen. Object permanence emerges simultaneously with a fear of strangers called stranger anxiety.

2. **Preoperational stage:** In the preoperational stage, lasting from 2 years to age 6–7 years, the child slowly learns the conservation principles and also slowly overcomes his egocentrism, perceiving the world from others point as well as his own. The child's thought are still primarily in terms of dominant characteristics of objects. He may think a tall narrow jar has more liquid than a flat vessel (**Fig. 3**).

The preoperational child cannot perform the mental operations to understand conservation. Closed beakers with identical volumes are seen suddenly hold different amounts after one is merely inverted (**Fig. 4**).

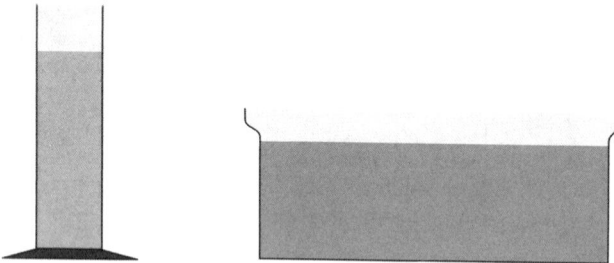

Fig. 3: Conservation principle: Only dominant characteristic.

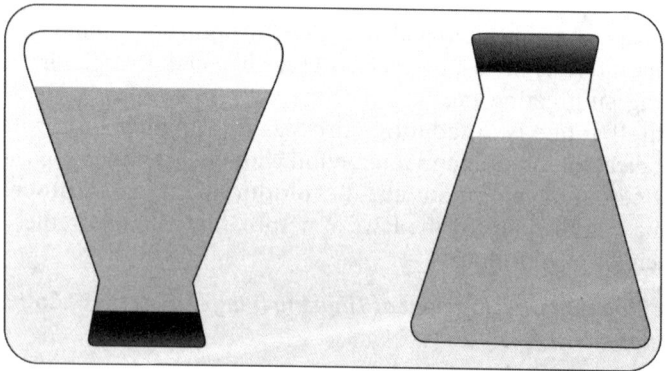

Fig. 4: Conservation principle: Closed beakers inverted.

When a child in the preoperational stage is asked "Do you have a brother? He answers "yes" What is his name? "Jim" but says "no" when asked "Does Jim have a brother". This illustrates his egocentrism.

3. **Concrete operational stage:** As concrete operations are achieved before 11 years, the child masters the operations required in solving concrete problems. The child is ordering and classifying things and understanding relations. They also enjoy jokes that allow them to use new concepts such as conservation:

   "Mr Jones went into a restaurant and ordered a new pizza for his dinner. When the waiter asked if he wanted it to be cut into 6 or 8 pieces, Mr Jones said Oh! You'd better make it 6, I can never eat 8 pieces.

4. **Formal operations (adolescence):** It involves capacity for solving abstract problems. Thinking, at this stage, involves imagining all the possible elements inherent in a given situation, formulating hypothesizes, and testing their validity.

The educational implications of Piaget's work are as follows:
- Keep the content of any teaching/learning in simple steps.
- Keep questions in single stages, so that they do not require elaborate multiprocessing.
- Stay within Piaget's framework but with the above in mind, expect considerable variations.
- Children are naturally inquisitive, so provide a "teaching" environment that allows slow and steady learning. Do not expect large jumps in understanding.
- 7–11 year olds can think, but they do better with concrete objects.
- Children learn by doing (rather than listening).
- The teacher's job is to provide an environment that creates curiosity and allows the child to discover.

Criticism of Piaget's Theory

1. American psychologists do not agree with Piaget's view that infants are born with some elementary mental structures to enable them to deal with the environment.
2. Gagne is of the view that stages described by Piaget are not a result of inborn "Time table" but as a result of later learning by the child which is complex, and progressive. Physical, and social environment also play an important role.

Bruner's Theory of Concept Formation

Jerome Bruner (1973) contrary to Piaget's biological approach theory believed that intellectual development does not follow any set patterns of stages. Children may follow different patterns as per their experience of thought development.

In Bruner's theory of concept formation, the usual course of intellectual development moves through three stages (a) Enactive, (b) Ionic, and (c) Symbolic, in that order. However, unlike Piaget's stages, Bruner did not consider that three stages were necessarily age related. Adults also use all these stages in acquiring language.

Infants, in the *enactive stage*, acquire knowledge by actively engaging in motor activities. This is similar to Piaget's sensorimotor stage. Young children need lots of opportunities to engage in activities with a variety of objects for effective learning. In this stage, knowledge is stored primarily in the form of motor experiences.

In the *iconic stage*, children learn through visual stimuli and knowledge is stored primarily in the form of visual images (mental imagery). At this stage (similar to Piaget's preoperational stage), children use visual representations to aid their thinking. Students' visual perceptions determine how they understand the world. When learning a new subject, it is helpful to have diagrams and illustrations to explain verbal information.

In the *symbolic stage*, children can understand symbols. The knowledge is stored primarily as words, mathematical symbols and or in any other symbol systems. Bruner's symbolic stage overlaps Piaget's stages of concrete and formal operations life. Like Piaget, Bruner emphasizes active learning. Students learn best by doing. Although extrinsic motivation, by the way of rewards and reinforces are helpful at the beginning of a lesson, Bruner stresses that meaningful learning depends on students' intrinsic motivation to know and understand. Therefore, teachers should encourage students' curiosity and desire to explore.

Information Processing Theories of Intelligence

These theories break intelligence down into various basic skills that people employ to take in information, process it and then use it to reason and solve problems. Robert Sternberg (1984) distinguishes between information processing "components" and "meta components". Components are the steps to solve a problem and the meta components are the basics of knowledge that one has to know to solve the problem. The information processing theory has often been compared with computers in which attention and memory have been designated as the intellectual hardware and Piaget's action schemes as the software. People's "software" grows more sophisticated as they mature, with their schemes expanding in complexity and their amount of mental energy increasing. Such changes promote the growth of intelligence.

Other Theories

Cattell's Theory of General Intelligence

RB Cattell (1971), on the basis of factor analysis, has divided general factor of intelligence (G) into two parts—(a) fluid intelligence (GF), and (b) crystallized intelligence (GC) the former being innate, biologically, or genetically determined and the later acquired based on cultural and educational experience. Fluid intelligence is the innate capacity for learning and problem solving. Crystallized intelligence is the fluid intelligence added with education, knowledge and learned skills. Though both are independent, they are interrelated to assume a person's general intelligence.

AR Jensen

Arthur Jensen (1969-70) splits intelligence into two levels (a) Associative abilities, and (b) Cognitive abilities. Associative ability is the capacity to learn, remember, and recall information. Cognitive ability is concerned with reasoning. Cognitive ability depends upon associative ability but not *vice-versa*. Jensen believed that both these abilities are largely hereditary.

HJ Eysenck (1973) distinguishes between speed, and power components of intelligence. Speed is measured by the time required to complete the task and power is measured through untimed test of reasoning.

ASSESSMENT OF INTELLIGENCE

Alfred Binet (1875-1911) was the first psychologist to devise an intelligence test. Binet and Theodore Simon developed their first intelligence scale in 1905. Their scale consisted of 30 items arranged in order of difficulty. Their method of calculating the mental age was based on the observation that intellectual performance of a child increased with age.

Stanford-Binet Tests

The test developed by Binet and Simon to identify mentally retarded children in French schools served its purpose well. Subsequently, several English language versions of the test were produced, e.g., by Lewis Terman of Stanford University in 1916 known as Stanford-Binet intelligence scale. In India, Binet-Kamath intelligence scale is widely used.

Table 3: Examples of age equivalent intelligence.

Age	Examples
2 years old	Name various parts of the body on a paper figure
3 years old	Copy drawing of a circle
4 years old	Explain correctly why we have houses or books
5 years old	Copy drawing of a square, define words like ball or stove
6 years old	Can deal with numbers
9 years old	Can rhyme simple words
Adult	Can describe the differences in meaning of abstract words.

Stanford-Binet can measure the age equivalent intelligence of individuals from 2 years of age to adult. It is administered to one person at a time. The test gives increasingly difficult questions for each age group, because it assumes that intellectual ability in a child increases with age. Thus, there is a different test for each age group. Some examples of what would be expected of each age are given in **Table 3**.

The score of the Stanford-Binet intelligence test will give the mental age (MA).

Intelligence Quotient (IQ)

William Stern, the German Psychologist introduced the concept of IQ. IQ is obtained when the mental age (MA) is divided by the chronological age (CA), which is the actual age of the person in years and multiplied by 100 (to avoid decimals):

$$IQ = \frac{MA}{CA} \times 100$$

Imagine a 10-year-old child scores a MA of 12. His IQ will be:

$$IQ = \frac{MA}{CA} \times 100 = \frac{12}{10} \times 100 = 120$$

If a 12-year-old child scores a MA of 12. His IQ will be:

$$IQ = \frac{MA}{CA} \times 100 = \frac{12}{12} \times 100 = 100$$

If two children both obtain an MA of 5 years, but one child is 4 years old and the other is 6 years old:

Child 1

$$IQ = \frac{MA}{CA} \times 100, IQ = \frac{5}{4} \times 100 = 125$$

Child 2

$$IQ = \frac{5}{6} \times 100 = 83$$

Thus, the bright child has an IQ of 125 while the slower child has an IQ of 83.

Any person will reach a maximum IQ at about 18 years. Depending upon favorable conditions, such as higher education and challenging learning experience, the IQ may increase slightly till age thirty. After 30 years, the IQ does not change except that it decreases slightly with old age. There is no difference between IQ of men and women.

When children grow into adults the CA will constantly increase, but MA will change very little. Thus, as per the formula:

$$IQ = \frac{MA}{CA} \times 100$$

Then, IQ will become lower and lower for a person growing older and older. Therefore, the results of IQ test for adults are compared with the test results of other adults of the same age and not with the same person's chronological age. This is called the deviation IQ.

Wechsler Tests

David Wechsler developed a family of tests for people at various age levels. The tests include the Wechsler adult intelligence scale revised (WAIS-R, 1981) the Wechsler preschool and primary scale of intelligence (WPPSI, 1967) for children between 6 and 16 years and the Wechsler intelligence scale for children revised (WISC-R, 1974) for children between 4 and 6.5 years. These are all individual tests made up of a variety of tasks. WAIS consists of 11 subjects made up of six verbal subjects and five performance (nonverbal) tests, which yield a verbal IQ performance IQ and a combined full scale IQ.

Wechsler scales have many advantages. The administration procedures for all the three tests are similar. Scores in the subsets of these scales enable the investigator to infer patterns of abilities from which localized brain damage can be identified. Wechsler scales have been found to have even cross cultural validation.

Another Indian Test

Wechsler's tests have been adapted for Indian population. *Bhatia's battery of performance* is also widely used. This test has five sub-tests namely: (i) Kohs block design test, (ii) Picture construction test, (iii) Pass along test, (iv) Pattern drawing test, and (v) Test for immediate memory.

TYPES OF INTELLIGENCE TESTS

According to the activities prescribed in them, the intelligence tests are of the following four types:
1. Verbal individual intelligence test,
2. Nonverbal individual intelligence test,
3. Verbal group intelligence tests, and
4. Nonverbal group intelligence tests.

Performance Tests

Some of the well known nonverbal (performance) tests are given below:
a. Alexander's pass along test,
b. Healey's picture completion test,
c. Cube construction test,
d. Kohs block design test,
e. Matrices test,
f. Picture arrangement test, and
g. Goddard form board test.

Different psychologists prefer different tests from this list. The modern tendency in intelligence testing is to have a composite battery of tests containing almost, e.g., equal number of verbal and nonverbal tests. This is an attempt to make sure that no factor of intelligence is left untested. One of the best known examples of this type of composite tests is the one devised by David Wechsler (WAIS) of BELLEVUE Hospital, New York. Stanford-Binet test is an individual verbal test. They have oral items.

The ability of individuals on concept like comprehension, reasoning, vocabulary, memory, etc., are measured by their verbal abilities.

When the individual tests are given to large groups, they are called group tests of the verbal type. When tests use very little language and focus on what people do with their hands they are called performance tests. These may be administered to an individual or to a large group. Individual tests are more sensitive than group tests.

Performance tests are useful when the person being tested cannot speak the language is deaf or dumb or has little educational background. Group testing is widely used when it is necessary to screen, many people such as those who seek admission to college, the military or various other kinds of employment. The patient's (subject's) cooperation is necessary for the proper assessment by these tests.

Uses of Intelligence Testing or Uses of IQ

Intelligence testing is used to predict how well a person will learn in a program of study. They help to classify students, so that the teacher

Chapter 9: Intelligence and its Measurement

knows the capacity of each student to learn. They help to separate the slower learner from the gifted learner, so that special methods can be adopted for training these two different groups. They are used in selection for admission into different courses of study and for awarding scholarships and vocational guidance. They are used in selection of candidates for different jobs.

Although intelligence tests are useful, they must be treated as guides to decisions rather than absolute statements. They do measure certain mental abilities but do not give any clue regarding a person's morals, character, emotions, general temperament and ability to work with other people. Also IQ is only a guideline and not a final verdict on intelligence.

LIMITATIONS OF THE CONCEPT OF IQ

The test scores in intelligence can give some idea about the grade of the intelligence of a person. IQ is an indication of the mental ability of the individual on the basis of which he can be directed about his future, remembering the limitation as given below:

1. IQ is not the quantity of a person's intelligence.
2. All the different intelligence tests do not yield the same IQ score. So the IQ revealed in one test only, cannot be completely depended on.
3. No person is completely devoid of intelligence. Hence, IQ should not start from zero.
4. IQ changes slightly at least once in three years.
5. As the IQ is the result of both heredity and environment, a change in environment may show of a difference up to 10 in IQ score.

Current Status of IQ

1. **Mental retardation:** One use of IQ scores has been to help identify individuals with mental retardation, which was Binet's original goal. However, psychologists caution against using IQ scores as the only test for mental retardation. IQ scores should be used in combination with observation of adaptive skills, which include social, home living, and communication skills. IQ defined and classified mental retardation into four subgroups.
2. **Academic achievement:** IQ scores are moderately good at predicting academic performance. But on its basis alone it will be difficult to predict specific person's academic performance, because performance is an academic field also depends on personal characters, such as one's willingness to study.
3. **Job performance:** IQ scores are weakly related to job performance. Hence, it would be very difficult to predict a specific person's job

performance solely on the basis of IQ scores. Job performance requires not only cognitive abilities which are measured by traditional intelligence tests, but also practical intelligence, such as how to solve problems and got the jobs done which are not measured by traditional IQ scores. Thus, IQ scores are relatively good at predicting academic performance but less successful as predicting job performance as they do not measure the various emotional; motivational are personality factors that also influence behaviors.

Binet had warned that intelligence tests should not be used to label people, for example "average", "genius", etc. Educational decisions especially about placing a child in a special education class, be made only after considering a wide range of information which may include IQ scores but also samples of the child's behavior from other situations. IQ scores should be used only as a guide and not as the last word.

It is an open secret that IQ scores and school/college grades are no direct pointer to success in life. A spectrum of skills is needed to tackle life's complexities. The keyword associated with intelligence today is multiple. Of many types of intelligence, it is the emotional intelligence that determines a person's ability to use his other intelligences (EIQ).

INDIVIDUAL DIFFERENCES

Individual difference is one of the most important characteristics of intelligence. Sir Francis Galton (1883) was the first scientist to study the individual difference in a systematic way. He found that people differed from one another in their intellectual ability. The fact behind individual differences is that the two individuals differ in their genetic makeup and also in the environment in which they are brought up.

Individual Differences in Intelligence

Intelligence (like many other psychological traits) seems to be distributed in the population in such a way that most people make score in the middle range while only a few people make very high or very low scores. This produces a bell-shaped distribution, the normal curve **(Fig. 5)**.

There exist wide individual differences among individuals with regard to intelligence. Not even identical twins or individuals matured almost in similar environment have equal intelligence (mental energy). Intelligence testing has indicated that not only there is difference in

Chapter 9: Intelligence and its Measurement

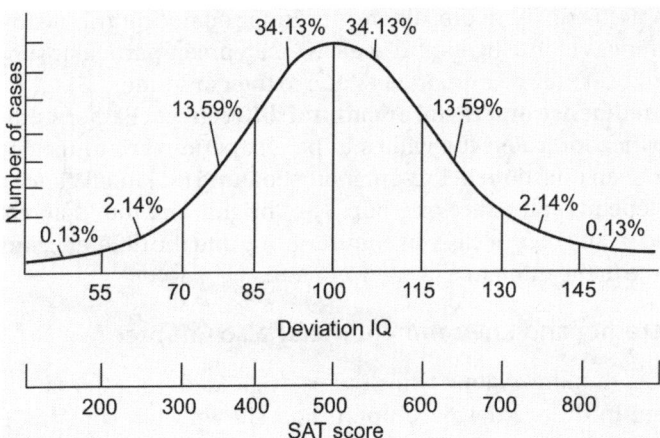

Fig. 5: Norms for IQ and SAT (Scholastic aptitude test) scores. Norms for large groups of measurements often approximate the normal curve (top). The numbers above the curve give the percentages of people in each of the indicated segments. For instance, 13.59% of the population obtain IQ scores between 115 and 130.

intelligence in different individuals, but intelligence varies in the same individual from time-to-time and situation to situation **(Table 4)**.

Intelligence and sex: Various studies have been conducted to find out whether there is any difference in the intelligence levels of males, and females. In most cases, no significant differences have

Table 4: Normal distribution of IQs with a standard deviation of 15.

IQ range	Descriptions (Educational classification)	% of Population
130 and above	Very superior gifted	2.2
120–129	Superior	6.7
110–119	Bright normal	16.1
85–109	Average	59.1
70–84	Borderline (slow learner)	13.6
55–69	Mildly mentally retarded (Educable)	2.1
40–54	Moderately mentally retarded (Trainable)	0.1
25–39	Severely mentally retarded (Trainable)	0.003
Below 25	Profoundly mentally retarded (Total care group)	0.0000005

been noticed. Therefore, differences in sex do not contribute toward differences in intelligence. If at all, women prefer particular subjects for study, it may be explained as due to their aptitude.

Intelligence and racial or cultural differences: Earlier studies in US, which indicated the whites to be a superior race to the blacks, have been questioned. Present indications are that intelligence does not depend on the race or group. The "bright" and the "dull" can be found in any race or caste or cultural group and the differences found are due to the influence of environment.

Heredity and Environment (Refer also Chapter 3)

Studies of monozygotic twins (twins originated from the same egg) reared in different environment had shown high similarities in behavior and intelligence, which emphasizes the role of heredity.

Emotional deprivation due to parental rejection, traumatic experiences like death of beloved ones and separation from parents can affect the mental functioning of individuals. Lack of opportunities affects language development, problem solving skills, and coping skills, which, in turn, affects intellectual functioning. Even malnutrition has adverse effects on mental functioning. All these suggest the influence of environment on intelligence.

Children from lower social class families generally perform less well on intelligence test than from higher social class. Greater parental attention received by children of smaller families and the first born may result in higher IQ scores.

Success of attempts through intensive stimulation and education to improve the IQ in high-risk children and mentally handicapped demonstrate the importance of environment.

Similarly, IQ scores have been found to increase when children are transferred from poor institutions (orphanages) to good foster homes.

Heredity has been compared to seed and environment to land. Just as fertile land and good quality seeds are required for good crop; both good heredity and stimulating environment are required for higher intelligence.

Causes of Mental Retardation or Subnormality (IQ below 70)

The causes of mental retardation are often unknown. About 25% of all cases are due to physical disorders, such as:
1. Birth injuries which are often due to lack of oxygen or caused by an extremely difficult birth.

2. Total damage as from use of drugs by the mother or infections of the mother before birth of the child or immediately after birth.
3. Metabolic disorders.
   a. Phenylketonuria (PKU), galactosemia.
   b. Cretinism.
4. Genetic abnormalities (Chromosomal abnormalities).
   a. Down's syndrome, Klinefelter's syndrome.
   b. Cerebral palsy.

Other physiological causes of retardation are environmental, not genetic. For example, pregnant women who contract rubella (German measles), scarlet fever, syphilis, or even mumps may give birth to infants who have suffered from brain damage as a result. Also injury to the brain or nervous system before or after birth may result in retardation. Such damages can be caused by X-rays, inappropriate drugs, severe pressure on the infants' head during birth, oxygen shortages during, or after birth or even severe maternal malnutrition.

Management of the Retarded or Mentally Subnormal (IQ less than 70)

Retarded individuals take longer time to learn new material and once they have learned something new, they usually forget more easily than do the normal persons. They need more sympathetic help from parents and teachers for learning skills. They often fail to learn by observation and, therefore, need more structured teaching. Help needs to be provided at an appropriate level for the child. It is useless to try and teach skills too far ahead of the child's present mental age. In the preschool period, the main task of professional teachers and speech therapists is in helping the parents to find ways to stimulate their child's development.

The Mentally Gifted Children

There are children with IQs 140 and above. In the early childhood, a gifted child is generally found to be a misfit in his class, because the level of teaching in normal classroom is for average child whereas the gifted child is able to comprehend much faster. As a consequence, they lose interest in studies and indulge in behavioral irregularities. They become gross underachievers and extremely unhappy. They find themselves intellectually misfit with children of their age and physically misfit with older children who are their intellectual equal. But things improve by adulthood and they appear to be happier and better adjusted than most others of their age.

It is important to recognize a gifted child. Parents and teachers should be aware of the child who wants everything explained, solves problems easily, has an exceptional memory, talks in complete sentences as early as 2 years of age, and is clever with the hands, such as mechanical, musical, and artistic abilities. With the right type of training, their superior potential should be channelized in constructive tasks. Some school systems provide special classes and programs for the mentally gifted as well as mentally retarded.

Intelligence and the Nurse

Knowledge of intellectual functioning is useful to a student nurse and later on for her as a teacher. Teaching methods, content of the subject matter and student expectations will be based on the intelligence level of the class.

Assessment and understanding of intellectual functions will be helpful to the nurse in her clinical work. She would be able to diagnose a patient with mental subnormality or with superior intelligence. Her explanations or guidance to the patients and their families would be according to their IQ. In diseases like neuropsychiatric disorders, epilepsy, psychiatric disorders, and in some endocrine disorders, assessment of intelligence is of great assistance in their management. Understanding the development of intelligence in babies and children is another challenge for the nurse. Babies and children should be closely observed for abnormalities and for very high or very low intelligence levels. When caring for older children, it is important to understand how the child's intelligence develops with years. The mildly mentally retarded will respond and accept responsibility for them, if they are given the right kind of encouragement, environment, and an opportunity to learn.

Recognizing individual levels of intelligence in your different professional colleagues and coworkers is also important in communicating with them. It will be your responsibility to know when communications or instructions can be given quickly in professional terms or when they must be given in simple terms and possibly repeated until well-understood.

The nurses can predict the behavior of their patients using their IQ. If the patient is mentally subnormal, she must be prepared to listens not very intelligent conversation from him. Similarly, if a person is very intelligent he is likely to be sensitive and demanding too many explanations about his disorder and will need a very considerate behavior from the nurse.

Chapter 9: Intelligence and its Measurement

Key Points ● ● ●

- There are factor and process theories of intelligence.
- Intelligence can be measured.
- Mental retardation is IQ below 70.
- IQ is calculated by MA/CA x100.
- Heredity and environment play a significant role in a person's intelligence level.

PRACTICAL EXPERIMENT

Intelligence Tests

Nonverbal Tests-Raven's Standard Progressive Matrices

Introduction

It is a nonverbal test of intelligence. There is no need of language and motor manipulation. These tests will consist of printed geometric forms, e.g., Raven's standard progression matrices designed by the British Psychologist JC Raven in 1938. Observation and clear thinking are measured. Test consists of 60 problems arranged in five sets. Each problem has a sample figure with a portion missing. Below the sample are given alternative answers of which only one is correct. This can be given also as a group test. It is a culture free test.

Problem

To measure the subjects' intelligence using Raven's progressive matrices.

Plan

Raven's progressive matrices are administered, responses are scored, and percentiles are determined.

Materials

1. RPM test booklet,
2. Data sheets,
3. Instruction manual,
4. Stop clock, and
5. Writing materials.

Procedure

The subject is seated comfortably and he is given the RPM test booklet and a data sheet. He is given the following instructions: "Open your booklet and get the first page. The upper part in the page has a pattern with a portion missing. In the lower part, there are six alternative bits out of which only one perfectly fills up the missing portion. Tell me the number of the alternative which will fit into the missing portion".

If the subject has understood the instruction, he will point out as the correct alternative. The instructions are continued "on every page of this booklet, there are similar problems. Go on writing the number of the correct alternative in the data sheet provided to you"

With these instructions the subject is allowed to answer and after he finishes answering all the problems in the booklet, the data sheet is collected and the time taken by the subject is noted down.

Analysis of the result

1. The score is determined by referring to the key provided in the instruction manual.
2. The score of the subject is converted into percentile points referring to the manual.

STUDY QUESTIONS

Long Essays

1. Piaget's stages in cognitive development.
2. Current uses of intelligence tests.

Short Essays

1. Spearman's two factor theory of intelligence.
2. Limitations of the concept of IQ.
3. Bruner's theory of concept formation.
4. Different tests for assessment of intelligence.

Short Answers

1. How will you as a nurse help the mother of a mentally abnormal child?
2. Definition of intelligence.
3. Define IQ.
4. Mentally gifted children.
5. Name types of intelligence.

Multiple Choice Questions

1. Spearman's basic assumption is that all mental tasks require two kinds of ability and these are:
   a. Crystallized intelligence and fluid intelligence
   b. Intellectual breadth and intellectual altitude
   c. Associative ability and cognitive ability
   d. General ability and specific ability

Chapter 9: Intelligence and its Measurement

2. Who developed the concept of "Primary Mental Abilities"?
   a. AR Jensen
   b. EL Thorndike
   c. JP Guilford
   d. LL Thurstone

3. Benito was born in 1937. In 1947, he scored 130 on an intelligence test. What was Benito's mental age when he took the test?
   a. 9
   b. 11
   c. 10
   d. 13

4. Rohan obtained a score of 85 on Wechsler's intelligence scale for Children –IV, he will be classified as having _____.
   a. Dull Normal
   b. Average
   c. Bright Normal
   d. Superior

5. Which of the following is not part of Howard Gardner's multiple intelligence theory?
   a. Naturalistic intelligence
   b. Body kinesthetic intelligence
   c. Musical intelligence
   d. Social intelligence

6. IQ is calculated as:
   a. The speed at which we process a piece of information.
   b. The ratio of mental age to chronological age.
   c. The number of items you get correct on intelligence test.
   d. How intelligent you are compared to an adult of the same gender

7. What is the range of IQ for superior level of intelligence?
   a. 71–79
   b. 101–109
   c. 90–109
   d. 120–129

8. Which are the two categories into which the subtests of the Wechsler's intelligence scales can be grouped?
   a. Performance and Numerical
   b. Numerical and Verbal
   c. Verbal and performance
   d. Numerical and memory

9. Theory of cognitive development given by _____.
   a. Jean Piaget
   b. Erickson
   c. Jensen
   d. Vygotsky
10. The term "g" refers to the idea that intelligence _____.
   a. Is made of genetically inherited abilities
   b. May be grouped into subcategories
   c. Has a basic general component
   d. Was developed by Sir Francis Galton

10. Aptitudes (Capacity or Innate Potential)

Chapter Outline

- Aptitude
- Scholastic Ability
- Differential Aptitude
- Clerical Ability
- Linguistic Ability
- Verbal Reasoning
- Numerical Ability
- Abstract Reasoning
- Mechanical Reasoning

Learning Objective

Students are introduced to aptitude and the ways in which it can be measured.

INTRODUCTION

In addition to general intelligence, man has aptitudes or special abilities or capacities which make him successful in spite of mediocre intelligence. Interests and aptitudes are two important personality characteristics. They are closely related to attitudes and ability.

APTITUDE

Aptitude means ability or a particular skill or a potential. While intelligence is a measure of general ability, aptitude is a special ability. It is the capacity to achieve on special lines. It is the special aptness or fitness for a special ability, such as mechanical, musical, artistic, scholastic, or religious. It is highly specific tendency or aptness due to special neural or muscular organization possessed by the individual, which sets him apart as being superior to the average in performance in that trait or activity. Different people have different aptitudes for different things.

Aptitude is neither completely inborn nor acquired. It is the outcome of both heredity, and environment. Aptitudes are talent potentials but can be improved by training in environment.

Aptitude Tests

A person who has aptitude for a particular skill needs only a minimum training for development. Thus, the use of aptitude test is important for vocational guidance and selection of jobs. Aptitude tests that are used to help to predict success in some particular course of study are called scholastic aptitude tests (SAT). The differential aptitude test (DAT) developed by George K Bennet, Harold G Seashor, and Alexander G Wesman measures verbal reasoning, numerical ability, abstract reasoning, spatial relationships, mechanical reasoning, clerical ability, and linguistic ability. Spatial relationships are the ability to visualize a constructed object from a picture and an ability to imagine how an object should appear, if rotated in various ways. It requires mental manipulations of objects in three-dimensional space.

PRACTICAL EXPERIMENT

Problem

To measure the differential aptitudes of the subject using the DAT battery (DATB).

Plan

The seven subtests of the DATB are administered one after the other and performance of the subject are recorded.

Materials

1. DATB booklet,
2. Answer sheets,
3. Key and norms,
4. Stop clock, and
5. Writing materials.

Procedure

Subtest I verbal reasoning: The subject is asked to read the instructions and examples given in the verbal reasoning test booklet. He is allowed 30 minutes to complete the 50 sentences as per instructions. The subject has to give his answer in the answer sheets.

Subtest II numerical ability: Here the subject is allotted 30 minutes to answer the 40 arithmetic problems.

Subtest III abstract reasoning: The subtest has 50 problem figures. The subject is allowed 25 minutes to find out the missing figures of the series from the alternatives.

Subtest IV space relations: The subject is given 30 minutes to answer the 40 problems.

Subtest V mechanical reasoning: To answer the 68 questions the subject is given 30 minutes.

Subtest VI clerical speed and accuracy: It has two parts—100 units of numbers, letters, and number-letter combinations in part I as well as part II. Each of the parts is allowed 30 minutes time.

Subtest VII (a) Language usage (Part I - Spellings): To identify the correctness or incorrectness of spelling 10 minutes are allowed.

Subtest VII (b) Language usage (Part II - Sentences): To find out the errors in 50 sentences the subject is given 25 minutes.

After all the subtests are administered, the answers are checked with the help of the key and the scores determined.

Precautions

1. The subject should not open the booklet until he is asked to do so.
2. The subject should be allowed sometime to understand the instructions.
3. The subject should not waste his time over any question but should go ahead with other questions.

Analysis of Result

The raw scores of each of the subtests are converted into percentiles.

Uses of Aptitude Tests

1. **Instructional:** Teachers can use aptitude test results to adapt their curricula to match the level of their students or to design assignments for students who differ widely. The test scores also help teachers form realistic expectations from students.
2. **Guidance:** Guidance counselors use aptitude test results to help parents develop realistic expectations for their child's school performance and help students understand their strength and weakness. These tests also help them in selection of special courses of instruction, fields of activities, and vocations.

3. **Administration:** Aptitude test scores can identify the general aptitude level of a high school. This can be helpful in determining emphasis to help identify students to be given extra attention for grouping in predicting role performance.

Aptitude and the Nurse

Nursing requires a certain number of special aptitudes. Manual dexterity is useful in practical bedside nursing. Speed is useful in all nursing tasks. Linguistic ability makes examination easier. Musical aptitude is useful in a nurse's home life. Some special aptitudes in sports, music, or art may be of great value to psychiatric nurses in the rehabilitation of patients.

Knowledge of the aptitudes, their measurements and conditions will be helpful to the nurse to develop a proper aptitude for her profession and to guide those around her in entering professions according to their aptitudes. This will also give her optimism in her own future success.

Key Points ● ● ●

+ Aptitude means ability or a particular skill or a potential.
+ Aptitude is the outcome of both heredity, and environment.
+ Aptitudes can be measured.

STUDY QUESTIONS

Short Answers

1. Aptitude
2. Differential aptitude test

MULTIPLE CHOICE QUESTIONS

1. _____ is the natural ability to do something.
   a. Aptitude
   b. Intelligence
   c. Attitude
   d. Motivation
2. Differential Aptitude test was developed by_____.
   a. Seashore, Westman and Benson
   b. Beck, Ellis and Jackson
   c. Bennet, Seashore and Wesman
   d. Bennet, Edward, Dieck

3. Numerical ability subtest of DATB consists of how many arithmetic problems?
    a. 35
    b. 40
    c. 45
    d. 50
4. Which subtest of DATB has two parts in it.
    a. Clerical speed and accuracy
    b. Abstract reasoning
    c. Mechanical reasoning
    d. Language usage

11

Motivation

Chapter Outline

- Arousal Theory
- Maslow's Theory of Needs
- Drive
- Motivation
- Drive Reduction Theory
- Need
- Goal
- Physiological Motives
- Instinct Theory
- Social Motives
- Incentive Theory
- Yerkes–Dodson Law

Learning Objectives

♦ Students will be introduced to the basic components of motivation and types of motives.
♦ Orients students to the various theories of motivation.

INTRODUCTION

Psychology deals with not only what people do but also why they do so. Motivation literally means to move, energize, or activate. Motivation is defined as "conditions within the organism which arouse, maintain, and direct behavior toward a specific goal". It is a driving or pulling force, which results in persistent behavior directed toward a particular goal. Motivation is a process of stimulating people to attain desired goals.

The main components of motivation are—need, drive, and goal.

For example, when we are hungry, there is a need for food because our earlier intake of food is used up. The need for food causes us to feel hungry, which is the drive which pushed us to find food and eat (goal). This is called the hunger drive. A biological need creates an aroused state (or drive). The physiological aim of drive reduction is homeostasis. This drive caused us to respond with some action, which in this case was finding food and eating (goal).

The word "motive" is commonly used to mean motivation. Generally, motivation is made up of motives or drives. Motives are expressions of a person's needs; hence, they are personal and internal. Incentives are external. Motives are not observed directly. Motives are inferences from observations of behavior. They are powerful tools for the explanation of behavior, and they allow us to make predictions about future behavior. Motives are the "dynamos" of human behavior **(Fig. 1)**.

TYPES OF MOTIVATION

1. **Extrinsic motivation:** A person performs an action, because it leads to an outcome that is separate from or external to the person. For example, selecting a major in college based on prestige and salary, rather than on personal interest.
2. **Intrinsic motivation**: A person performs an action, because the act is rewarding and satisfying in internal manner. For example, writing poems, painting, reading nonfictional books for fun.

MOTIVE

A motive is a specific need or desire that arouses the organism and directs its behavior toward goal. Motives are triggered by stimulus. For example, a bodily condition-like low blood sugar. Most of our day-to-day explanations about behavior are given in term of motives.

Types of Motives

There are two kinds of motives—(a) Primary, and (b) Secondary. Primary motives are called physiological or basic needs as they are

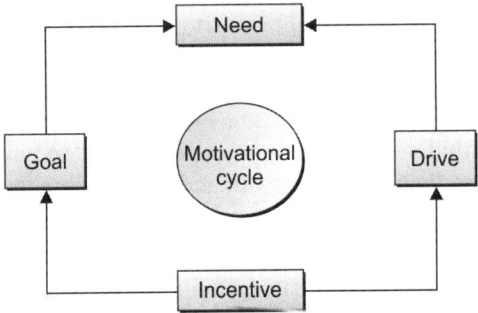

Fig. 1: Motivational cycle.

necessary for survival of any organism—human, animal, or plant. They are caused by the needs of our bodies. The main primary motives are hunger, thirst, avoidance of pain, need for air and sleep, elimination of wastes, regulation of body temperature, and sex. All these are unlearned motives inborn in the organism.

Primary/Physiological Motives

Primary motives are essential for survival. They must be satisfied first before we can take up any other activity. Primary motives come to action when the physiological balance of the body is upset. This balance is called homeostasis.

Homeostasis: A body's tendency to maintain a steady internal state.

Examples:
1. Maintaining blood glucose at a particular level to maintain body chemistry.
2. If our body temperature cools, blood vessels constrict to conserve warmth and we feel like wearing more clothes or seek a warmer environment.

Hunger drive: Early experiments showed stomach contraction leads to hunger but later people also reported normal feelings of hunger even when nerves of stomach are cut or stomach removed. Therefore, other mechanisms are also involved in hunger. When the food supply of the body has been exhausted, certain biochemical changes take place in the tissues of the body. This causes the stomach to contract which gives hunger pains. The hunger must be satisfied in order to help the body to return to a physiological balance or homeostasis. Hypothalamus plays a main role in motivation to hunger. Lateral hypothalamus is the center for eating, damage to this area person refuses food and water, and may starve to death unless forcefully fed. Ventro-medial hypothalamus is the center for stop eating and damage to this area person overeats. Few of the hormones like CCK, Ghrelin, Insulin and Leptin have a major role in the hunger drive. The CCK limits the meal size by closing the sphincter muscle, the one between the stomach and duodenum causing the stomach to hold food. Ghrelin acts on hypothalamus to decrease appetite. Insulin helps glucose to enter cells. Leptin signals the brain about the body's fat reserves.

Thirst drive: Two conditions that can trigger thirst are loss of water from cells and reduction of blood volume. When water is lost from bodily fluids, person dehydrates. Osmo receptors in hypothalamus generate nerve impulses when cells are dehydrated. Loss of water from body decreases blood volume, thus BP drops and kidneys release an enzyme renin, which, in turn, forms angiotensin II. This circulates in the blood and triggers drinking.

Respiratory drive is the drive for air and oxygen. One cannot survive for long without a regular supply of air or oxygen. If oxygen is not supplied even for a short time, it is possible to experience brain damage, loss of memory, and control over one's body.

Sleep drive usually occurs at regular intervals for each person. When the body continues activities without rest or sleep for a long time, it is possible to experience confusion, inability to pay attention, droopy eyelids, staring, muscle tremors, and increased sensitivity to pain. The body temperature and metabolism drop enough during sleep, saving up energy.

Drive for elimination of wastes: When the bladder or intestine becomes distended with waste material, they cause pressure and discomfort. The person becomes restless until the waste materials are disposed of and pressure relieved.

Sex drive is considered a biological drive, since it is dependent on physiological conditions. Unlike hunger and thirst, sex is not essential for the survival of the individual but is necessary for the survival of the species. The initial drive to sex activity comes from nervous tensions within the body set up by various sex hormones. Limbic system plays an important role in sexual excitement. Other than biological factors cultural and environmental factors also influence sexual behavior like pornographic movies, magazines, sight of a partner, clothing style, voices, and body shapes.

Maternal drive is a physiological motive. Maternal behavior is instinctive in nature. It is unlearned. Physiological drive causes maternal behavior. Maternal drive is caused by prolactin, a hormone secreted by the pituitary.

Social/Learned/Secondary Motives

Human beings are not only biological but also social. Therefore, human behavior is activated by the following social motives:
- Achievement motives,
- Affiliation motives,
- Aggression motives, and
- Power motives.

These are called social motives, because they develop through relationship with people.

According to David McClelland, people are motivated by their three important needs: (a) Need for achievement (N ach), (b) Need for affiliation (N aff), and (c) Need for power (N pow). These motives are known as social motives.

Need for achievement: Achievement motivation refers to a drive toward some standard of excellence. People with high need for achievement prefer tasks that would promise success and are moderately difficult. David C McClelland has found that while high achievers tend to succeed, low achievers tend to avoid failures. High achievers challenge failures and work harder while low achievers accept failures and go for less difficult tasks. High achievers prefer personal responsibility and like to get feedback about their work. When these people are successful, they raise their levels of aspiration in a realistic way and move on slightly more challenging tasks.

Children whose parents have accepted their independence tend to become high achievers. Children of overprotective parents become low achievers. Children learn by copying the behavior of their parents and other important people who serve as models. Through such observational learning, children adopt the characteristics of the model, including the need for achievement. The expectations that the parents have for their children also develop achievement motivation in children.

Affiliation motives (Affection, gregariousness). Man cannot exist in isolation. The need to be with other people is referred to as affiliation need. This need is revealed by a need to be attached to others through friendship, sociability or group membership. They make more local phone calls, visits, and seek approval of others. Need to rely on others which is called dependency motive is one form of the need for affiliation. When little children are frightened, they seek others to comfort them. This kind of experience in early life makes one seek the friendly company of others when faced with anxiety and fear.

Aggression motives: Intense frustration after high expectations, verbal and nonverbal insults, fear and anxiety can trigger aggression. Television and cinema depicting violence can make youngsters model themselves to aggressive behavior.

Psychoanalysts maintain that each individual, as part of his biological inheritance, possesses destructive death urges as well as constructive life urges. In most of us, a favorable balance exists between life and death urges, so that kindness triumphs over cruelty. Social learning (modeling), classical conditioning, and instrument conditioning are ways in which hostile aggression may be learned.

Power motives: Social power is defined as the ability or capacity of a person to produce intended effect on the behavior or emotions of other people. Persons with power motives will be concerned with having impact, reputation, and influence. They exercise their power by joining political parties, voluntary organizations and associating with prominent and popular men. They select jobs which have an impact on others and dominate weaker sections of the society. They often try to convince others, play more competitive sports and drink more heavily.

Achievement-oriented people actively focus on improving what is—they transform ideas into action and wisely, taking risks when necessary. In contrast, affiliation-oriented people focuses their energies on families and friends, their overt productivity is less because they view their contribution to society in a different light from those who are achievement-oriented. Research shows that women generally have greater affiliation needs than men. Nurses have high affiliation needs.

Power-oriented people are motivated by power that can be gained as a result of specific action. They want to command attention, get recognition and control others. McClelland theories that managers can identify achievement, affiliation, or powers needs of their employees and develop appropriate motivational strategies to meet those needs.

Need Deprivation

When needs are not satisfied, it is called need deprivation. Deprivation of the need to be loved makes it very difficult to express love to others. Most cases of child abuse come from parents who received no love and security in their own childhood. When deprived of the need of self-esteem or social status, people respond with tremendous frustration and aggressive harmful behavior. Riots, violence and murder follow. Sensory deprivation or lack of stimulation through the senses causes abnormalities in behavior. Experiments have been conducted by placing a person in an isolated room with no light or sound. The results of these experiments showed that severe sensory deprivation can cause disorientation, confusion, restlessness, irritability, emotional upsets and loss of concentration.

THEORIES OF MOTIVATION

Theories of motivation are classified mainly into two types:
1. Biological theories
    a. Instinct theory
    b. Drive reduction theory
    c. Arousal theory

2. Psychological theories
   a. Incentive theory
   b. Maslow's hierarchy of needs

Biological Theories

Instinct Theory

Instincts are inborn patterns of behavior that are biologically determined rather than learned. According to instinct approaches to motivation, people and animals are born with sets of behaviors essential to their survival. Those instincts provide the energy that channels behavior in appropriate directions.

Motivation is due to a combination of biological factors, external force, and unconscious phenomenon.

Our actions are determined by the inner forces or impulses, often operating below the level of consciousness. Freud believed that all behavior stemmed from two opposing groups of instincts, the life instincts (Eros) that enhance life and the death instincts (Thanatos) that push toward destruction. Activities to satisfy hunger, thirst, sex, etc., are life instincts. Activities to satisfy aggression and destructive tendencies are death instincts. Life activities are interaction of life and death instincts. The energy of the life instinct is the libido which involves mainly sex and related activities. The death instincts can be directed inwards in the form of suicide or self-destructive behavior or outwards in the form of aggression toward others.

Freud also emphasized the powerful role of unconscious motives in human behavior. He pointed to several forms of behavior through which unconscious motives are expressed:
a. In dreams, we often express wishes and impulses of which we are unaware.
b. Unconscious mannerisms, slips of pen and tongue, our irrational fears of specific objects or phobias reveal hidden motives.
c. Our chronic headaches, insomnia, gastric troubles for which there are no physical or organic reasons, show the unconscious needs of the person.

Drive Reduction Theory

It is also called as "push theories of motivation". According to Clark Hull (1952), human beings have internal biological needs which motivate us to act in a particular way. Behavior is pushed toward goals by driving states within a person or animal. This approach states that a physiological need creates an aroused tension state (a drive) that motivates an organism to satisfy the need **(Fig. 2)**.

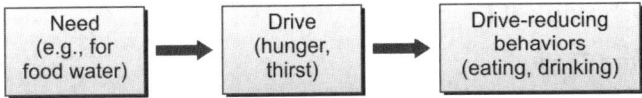

Fig. 2: Drive reduction theory.

According to this theory, we are drivers to reduce these drives, so that we may maintain a state of internal calm. Humans and other animals are motivated by four drives: (a) Hunger, (b) Thirst, (c) Sex, and (d) Avoidance of pain. They are responsible for initiating and maintaining our primary responses.

Arousal Theory
Arousal theory states that each person has a unique arousal level that is right for them. When the arousal levels drops below the individuals mandated levels, they seek stimulation to elevate them.

Yerkes-Dodson Law
The law states that increased levels of arousal will improve performance, but only up until the optimum arousal level is reached. At that point, performance begins to suffer as arousal levels increase **(Fig. 3)**

For example, students when taking final exams, increased arousal can lead to better test performance by helping them to stay alert, focused, and attentive. Excessive arousal can lead to test anxiety, nervous, and unable to concentrate on the test. When arousal levels are very high or very low, performance tends to be worse.

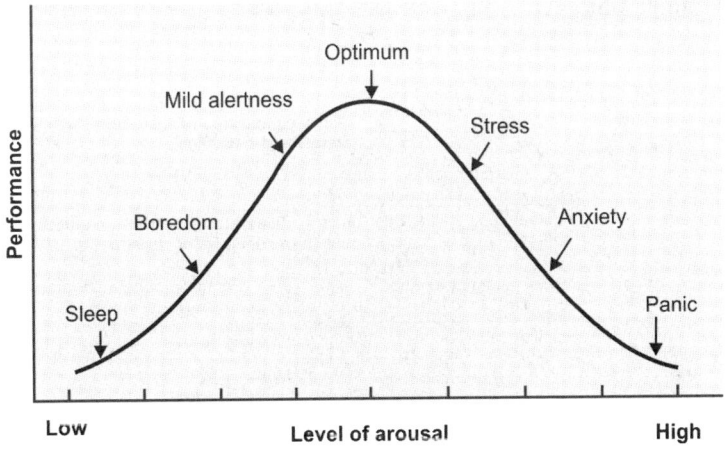

Fig. 3: Yerkes–Dodson law.

Psychological Theories

Incentive Theory

An incentive is a positive or negative environmental stimulus that motivates behavior. *For example,* we choose to an incentive (such as a mouthwatering dessert) even though we lack internal cues (such as hunger).

It is not only "need" that pushes us to reduce drive, but we are also pulled by incentives. In contrast to the push of drive theories, incentive theories are "pull theories" of motivation. Individuals expect pleasure from the attainment of positive incentives and from the avoidance of negative incentives, e.g., wages, bonuses, etc.

Abraham Maslow Hierarchy of Needs Theory

Abraham Maslow (1908–1970) classified motives into five categories and arranged them in a hierarchical fashion. Basic (responsible for imitating) biological needs form the base of this hierarchy. In an ascending order, the five needs are arranged according to their importance **(Fig. 4)**. They are as follows:
1. Physiological motives (hunger, thirst, etc.),
2. Safety needs (protection from harm or injury),
3. Social/love needs (affection, warmth, belongingness),
4. Esteem needs (self-respect, self-approval, prestige, autonomy, and attention), and
5. Self-actualization (achieving maximum development of one's potentialities).

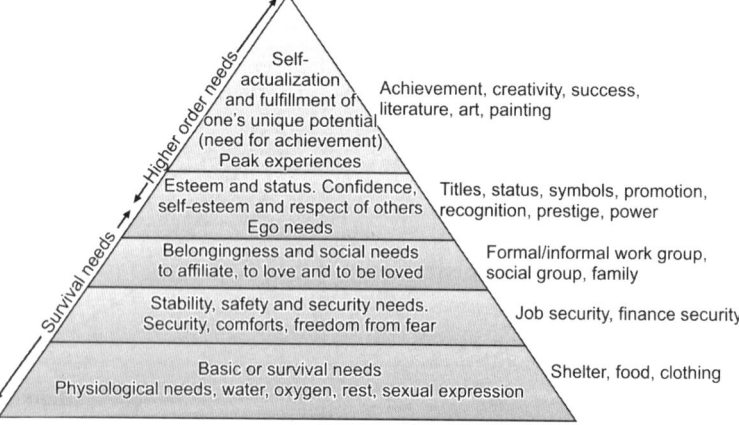

Fig. 4: Abraham Maslow hierarchy of needs theory.

Maslow's hierarchy of needs showing how a person moves from fulfillment of basic needs to high level of needs with the ultimate goal of integrated human functioning and health.

Motivation is based on both physiological and psychological factors. The needs at one level should be at least partially satisfied before the needs at the next level become active. For example, when food and safety are difficult to obtain, the satisfaction of these needs will dominate a person's actions and the higher motives (growth or learned needs) will not have any significance. Only when the biological needs are satisfied, the individual will have the time and energy for aesthetic and intellectual pursuits. The need in the highest level of hierarchy is the need for self-actualization. Self-actualization is the ultimate goal of life. This is the need for the fullest development of one's potential and achieves something. It means becoming all one is capable of becoming Maslow's hierarchy of needs is somewhat arbitrary. People have starved themselves to death to make a political statement. Motivation affects people as a whole, rather than just a part. Maslow believed that people are motivated to seek personal goals, which makes their life rewarding and meaningful.

People go up pyramid as they go through life gaining wisdom and knowledge on how to handle many different situations. A shift in a life's circumstances can lead down to a lower need. A person at the stage of belonging needs may lose job and get down to securing safety needs by trying finding a new job to survive.

MOTIVATION AND THE NURSE

The knowledge of motivation process will help the nurse in her profession as follows:
1. It will help her in maintaining her own mental health.
2. It will be helpful in her adjustment with doctors, patients, and their relatives.
3. It will give her an etiology of patient's behavior leading to better understanding.
4. It will help her in the diagnosing of the disease.
5. It will facilitate faster cure of the disease.
6. It will give her job satisfaction.
7. It will improve her relations with her colleagues.
8. It will be useful in solving most of the problems in interpersonal relationships.

The nurse has to remember that motives are at work in the life of patients, colleagues and her own daily relationships. Understanding own motives and motives in the patient will help the nurse to build a cooperative relationship between the patient and the health care team.

Nurse and Needs of the Patients

The nurse should always be aware of the need for the satisfaction of the primary needs. The patient's need for proper food, water, or fluids and a constant supply of air or oxygen should be met. She must feed patients who are unable to eat by themselves. Similarly cover them with blankets and also help them in their elimination needs.

Patient, on admission to the ward, does not know the do's and don'ts of the ward. He is anxious about what will happen to him. In uniform all nurses look alike even though uniform will provide authority and assurance. The nurse must introduce herself as the nurse concerned with his care. Also give him as much information especially the location of toilets and general geography of the ward. A regular ward routine, with fixed timings for meals, drugs, visitors, and doctors rounds with which the patient can quickly become familiar also will add to security. Patients should be helped to retain intact their family and social links. For small children, it is particularly important that the bond with their parents remains intact.

Relatives and friends demonstrate their love and affection by bringing flowers and presents and by sending cards and letters. These symbolic acts should be treated with respect by the nursing staff. The nurse's help may be needed during visiting time to ensure privacy.

The very fact that one has fallen ill and is unable to work or cope with the home and family is a threat to self-esteem. The stigma attached to certain illnesses like tuberculosis and leprosy and to certain types of hospitals like cancer hospitals adds to this problem. It may not be possible to avoid all the practices known to lower self-esteem, e.g., asking a patient to undress and expose his body for physical examination, but nurses should recognize that this is humiliating to the patients and therefore should be minimum.

It is particularly distressing to the adolescent who has only recently established his independence to have his bodily needs attended to by nurses who are not much older than himself. Nurses should restrain from "talking down" to patients when giving instructions or information. The nurse should avoid intrusive history-taking and should keep all information strictly confidential.

There is a skill involved in conveying to a patient unconditional respect and acceptance when his sickness has reduced his value as a human being.

Though it is difficult for the nurse to contribute to the self-actualization needs of patients, she should remember that some patients discover their artistic, literary or musical talent through various forms of art and occupational therapy. Patients may have "peak experiences" or heightened religious faith through suffering, tragedy, and a contemplation of impending death.

The need to avoid pain or seek relief from pain is very important for the patient. Illness or injury always produces pains and aches. The nurse must be on alert to recognize the discomfort of her patients and help in whatever way possible to alleviate the pain. Patients must be protected from cold and injury.

Secondary needs of patients: The nurse has to recognize the mores customs and codes of the society resulting in the meaningful behavior of patients. What clothes to wear, what religious duties and symbols are important, who is welcome with the patient, how much of privacy should be recognized by the nurse. In some societies, privacy is very important, in others not so much.

Key Points

- Motivation literally means to move, energize or activate.
- Motives are not observed directly, they are inferred from observing behaviors.
- Motives are mainly classified into physiological and social motives.
- Theories of motivation are classified into biological and psychological theories.
- Instinct theory of motivation says people are born with behaviors essential for survival.
- Drive theory of motivation is also called "Push theory of motivation".
- Arousal theory states that each person has a unique arousal level that is right for them.
- Incentive theory of motivation is also called "Pull theory of motivation".
- Abraham–Maslow classified motives into five categories and arranged them in a hierarchical fashion.
- Nurses should understand their own motives and motives in the patient, thus helping the nurse to build a cooperative relationship between the patient and the health care team.

STUDY QUESTIONS

Long Essays

1. Describe Maslow's need hierarchy theory.
2. Distinguish between primary and secondary motives. Describe briefly the physiological motives that determine our daily behavior.
3. Explain the concepts and theories of motivation.
4. What is motive? Classify motives. Describe, in detail, the physiological motives.
5. Explain biological and social motives with one example for each.

Short Essays

1. Classify need drives and motives.
2. What is the effect of personal and social motives on behavior?
3. What are personal motives?
4. Discuss the importance of unconscious motivation.
5. What are the nursing applications of motives?

Short Answers

1. What are the biological motives?
2. Define social motives.

Multiple Choice Questions

1. Which of the following is not considered as a primary drive?
   a. Sex   b. Social approval
   c. Hunger   d. Thirst
2. Who proposed the human motives in a hierarchy of potency?
   a. Singer   b. Miller
   c. Maslow   d. Beck
3. Motives are not directly observed; but inferred form:
   a. Tension   b. Behavior
   c. Conflict   d. Stimulus
4. _____ is called the "pull theory" of motivation.
   a. Drive reduction   b. Instinct
   c. Arousal   d. Incentive
5. Motivation due to factors within the individual is_____.
   a. Intrinsic   b. Extrinsic
   c. Amotivation   d. Behavioral motivation

12 Frustration and Conflicts

Chapter Outline

- Motivation
- Frustration
- Conflict
- Task-oriented Mechanisms
- Defense Mechanisms

Learning Objectives

◆ Students will be aware about the differences between frustration and conflicts.
◆ Orients students to various frustration and conflict coping mechanisms.

INTRODUCTION

Motivation is an internal urge to act toward a particular goal. When motives are hindered or blocked, frustration occurs. People, who cannot achieve their important goals, feel depressed, anxious, fearful, guilty, or angry.

Frustration is a negative feeling when one is prevented from reaching a goal (**Fig. 1**). For example, one will be frustrated if:
a. After getting up early to bath before most others, one finds that there is no water.
b. After reaching the bus stand well in time, one finds that the bus had left earlier than the scheduled time.
c. After studying very hard, one fails in the examination.

Definitions of Frustration

1. *Frustration means emotional tension resulting from the blocking of a desire or need.*

—**Carter V Good**

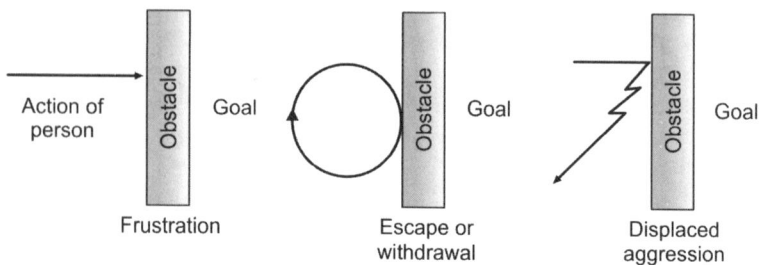

Fig. 1: Results of frustration.

2. *Frustration is the feeling of being blocked or thwarted in satisfying a need or attaining a goal, the individual perceives as important.*
—**Kolesnik**

SOURCES OF FRUSTRATION

1. **Environmental forces** that block motive fulfillment. The obstacle may be something physical, e.g., a locked door, lack of money, or it may be people—parents, teachers, or policemen. The restrictions placed on behavior by the rules of the society are another source of frustration.
2. **Personal inadequacies** that make it impossible to reach goals. For example, some people are handicapped by blindness or paralysis. As children grow into adulthood, the unattainable goals bring more and more frustration. These are mainly learned goals that cannot be achieved, because they are beyond the person's abilities. A boy may learn to aspire for too high an academic achievement but is neither very intelligent nor hardworking. He gets only low marks because of his level of performance.

   Most individuals have somewhat similar desires, but they are not equally equipped to satisfy them. In life's struggle for health, marital partners, and other values, the more gifted encounter fewer obstacles than the less endowed. All things being equal, some perform better than the less privileged.
3. **Conflict between motives within the individual:** The most serious and deep-rooted frustration occurs due to conflict between motives. These conflicts are of four basic forms. In each of these conflicts, attainment of a goal, for a time, is hindered. Depending, on the type of conflict, various emotional and behavioral reactions may occur, e.g., conflict between independence and affiliation.

Personal Frustrations

Characteristics of body, personality, and intelligence may cause frustration. It is called "personal". A boy wants to take up engineering but he cannot do so, because he has not been able to make the grade in mathematics. An adolescent feels that his life is ruined because of acne and he keeps away from society. Illness of any sort causes frustration, because it comes in the way of our desires.

Frustration produces an emotional state, which is always unpleasant. It creates tension or stress, which varies from simple annoyance to heated anger. But frustration is inevitable. It begins at birth. The process of birth itself is a frustrating experience for the baby. When the child is hungry it gets frustrated, if the mother delays in getting the bottle of milk ready. As the child grows, there are many parental demands which come in the way of his natural desires.

Frustration creates uncomfortable emotional tensions and so the individual tries to reduce the tension in a variety of ways. The important reactions are as follows:

Direct approach: Two direct methods of overcoming obstacles are increased effort and changing the mode of attack. If both the methods fail, the third alternative is in changing the goal to one that is more attainable.

Feelings of inferiority: When increased effort and variation of attack fail and substitute goals are unavailable, individual often react by developing feelings of helplessness and inadequacy. This emotionally distressing state of the mind is referred to as inferiority complex. An inferiority complex is the form of self-criticism usually involving fear of social disapproval. The common reactions are fear of competition, extreme sensitivity to criticism, suspicion, envy, self-consciousness, worry and extreme self-analysis.

Aggressiveness: Instead of adjusting passively to obstacles with a defeatist attitude, many react aggressively toward the source of frustration. Aggressive reaction is very common when some external obstacle is the cause of frustration. The target of attack is usually some other person or object and the intensity of attack is proportionate to the amount of frustration.

Conflict

Conflict is a special type of frustration. The existence of frustration in life is unavoidable, without which development is not possible when conflicts become excessive, they become harmful. Excessive conflicts indicate a weakness of determination. Strong will power is required to get rid of conflicts.

When you are unable to resolve the conflict, obstacles cannot be overcome and delays will have to tolerate. Too much of conflict may make people neurotic.

Types of Conflicts

Conflicts are of four basic forms:

Approach-approach conflict (Fig. 2)

This is the simplest kind of conflict and occurs between two positive goals that are equally attractive. The person is attracted at the same time by two goals that are incompatible.

A physiological conflict arises when a person is both hungry and sleepy at the same time, choosing between two cinemas or to go for a cinema or a party scheduled for the same night. A man who wishes to get married and settled in his homeland is offered an attractive job abroad. The proverbial donkey is supposed to have starved to death, because it stood halfway between two piles of hay and could not decide which to choose.

When one is able to make up one's mind quickly and easily, the conflict is resolved. Even more serious approach-approach conflicts, such as choosing your place of work after graduation can be resolved more quickly than other types of conflicts.

Avoidance-avoidance conflict (Fig. 3)

It takes place when one is forced to choose between two negative goals. An individual is caught between the devil and the deep blue sea because of personal needs and moral values. The individual is caught between two threats, fears or situations that are equally repelling. One has to choose between a toothache and going to the dentist. One may dislike studies and also failure and has to choose between the two. Another avoidance conflict is between unhappy employment and loss of income. These conflicts are not resolved quickly but often go on for a long time.

An example of an avoidance conflict, which reflects one's personal belief, is having to choose between abortion and unwanted pregnancy.

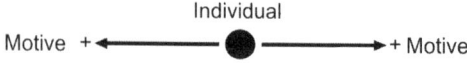

Fig. 2: Approach-approach conflict.

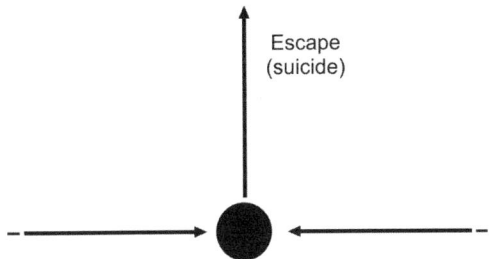

Fig. 3: Avoidance-avoidance conflict (from fire to frying pan).

The avoidance conflict is the worst type of conflict and is stressful. It leads to indecision, vacillation, inaction, and sometimes "freezing" and "escape"—leaving the field (vertical arrow in **Fig. 3**).

Theoretically, a person might escape the avoidance conflict by running away from the field and people try this. In practice, however, there are additional negative forces in the periphery of the situation that prevent them from running away. For example, a girl who does not want either to do her arithmetic or get a spanking might think of running away from home. But the consequences of running away are even worse than her other alternatives, and so she does not do it. A man must undergo preventive surgery or run the risk of later illness. A student has to sell his car to pay his fees or leave the college.

People in avoidance-avoidance conflicts, may try different means of running away. They often rely on imagination to free them from the fear and anxiety generated by the conflict. They may spend much of their time in day-dreaming, conjuring up an imaginary world where there are no conflicts or they may recreate in their minds the carefree world of their childhood before the unpleasant tasks and avoidance-avoidance conflict existed. This way of leaving the conflict is called regression.

Approach-avoidance conflict (Fig. 4)
It is the most difficult to resolve because in this conflict, a person is both attracted and repelled by the same goal object.

Ice cream is delicious but also causes obesity. A man wants to marry a girl for her beauty but, at the same time, her educational level is too low. A girl wants parental protection but, at the same time, does not want parental domination. A child starts to pat a dog, but is afraid and pulls back his hand. A lady picks up a telephone and dials a number but fearing the other person's response, puts the receiver back.

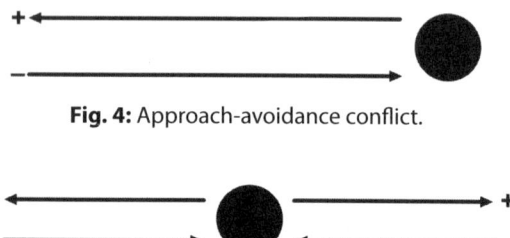

Fig. 4: Approach-avoidance conflict.

Fig. 5: Double approach-avoidance conflict.

Multiple approach-avoidance conflicts (Fig. 5)
Many of life's problems involve many positive and many negative goals.

Consider the student who experiences a conflict between making good grades and making it to the college football team. Superficially this appears to be a simple case of approach-approach conflict, between two positive goals. But the obedient boy experiences considerable social pressures from his family and friends to achieve both the goals. He may incur the disapproval of his parents, if he fails to make good grades in studies. He will lose the esteem of his friends, if he does not make it to the college football team. This failure at either end carries a threat.

Another example is a career woman engaged to be married. The goal of marriage has a positive value for her because of the stability and security it will provide and because she loves the man she will be marrying. But marriage is repellent to her, because it will mean giving up an attractive offer of job in another city. If the over-all sum of marriage values is greater than that of the career, she might hesitate for a while, vacillate back and forth, and then get married.

In still another example, a man may be in conflict not only about whether to get married but also about which of the several girls would make the ideal wife. Internal obstacles are harder to resolve than the external ones.

People may find ways to getting around environmental obstacles, but they find it very hard to escape from obstacles within themselves, i.e., from personal inadequacies and conflicts between motives. The emotional reactions due to approach-avoidance conflicts in which internal obstacles are involved cause several behavioral problems. Conflicts are resolved through the use of certain methods of thinking and acting, which either eliminate the conflict or reduce its severity (defense mechanisms like sublimation, compensation).

REACTIONS TO FRUSTRATION

Pent up frustrations lead to different reactions in people. Some have frustration tolerance to the extent that they bear the consequences with no injury to themselves or to the society, while others become violent and aggressive.

Simple Reactions

a. **Increasing efforts and trials:** During frustration, some individual become introspective for overcoming the obstacles by putting in more efforts or bring about improvement in their behavior or processes.
b. **Compromise:** Repeated failure in one direction may lead the individual to lower or change the aim. A student who is not able to cope with BSc (Nursing) course may join for GNM or may change to physiotherapy course.
c. **Submissiveness:** The individual surrenders himself and accepts his defeat as inevitable.

Violent Reactions

In addition to simple reactions, the individual becomes emotionally tense and the frustration causes aggression. Studies conducted by social psychologist Bandura have shown the relationship between frustration and aggression which are of two types:

a. **External aggression:** This aggression may be directed toward either the person or persons who caused the frustration or toward softer targets as substitutes. For example, an employee denied promotion may quarrel with his supervisor or rebuke his wife or beat his children. When deprived of social needs, people respond with tremendous frustration resulting in aggression and harmful behavior. Riots and violence may follow.
b. **Internal aggression:** Instead of relieving emotional tension by attacking others, the aggression may be directed toward self by blaming self. Eventually, the person becomes neurotic or tries to find escape through suicide. Internal aggression is worse than external reactions for the individual.

Task-oriented Reaction Pattern

Task-oriented reactions may involve making changes in oneself or in his environment or in both depending upon the situation. The reaction may be:

1. Attack,
2. Withdrawal, and
3. Compromise.

Attack

In attack behavior, the individual tries to remove or overcome (surpass) the obstacle to his goal. The type of stress influences his action, such as:

a. **Frustration and direct action:** In frustrating condition, a person tries to take a direct action in an effort to solve the problem and remove the obstacles. For example, when failing in a particular job, one may exert greater effort and try systematically to improve his skills thereby to overcome his frustration.
b. **Conflict and choice:** In a conflicting situation, the individual may face the problem by analyzing the advantages and disadvantages of various options and making an objective direction (choice).
c. **Pressure and resistance:** Usually, the individual resists pressure especially when pressure is perceived as arbitrary and unwanted. Defiance and rebellion are active forms of resistance.

Withdrawal

Whenever an individual suspects that he is likely to be criticized, ridiculed, or disgraced on account of some poor unfortunate experience or failure, he resorts to withdrawal. Such a person will be seen avoiding all work saying that he is unable to do the same. Withdrawal serves to remove the organism from dangerous situation, which he cannot overcome. The most common emotion accompanying withdrawal is fear.

Compromise

When the stress and withdrawal do not work, some sort of compromise is required, e.g., defense mechanisms. Some methods of developing a compromise and relieving tension and anxiety are needed. The human being is usually able to resolve the conflict by utilizing certain forms of adaptation which are called defense mechanisms, adjustment mechanisms, or mental dynamisms.

Defense-oriented Reaction Pattern

Kindly refer Chapter 14 Defense mechanisms.

Adjustment Mechanisms

The different kinds of habits that people acquire to satisfy their motives are called adjustment mechanisms.

The good adjustment is one which fully and directly satisfies a person's desires (motives) and forms an integrated system. A good adjustment is one that manages to satisfy subsistence, social and other motives simultaneously through effective behavior in the real world.

A mature person is more interested in correcting his failures from it rather than blaming others for his failure. He feels secure and confident. He has full faith in his environment and has self-respect. But, for a maladjusted person, the environment appears hostile and he is very diffident about himself.

Coping with Frustration and Conflict by the Nurse

Frustration and conflict cause stress and anxiety causing harm to the body. Some common reactions to frustrations are persistence, escape, and aggression. Some methods of relieving frustration are:

1. Identify the source of your frustration. Can you change it or control it. If you cannot, learning to accept the situation might be the right answer.
2. Decide important things carefully. Check everything out carefully before making a change in your job or residence.
3. Try to find compromises. Look for positive things when all choice seems negative. Every cloud has a silver lining.
4. Seek reliable help from advisors, teachers, and other counselors.
5. Avoid indecision. Stick with your decision and forget about the other choices unless you are clearly in the wrong.
6. Substitute your goals by others, which are equally satisfying but are different and attainable.
7. A student nurse is likely to be frustrated in the course of education:
   a. Failure to be relieved from duty for an interesting lecture.
   b. Failure to get adequate exposure, e.g., lack of opportunity to make as an assistant in an operation theater posting.
   c. Inability to attend some social function due to duty.

She has to understand that there will be sufficient opportunities of the same kind again in the future and there is no need for frustration. She must also realize that 100% success is not possible in treatment of some diseases.

Key Points ● ● ● ●

- Frustration occurs when motives are blocked.
- Conflict is a special type of frustration.
- Approach: Approach conflict occurs when two positive goals are equally attractive.
- Avoidance: Avoidance conflict occurs when one is forced to choose between two negative goals.
- Approach: Avoidance conflict occurs when a person is both attracted and repelled by the same goal object.

STUDY QUESTIONS

Long Essays

1. How do we resolve conflicts? Explain any two ways of resolving conflicts.
2. What is conflict of motives? Explain the various types of conflicts.
3. Define frustration. Briefly discuss the sources of frustration.
4. What are conflicts? Explain the different types of conflicts with examples for each.

Short Essays

1. What do you understand by conflict resolution?
2. Define frustration and its sources.
3. How will you cope with frustrations and conflicts?
4. What is frustration? Describe the role of nurse in conflict resolution.

Short Answers

1. What are conflicts?
2. Define avoidance. Describe an avoidance conflict.
3. Conflict.
4. Define conflict in motives.
5. Name the different types of conflicts.
6. What is approach-avoidance conflict?
7. Describe the resolution of a conflict.
8. What is the role of frustration in nursing?
9. What is the relationship between conflicts and nursing?

Chapter 12: Frustration and Conflicts

Multiple Choice Questions

1. The blocking of behavior directed toward a goal is called_____.
   a. Frustration
   b. Stress
   c. Pressure
   d. Strain
2. Shyam does not like to be in family gatherings but his mother has asked him to attend it. He decides to tell a lie that he has examination on that day however he finds it very distasteful. Shyam is experiencing _____.
   a. Double-avoidance conflict
   b. Double approach conflict
   c. Approach-avoidance conflict
   d. Double approach-double avoidance conflict
3. Conflict is:
   a. an unavoidable fact of life
   b. sometimes constructive
   c. a destructive force in relationships, if continually avoided
   d. All of the above
4. When we speak of "multiple conflict", generally we mean:
   a. Avoidance-avoidance conflict
   b. Approach-avoidance conflict
   c. Double approach-avoidance conflict
   d. Approach-approach conflict
5. What type of defense mechanism is used by a person when he gets angry at the child or spouse because of a bad day at work?
   a. Denial
   b. Repression
   c. Projection
   d. Displacement

13
Stress and its Management

Chapter Outline

- Stress
- Crisis Intervention
- Pressure
- Frustration
- General Adaptation Syndrome
- Psychosomatic Diseases

Learning Objective

Students will be familiarized with sources, symptoms and management of stress.

INTRODUCTION

The following factors are responsible for the health of any individual **(Flowchart 1)**.

Stress refers to the widespread, generalized responses of the body to various environmental, physical, or social situations. Any interference, which disturbs the homeostasis of an organism, is called stress. The causative factors are called stressors. Stressors are biopsychosocial in origin. It is a force that effects our emotions and motives. It is the wear and tear of life. It is called the disease of modern civilization. It affects people of all ages and can be both good and bad. Each person reacts differently to stress, but we all need some stress in order to be active, happy, and productive.

It is the pattern of specific or nonspecific responses an organism makes to stimulus events that disturb its equilibrium and tax or exceed its ability to cope. The stimulus events include a large variety of external and internal conditions, collectively called stressors. A stressor is a stimulus event that places a demand on an organism for some kind of adaptive response.

Flowchart 1: Determinants of health.

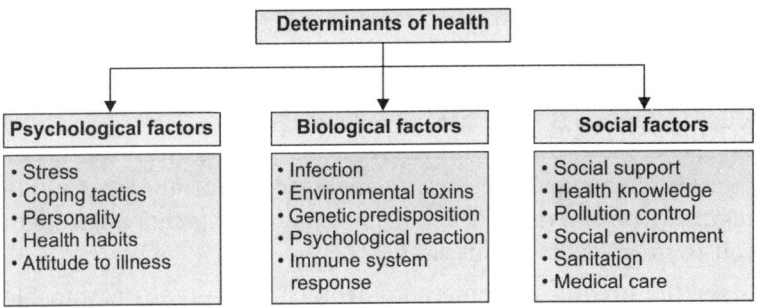

SYMPTOMS OF STRESS

Symptoms of stress appear in many forms. Some symptoms only impact the person who is experiencing stress, while other symptoms may have an impact of our relationship with others.

Physical Symptoms

a. Muscle tension,
b. Colds or other illnesses,
c. High blood pressure,
d. Indigestion,
e. Ulcers,
f. Rapid breathing or pounding of heart,
g. Difficulty in sleeping,
h. Fatigue,
i. Backaches,
j. Headaches, back or neck problems,
k. Increased smoking or drinking alcohol, and
l. Being more prone to accidents.

Cognitive Symptoms

a. Forgetfulness,
b. Unwanted or repetitive thoughts,
c. Difficulty in concentration,
d. Fear of failure, and
e. Self-criticism.

Emotional Symptoms

a. Irritability,
b. Depression,

c. Anger,
d. Fear or anxiety,
e. Feeling overwhelmed, and
f. Mood swings.

SOURCES OF STRESS

Stress and change are closely related. Any important event in life requires a person to make major adjustment. Any major adjustment causes stress leading to diseases.

Major life stressors: Naturally occurring changes are an unavoidable part of life. We attend college, succeed, fail, get new jobs, leave home, get married, etc. Even welcome events also require change in routine and adaptation.

Factors which introduce stress: Thomas Holmes (1984) studied 5,000 patients to determine how the stress of change affects our bodies. He assigned scores of "life changing unit points" to each life event as listed in **Table 1**. He predicted the possibility of person becoming ill by how high that person scored. Life changes intensity as measured by life change units (LCU) scale raises sharply before the onset of an illness, e.g., cardiac death, tuberculosis, multiple sclerosis, diabetes, complications of pregnancy, and birth.

According to Holmes, the person is to list each major event experienced during the past one year and add the points together. As the severity of life crises increases from mild (150–199 LCUs), to moderate (200–299 LCUs) to major (over 300 LCUs), susceptibility to illness rises progressively in the next 2 years.

Catastrophic events: Natural and man-made catastrophes include flood, earthquakes, violent storms, fires, and plane crashes.

Life's little hassles: Much stress arises from nonevents like boredom, continuing tension on a family relationship, lack of occupational progress, loneliness, absence of meaning, and commitment.

Other sources are conflict, unemployment, divorce, and separation.

TYPES OF STRESS

1. **Eustress:** Good stress, e.g., winning lottery, job promotion, having a child, taking vacation, etc.
2. **Distress:** Stress from bad source, e.g., loss of job, worry about family, death, conflict in interpersonal relationships, etc.

Table 1: The social readjustment rating scale (student's version).

Life event	Life change units
Death of close family member	100
Death of close friend	73
Divorce between parents	65
Jail term	63
Major personal illness or injury	63
Marriage	58
Being fired from job	50
Failing an important course	47
Change in health of family member	45
Pregnancy	45
Sex problems	44
Serious argument with close friend	40
Change in financial status	39
Change of major academic subject	39
Trouble with parents	39
New girl or boyfriend	38
Increased workload at school	37
Outstanding personal achievement	36
First quarter/semester in college	35
Change in living conditions	31
Serious argument with instructor	30
Lower grades than expected	29
Change in sleeping habits	29
Change in social activities	29
Change in eating habits	28
Chronic car trouble	26
Change in number of family get-togethers	26
Too many missed classes	25
Change of college	24
Dropping of more than one class	23
Minor traffic violation	20

Chronic Societal Sources of Stress

Pressures

Pressures occur when we feel forced to speed up, intensify or shift direction of our behavior, or to meet a higher standard of performance. We are taught to see failure as a shame.

Frustration

Frustration occurs when a person is prevented from reaching a goal because of someone or something being in the way. The sources of frustration are as follows:
a. Delays,
b. Lack of resources,
c. Losses such as end of an affair, friendship,
d. Failure, guilt, and
e. Discrimination on account of sex, age, religion, caste, etc., in spite of qualifications.

Individual differences in the reactivity of the autonomic nervous system.

A person who characteristically responds to stress with increased secretions of stomach acid (HCl) may eventually develop ulcers; one who reacts with a rise in blood pressure may develop heart disease.

Personality Types and Heart Disease (The Stress of Adjusting to Change: Type A and Type B Persons)

Each individual adjusts to change differently. The type A person is ambitious, self-driving, self-demanding, and controlled by the clock. The type B person is less concerned with success and achievement, less self-demanding and much less controlled by the clock. The type A person is believed to have a risk of heart disease seven times greater than that of a type B person.

Stress of Hospitalization

There are two main sources associated with admission to hospital:
a. Problems arising from illness, i.e., the stress attached to the illness itself and its implications.
b. The hospital environment, i.e., the stress bought about by the aspects of the hospital environment, e.g., admission procedure, staff behavior and communication, the various investigation and treatment procedures, and the need for privacy.

EMOTIONAL REACTIONS TO HOSPITALIZATION

Adverse emotion can complicate the course of recovery from illness, reduce the effectiveness of treatment, and even cause illness. This should be recognized by the health care team. There are four kinds of emotion or manifestation of distress noticed during hospitalization:
a. Anxiety/fear,
b. Depression,
c. Irritability/anger, and
d. Dependence/submissiveness.

The patient's anxiety can be relieved and ability to cope can be increased, if nurses learn to increase communication with the patient and if they give the patient the relevant information. Patients and relatives have difficulties in coping with the fear of a diagnosis of cancer or with having these fears confirmed. Any illness or treatment, which results in disfigurement and consequent change of body image, provokes stress. People need to talk about stressful life events. By doing so, they learn to cope with the feelings of helplessness and despair. Nurses can be of help if they can find time to listen often to stories repeatedly told.

In order to cope with their own emotional distress resulting from empathy with the patient, nurses need the support of their colleagues.

ADAPTATION THEORY (DR HANS SELYE) (1945)

All stresses tend to produce a homeostatic change in the body. Though stress itself cannot be perceived, it can be measured by the structural and chemical changes that it produces in the body. These manifest themselves as the general adaptation syndrome (GAS) when affecting the whole body and as local adaptation syndrome (LAS) when only a limited part of the body is exposed to stress. A syndrome is a particular pattern or grouping of symptoms.

General Adaptation Syndrome

The general adaptation syndrome occurs in three stages:
a. **Alarm reaction fight or flight response:** The alarm reaction is essentially the emergency response of the body. It is the body's initial reaction to a stressor. The stress responses, which characterize the alarm reaction include:

1. Heart rate and strength of cardiac muscle contraction increases. This circulates blood quickly to areas when it is needed to fight the stress.
2. Blood vessels supplying to the skin and viscera, except heart and lungs constrict; at the same time, blood vessels supplying to the skeletal muscles and brain dilate. These responses route more blood to organs active in the stress responses, thus decreasing the blood supply to organs, which do not have in immediate active role.
3. RBC production is increased, leading to an increase in the ability of the blood to clot. This helps control bleeding.
4. Liver converts glycogen into glucose and releases it into blood stream. This provides the energy needed to fight the stressor.
5. The rate of breathing increases and respiratory passages widen to accommodate more air. This enables the body to acquire more oxygen.
6. Production of saliva and digestive enzymes reduces. This reaction takes place as digestive activity is not essential for counteracting stress.

b. **Stage of resistance:** A major feature of the stage of resistance is that certain hormonal responses—especially in the adrenocorticotropic (ACTH) axis—an important line of defense in resisting the effects of stresses. Prolonged activity of the adrenocorticotropic axis (or other hormonal systems) can impair the body's ability to fight infection and can have other harmful effects.
c. **Stage of exhaustion:** The body's ability to respond to stresses has been seriously affected. At this stage or late in the stage of resistance, various psychosomatic (mind-body) disorders may occur.

Crisis Intervention

When people face problems which they are unable to resolve by well-tried defense mechanisms, a brief psychotherapeutic intervention which focuses on the immediate crisis can be of great assistance.

The greatest need for an individual in a crisis is to find some significant person who will stand by him, at least for the time being while he begins to plan his new life.

Quite often the nurse may be this significant person for the patient, because she will be around when the patient needs help most.

Psychosomatic Diseases (Psyche = mind, soma = body)

Psychosomatic problems arise from stress—when there is more stress than that which the body can cope. Stress is the fastest growing disease in the modern industrialized society.

Stress alone may not cause disease, but is appears to be a key factor. There is a relationship between stress and diseases, such as cancer, heart ailments, headaches, arthritis, high blood pressure, and even injuries from accidents.

The term psychosomatic disorders are used to refer to both symptoms—rapid pulse rate, high blood pressure, and actual tissue damage that may be the result. It is estimated that about half of the patients, who visit doctors, have symptoms caused by emotional disturbances. Pent-up emotions may lead to physiological changes in the stomach, resulting in peptic ulcer, high blood pressure, colitis, migraine, back pain, obesity, and asthma.

In the psychosomatic diseases, both symptoms and cause need treatment. People with psychosomatic diseases are often hospitalized for physical symptoms and then treated with medicines. They are discharged when the physical symptoms are gone. The psychological and emotional causes, however, remain and the patient eventually returns with the same symptoms.

How People Cope with Stress

Adaptation to stress is called coping, whatever its source, stress calls for adjustment either by direct coping or by defensive coping.

Direct Coping

Confrontation

Confrontation means facing the problem forthrightly acknowledging to one that there is a problem for which a solution must be found; attacking the problem head on.

Compromise

We often realize that we cannot have everything we want and that we cannot expect others to act as per our wishes. In such cases, we may decide to settle for less than we originally wanted. If we cannot get what we like, we must like what we get.

Withdrawal

When we realize that our adversary is more powerful than we are or that there is no way we can change ourselves, alter the situation or reach a compromise. The most effective way of coping with stress is to withdraw from the situation.

Defensive Coping: Defense Mechanisms

In all the above cases, we were dealing with stress from a recognizable source. In other cases, when we cannot identify the source of stress, we make use of defense mechanisms like denial, repression, projection, identification, reaction formation, displacement, and sublimation.

Altering Bodily reactions during Stress/reducing Stress reaction (*Yoga* or meditation)

The relaxation response is a condition in which muscle tension, cortical activity, heart rate and blood pressure, all decrease and breathing slows. There is reduced electrical activity in the brain and the input to the central nervous system from the outside environment is lowered.

Four conditions needed to produce relaxation response are as follows:
a. Quiet environment,
b. A comfortable position,
c. Closed eyes, and
d. A repetitive device (manthra).

The first three lower inputs to the nervous system while the fourth lowers its internal stimulation.

Yoga, is a way of life, a philosophy, which aims at attaining a higher state of conscience known as "samadhi", which is a stage of inner tranquility. *Yogis* have performed remarkable feats: reduction of heart rate, oxygen consumption, blood pressure, body temperature and many other responses under the control of the autonomic nervous system, and hence beyond any voluntary control.

Coping with Stress by the Nurse

Nursing is one of the four most stressful professions the others being medicine, army, and police. Stress is a part of everyday life and cannot be eliminated altogether. The following steps will help you to cope with stress in life:

1. Balance your life activities with work and play, family and friends, and time for yourself.
2. Exercise your body every day or at least four times a week. Sports, yoga, dancing, or walking will relieve the body from physical tensions.

3. Meditate to promote relaxation.
4. Relax your body regularly through a systematic method of tensing and relaxing all your muscles.
5. Slow down your pace of life.
6. Make your goals realistic. Understand and accept what you can and what you cannot do or be.
7. Organize your life with priorities, so that you will always accomplish what must be done at the right time.
8. Develop healthy social relationships. People will support and help you in stressful situations.
9. Practice coping statements. These are statements you say to yourself in stressful situations. When going for an examination, your thoughts may be, "I am stressed", "I do not remember the right things". These are negative thoughts and should be replaced by coping statements like "I will do my best", "if I forget something, I will just wait for a moment", "we can, if we think, we can".

Key Points

- Stress occurs when pressure is greater than resources.
- The general adaptation syndrome occurs in three stages.
- Psychosomatic problems arise from stress.

STUDY QUESTIONS

Long Essay

1. Enumerate different stressors and explain Selye's theory of stress.

Short Answer

1. Define stress.

Multiple Choice Questions

1. Aches, shallow breathing, and sweating, frequent colds are:
    a. Physical symptoms of stress
    b. Behavioral symptoms of stress
    c. Emotional symptoms of stress
    d. Cognitive symptoms of stress

2. _____ is defined as the optimal amount of stress that helps to promote growth and health,
   a. Prostress
   b. Eustress
   c. Neostress
   d. Austress
3. In the context of stress research, GAS stands for:
   a. Generalized anxiety symptoms
   b. General adaptation syndrome
   c. Gustatory alimentary system
   d. Generic adrenal sensitivity
4. According to Selye's GAS model, we respond to stress with alarm, then with resistance and, finally, with _____.
   a. Adjustment
   b. Eustress
   c. Commitment
   d. Exhaustion
5. In response to stress, levels of adrenaline _____ and levels of cortisol _____.
   a. Rise, rise
   b. Fall, fall
   c. Rise, fall
   d. Fall, rise

14

Defense Mechanisms

Chapter Outline

- Defense Mechanisms
- Successful Mechanisms
- Unsuccessful Mechanisms
- Compensation
- Conversion
- Denial
- Displacement
- Fantasy
- Identification
- Intellectualization
- Projection
- Rationalization
- Reaction Formation
- Regression
- Repression
- Suppression
- Sublimation
- Withdrawal

Learning Objectives

♦ Orients students to different defense mechanisms.
♦ Students will be familiarized with the characteristics of defense mechanisms.

ANXIETY AND FEAR

Fear is the feeling aroused by accurate perception of a genuine external danger. The intensity of fear is proportionate to the degree of that danger. For example, one feels fear when one is left alone on a dark city street late at night. One's apprehension about being attacked is realistic in view of the high urban crime rates.

Anxiety, on the other hand, is not objectively realistic. It is an unexplained discomfort. Anxiety is produced by any situation that threatens the individual's identity or self-esteem or causes one to feel helpless, isolated, and insecure. The reason behind anxiety is subjective. It is caused by personal fears rather than by actual danger.

ADJUSTMENT MECHANISM OR DEFENSE MECHANISM

Adjustment is the process by which an individual maintains a balance between needs and circumstances that influence the satisfaction of these needs. Defense mechanisms are adjustment mechanisms.

Freud, in 1904, used the term "defense mechanism" to refer to the unconscious process that defends a person against anxiety. When the primitive Id drives are in serious conflict with the controls imposed by the Ego or the Superego, the individual suffers from tension and anxiety. This uncomfortable situation is reflected in the individual's behavior. The human being is, usually, able to relieve the conflict by utilizing certain protective forms of adaptation, which are called ego defense mechanisms, adjustment mechanisms, or mental dynamisms.

The different kinds of habits that people acquire to satisfy their motives are called "adjustment mechanisms".

The good adjustment is one which fully and directly satisfies a person's motives and forms an integrated system.

Defense mechanisms enable a person to "resolve the conflict" and reduce the "stress and anxiety" associated with it. Of course, many of these strategies are self-deceptive in nature. When more adaptive measures to resolve the conflicts are not available to the individual, these mechanisms help him to live comfortably without having to face very difficult problems. For instance, individuals who suffer from a disease such as cancer and are sure to die may deny such a state of affairs to themselves and others and they may plan their future projects as if they have many years of life before them. Such a denial of fact rids the individual of the agony of thinking about his impending death.

Mental mechanisms are a means of compromising with forbidden desires, feelings of guilt or an admission that one is inadequate in facing certain problems. They salvage the individual's self-respect avoid an open admission of failure and save psychic energy. With the exception of sublimation, all defense mechanisms indicate an inner conflict.

Characteristics of Defense Mechanisms

1. They protect persons from anxiety.
2. They protect persons from insult by boosting self-esteem or through self-enhancement.
3. Defense mechanisms are not used deliberately; they are unconscious or partly so.
4. Defense mechanisms operate by:
    a. Masking or disguising our true motives.

Chapter 14: Defense Mechanisms

b. Denying the existence of impulses, actions or memories within ourselves that might provoke anxiety to us.

All of us use defense mechanisms sometimes or the other in our normal behavior. When used moderately, they are harmless and help us face conflicts and frustrations easily and protect our ego. However, excessive and persistent use of these mechanisms is harmful as they do not solve conflicts and frustrations basically, but only help the individual to make adaptations to distressing experiences.

Defense mechanisms can be divided into successful and unsuccessful mechanisms is given in **Table 1**.

Successful Mechanisms

Commonly used defense mechanisms that help an individual to deal with reality.

Compensation

Compensation means something given to replace a loss or to make up for a defect. Just as nature compensates for disease in our bodies (as when a blind person develops extraordinarily keen hearing), so we develop personality traits to compensate for various inadequacies. When people are frustrated in their desires in one direction, they compensate for it by attaining success in other directions. A student who fails in his studies may compensate by becoming the college champion in athletics. A student with physical handicap works very hard and achieves scholastic distinction. A plain girl who cannot compete with her more beautiful sisters may compensate by studying hard and come first in her class. Rivalry often leads to compensation. A mother is over-protective of and over-indulgent to a child whom unconsciously she rejects. When carried to excess, it is called over compensation. Students practice compensation when they excel

Table 1: Types of defense mechanisms.

Successful	Unsuccessful
Compensation	Conversion
Identification	Denial
Intellectualization	Displacement
Rationalization	Fantasy
Repression	Projection
Sublimation	Reaction formation
	Regression
	Suppression
	Withdrawal

in objective and practical exams after doing poorly in essay type questions. Helen Keller was born blind and deaf but her determination overcame these handicaps and she won world fame. Similar in the case of Scientist Stephen Hawking, the cosmologist.

Identification

By this adjustment, the individual feels the personal satisfaction in the success and achievements of other people and groups. Thus, the little boy takes the masculine attributes that he admires in his father. Girls identify with their mother, later perhaps with their teacher, and later still perhaps with a film star. Young nurses identify with the ward sister. Hero worship is an obvious form of identification.

Parents may identify themselves with their children. An illiterate father often takes his son's higher education as his own achievement. A dignified mother takes her daughter's failures as her own degeneration. Many people, while watching a film identify with the hero and heroine to the extent that they burst into tears when the hero/heroine is shown mercilessly attacked by villains.

Much of the learning process in childhood is through identification. As we grow a little older, we identify with our teachers, legendary figures, heroes, and idols.

A very common age for practicing identification is in the teens. Adolescents often will identify with successful people in the movies. Identification with a hero either in fiction or in real life is called hero-worship.

Identification is quite normal and healthy, since it plays a large part in the development of a child's personality and in the process of acculturation. Through the process of identification, a child takes on desirable attributes found in the personalities of people in his environment for whom he has admiration and affection. If the object with which we identify is good, their effect on us will be constructive; if it is bad, the effects can be destructive. Also, we cannot grow and mature, if we are completely satisfied by identifying with the experiences and successes of others. We must have our own identity for our growth.

Intellectualization

Related to rationalization is intellectualization, another defense mechanism, which involves reasoning. It is the distancing from an emotional or threatening situation by talking or thinking about it in intellectual terms. A nurse, doctor, or paramedical worker cannot afford to become emotionally attached to each patient. So, they use the technique of detaching themselves from emotions through calm abstract statements about the situation. As a student nurse, probably you use this most of the time when working with patients who are acutely or terminally ill. You may speak calmly and intelligently rather than emotionally with patients and their families. For example, if there is a patient who is acutely ill, calmly tell the family members rather than saying "I am so sorry", etc.

This is a helpful defense mechanism to separate yourself from professional crises. But to go on using it in all your relationships and experiences is to become a very cold and detached individual without healthy emotional experiences.

Rationalization
In rationalization, we "make excuses" giving a reason different from the real one for what we are doing. It is a defense mechanism in which an individual justifies his failures and socially unacceptable behavior by giving socially approved reasons. For example, students who fail in the examination may complain that the hostel atmosphere is not favorable for study. A tense father who beats his child may rationalize that it is for the child's good. A scientist who is unable to carry out research of high order may blame the lack of facilities in his laboratory. An employee who fails to get promotion may blame the employer's partiality.

Rationalization is not lying. We believe in our explanations. It is like a blanket to cover the human weaknesses. It operates in two forms:

1. **Sour grape (from Aesop's fable of the fox and grapes):** A young man who fails to get a beautiful wife may remark that a beautiful wife is a liability. A doctor without a vehicle "does not want to risk his life" by driving a scooter or a car. A girl who fails to get admission for the nursing course may point out a number of difficulties of the nursing profession. "An unskilled worker always quarrels about his tools".

2. **Sweet lemon** form is an extension of the "sour grape" type. The individual justifies his lower achievements by pointing out their merits. For example, a poor, idle man "does not want to earn more money" because "money is the root cause of many evils". People living in small houses due to limited financial resources may point out many virtues of small houses. A husband who fails to get a highly educated wife may enumerate a number of virtues in an uneducated woman.

Repression
According to Freud, repression is basic to all other forms of defense mechanisms. Repression refers to the process by which an individual strives to keep unacceptable, painful, unpalatable, and anxiety provoking needs, urges and feelings associated with them in the

unconscious layers of the mind. The occurrence of the process of repression is itself unconscious, and hence, the individual is unaware of such urges. We forget and then forget that we forgot.

When we cast a discomforting idea or desire deliberately out of our mind or field of attention, we call it suppression. Suppressed material is easily recalled and is, thus, available to the conscious mind. When this process takes place unconsciously, we call it repression. A group of repressed desires and ideas, strongly emotionally toned, forms a complex.

In terms of psychic energy, repression is an expensive defense mechanism. If it operates smoothly and prevents feelings of anxiety, it may help promote a well-adjusted life. However, it is a sort of "burying alive" mechanism. The repressed material is always active and the unconscious memories or urges continue to seek expression and may emerge in the form of accidents (e.g., "slips of the tongue or pen") or neurotic symptoms. Many painful experiences are repressed during early childhood and become unconscious sources of emotional conflict in later life. Selfish, hostile feelings, and sexual impulses are frequently repressed. These may later escape through conversion into obsessions and into morbid anxiety that arises without apparent reason.

Repression is a process of unconscious forgetfulness of our unpleasant and conflict producing emotions and desires. If these experiences were to remain in the conscious, they would cause a person to feel ashamed, guilty, and unworthy.

Examples:
- People may forget to turn up for an appointment for a treatment they do not like.
- Mistakes made in nursing patients may be forgotten.

The repressed material forms part of the unconscious level of the mind and may affect behavior without the person being aware (unconscious motivation). For example, a child may feel angry with his mother because she had punished him. If he feels too guilty about his anger, he may repress it and may still be unconsciously angry. This may be shown by the accidental breaking of his mother's favorite things or in his bed wetting or refusal of food.

Sublimation

It is the channeling of a strong and socially unacceptable drive or urge into a form that is acceptable to society. The most important of these are sexual desires. Others are aggressive feeling, greed, and even lying.

Sublimation is one of the more positive mechanisms of adjustment and is responsible for much of the artistic and cultural achievements of the civilized people. An unmarried woman can express repressed sexual desires, by becoming a nursery school teacher. A young man who has lost his lover may turn to write poetry about love. A person who has aggressive feelings may not be able to express these in society but can become a boxer or soldier. A person with greed can become a successful businessman. A person who needs love can re-channel these energies into fiction writing.

The unfulfilled need to give maternal care may find gratification in the care of the sick. Some lonely people give much love and care to cats and dogs when no opportunity occurs for giving their affection to human beings. One positive result of sublimation is personal satisfaction experienced by the individual. Society also profits as activities like creative writing, music, painting, and sculpturing as a result of sublimation are enjoyed.

Unsuccessful Defense Mechanisms

These when used in moderation and are adaptive they are also called compensatory type defenses. If used excessively it creates emotional problems. These defenses are considered to be deviations and are looked a symptoms of emotional problems.

Conversion

Conversion is a defense mechanism by which strong emotional conflict is expressed as a physical ailment for which there is no demonstrable organic basis. A student nurse, very anxious about her exam, may develop a headache. A woman invited for a party which presents an upsetting situation to her may develop gastrointestinal symptoms and may excuse herself from the party. Usually, when the party time is over, her symptoms resolve themselves.

Another example of this mechanism would be that of a small boy who hated his father so deeply that he wished to strike him. He could suddenly develop complete paralysis of his right arm which would do two things for him:

a. Resolve the conflict (he cannot strike his father even if wished to do so).
b. Bring him a great deal of attention and sympathy.

Denial

Denial of reality is when we refuse to accept or believe the existence of something that is very unpleasant to us. We use denial most often when faced with death, serious illness, or something painful and threatening. A patient often practices denial, at least for a period of time, when he knows he has a fatal illness but cannot accept his impending death.

Parents of fatally ill children will also deny the serious nature of illness for sometime. Many old people will not easily accept that their mental and physical powers are on the decline as they advance in age. Backward students do not find any reliability in the intelligence tests. When some very near and dear one dies in the family, some people try to keep up the pretense that he is still alive. At the dining table, his place is left empty. A patient admitted to the psychiatric ward may say that he just "needs rest". An alcoholic denies the amount he consumed. A student who spends beyond his means is denying his lack of money. Often, nurses protect themselves from the impact of the numerous traumatic experiences of emergencies, suffering and death by developing an unfeeling and apparently callous attitude.

Denial is quite harmless, if practiced in moderation, but can lead to serious difficulties in health and life style, if practiced to excess.

Displacement

Displacement means to substitute the real object of one's feelings, which are often aggression, with another object. A person who is angry with his boss, but cannot show it for fear of losing the job may fight with his wife and children on return from the office or kick his dog. Anger against the ward sister may be displaced on to a more junior nurse or a patient. When a new baby is the center of attraction, an older child may become jealous; prevented from harming the baby, the child demolishes a doll.

Fantasy or Day-dreaming

The motives that cannot be fulfilled in reality are fulfilled by resorting to wishful thinking. Wishful thinking means thinking as one wish to. It is a kind of withdrawal when faced with real problems of life. We retire to a make belief world, where everything is possible, where we are victors or conquerors. The tendency to day-dreaming is most pronounced during adolescence.

Day-dreaming is a pleasant thing. It may help us to escape during times of stress. For example, when one is having financial problems, one can escape from them temporarily by planning how to spend an imaginary fortune. Patients who are very ill may fantasize that when they recover, many good things will happen to them.

Fantasy may offer temporary relief from pressures. But excessive day-dreaming may lead to loss of contact with realities and may lead to a psychotic disorder called schizophrenia.

Projection

Projection is a frequently used unconscious mechanism that relieves tension and anxiety by transferring the responsibility for unacceptable ideas, impulses, wishes, or thoughts to another person. It is an attempt to deal with our own shortcomings, by seeing them in others and denying them in ourselves.

The student who believes that everybody cheats in examinations may also cheat in the same way. People who are dishonest often attribute dishonesty to others. An adulterer blames his wife that she is an adulteress. When we feel guilty about our dislike of another nurse, we complain that she is the one who dislikes us. The nurse who is poor in clinical practice may claim that all of the health care team members are giving poor patient care. The surgeon who bungled an operation may insist that it happened because the theater nurse and ward boy did their task badly. Carried to the extreme, projection is the mask of a behavior disorder known as paranoia.

When you practice projection, your relationship with others will be strained. Firstly, you will not see or understand your own failings. Secondly, you will find others relating poorly with you because of your negative attitude towards them. Thirdly, you will find it very difficult to accept responsibilities for your own behavior because you blame others for anything that goes wrong.

Overcompensation or Reaction Formation

It is sometimes possible to conceal a motive from ourselves by giving strong expression to its opposite. Such a tendency is called reaction formation. The mother of an unwanted child may feel guilty and so becomes over-indulgent and over-protective of the child to assure herself that she is a good mother. A nurse may request the doctor's special care for a patient whom she does not like. A mother-in-law may claim that she loves her daughter-in-law more than her daughter and vice-versa.

People, who are extremely friendly, overly polite and very socially correct, frequently have unconscious feelings of anger and hatred towards many people.

Regression

To regress in behavior means to behave in a less mature way, i.e., go backward. An adult behaving like a child is practicing regression. When faced with difficulties of life, the individual reverts to a less mature form of behavior, where he finds less conflict, and hence less anxiety. Such a person becomes indecisive and dependent forever.

Faced with the unwelcome arrival of a new baby or going to school for the first time, a 5-year-old may have toilet accidents, revert to "baby talk", demand cuddling, etc. "Crying on someone's shoulder" is symbolic of the infants seeking comfort at the maternal bosom. You may practice regression when faced with pressures of an examination.

Another example is when the nurse makes an error in giving medicines or nursing care and then starts crying.

Adults too, may regress to the oral stage of development and suck their thumbs when life gets stressful. One may regress so profoundly that he will curl up in the fetal position and remain in it without moving. Any retreat into a state of dependency or other to avoid facing acute problems is called a regressive trait.

Some regressions, such as tears on becoming very emotional are quite normal while facing serious problems in life. Extreme forms and degrees of regression result in psychosis.

Suppression

Suppression is an intentional pushing away from awareness of certain unwelcome ideas, memories, or feelings. We merely push them into the background, into our subconscious mind, where they are accessible to us whenever we wish to remember them. Because it is conscious, it is not a defense mechanism in the strict sense of the term. For example, a student consciously decides not to think about her weekend, so that she can study effectively. A patient may refuse to consider his difficulties by saying that he does not want to talk about it. Suppression is easier to deal with, because the material remains conscious.

Withdrawal

Whenever, an individual suspect that he is likely to be criticized, ridiculed or disgraced on account of some prior unfortunate experience or failure, he resorts to withdrawal. Such a person is seen as avoiding all work saying that he cannot do this or he cannot do that. It is a protective device by which the individual prevents further hurt and damage to his security by withdrawing from people and avoiding all close interpersonal relations. It may occur as a temporary pattern. They make no real friends.

Withdrawal is one of the dominant personality traits of the schizophrenics. These patients not only have an inability to relate well with people emotionally but they also use "regression".

Defense Mechanisms and the Nurse

Understanding defense mechanisms will enable the nurse to support the patient and his family. Denial, for example, is a common reaction to a serious diagnosis or at the time of death. The patient and his family should be allowed to deny the situation until they are prepared to face the reality. The patient will often practice regression through tears, trembling or demanding special treatment. Some patients may also practice withdrawal and should be allowed to do so. Many patients intellectualize about a serious sickness or prognosis just like the nurses and other members of the health team.

Rationalization may actually lead to rational conduct in future because of the tendency to search for reasons. The tendency to justify behavior that we have found satisfying may lead to false reasons, but it may also lead to a careful analysis of cause and effect relationships.

Moderate and intellectual use of mental mechanisms, provides a temporary relief to stress and contributes for a healthy living.

Overuse and abuse of ego defense mechanisms give rise to psychological disorders.

Identification can be seen in patients who rely heavily on the nurse's advice and support. They expect that all of their needs will be met and that nothing will be expected of them. It is important for the nurse to recognize that identification can be used constructively to teach proper health care.

Patients who must deal with the stress of serious illness may shift the blame for their condition onto the nurse (projection). They may complain of poor nursing care to a nurse who is actually very skillful. Nurses should not show anger and retaliate but should encourage the patients to explore the realistic aspects of their situation.

Both well-adjusted and maladjusted individuals make use of the defense mechanism in their daily life. The well-adjusted individuals use them sparingly and in socially desirable ways, whereas the maladjusted individuals including psychotics and neurotics use them too frequently and inappropriately.

Key Points ● ● ● ●

Defense mechanisms	Definitions
1. Repression	Unconsciously forgetting unpleasant experiences
2. Reaction formation	Strongly expressing the reverse of what one feels
3. Projection	Pretending that others have your own failings
4. Rationalization	Making excuses giving a reason different from the real one for what we are doing
5. Intellectualization	Distancing oneself from emotional situations by abstract talking or thinking
6. Displacement	Discharging pent-up feelings on persons less dangerous than those who initially aroused the emotion
7. Regression	Acting immaturely
8. Sublimation	Directing unacceptable desires into socially acceptable behavior

Contd...

Contd...

Defense mechanisms	Definitions
9. Identification	Finding satisfaction through what another person does
10. Compensation	Working hard to make up for a weakness or deficiency
11. Denial	Refusing to believe that something unpleasant exists
12. Fantasy	Withdrawal to a make belief world when faced with real problems
13. Withdrawal	Avoiding all close interpersonal relationships
14. Conversion	An emotional conflict is expressed by a physical illness or a physical symptom without any organic cause
15. Suppression	Intentional pushing away from awareness of certain unwelcome ideas, memories and feelings

EXERCISES

Name the ego defense mechanism involved in the following:
a. Demanding extreme degrees of health care for patients whom you always disliked (2).
b. Excelling in drama when weak in studies (10).
c. Saying you are fine when you are in severe pain (11).
d. Staying in your room when your friends are at a party (13).
e. Pretending that everybody is a liar (3).
f. Day-dreaming about being the best student in the science class (12).
g. Forgetting that you failed in the fifth standard (1).
h. Excelling in orphanage work when unmarried (8).
i. Dressing up like a popular film star (9).
j. Crying or pouting when you make an error (7).
k. Arguing with a junior student when angry with the principal (6).
l. Studying very hard after your classes are over (10).
m. Believe or pretend to believe that psychology is not important (11).
n. Cultivate the friendship of the best student of science (9).
o. Without working hard, bask in the best student's reflected glory (9).
p. Blame the lecturer for not being able to teach well or to arouse interest in the subject (4).
q. Talk about other students who are having difficulty in anatomy and physiology (3).
r. Become ill or feel sick and cut classes and tests (14).
s. Saying "I don't like the prize anyway" when failing to win a prize (4).

Chapter 14: Defense Mechanisms

STUDY QUESTIONS

Long Essays

1. What is ego defense mechanism? Explain any two with suitable examples.
2. Explain the various types of adjustments (defense mechanisms).

Short Answers

1. What do you understand by defense mechanism? Define identification.
2. What is adjustment mechanism?

Multiple Choice Questions

1. To prevent itself from being overwhelmed by excessive demands from the id and superego, the ego relies on:
   a. The Oedipus complex
   b. Defense mechanisms
   c. The reality principle
   d. The pleasure principle
2. The defense mechanism that involves banishing threatening thoughts, feelings, and memories into the unconscious mind is known as:
   a. Repression   b. Conversion
   c. Suppression   d. Rationalization
3. Anna's husband dies, and she continues to set a place for him at the dinner table. This is an example of:
   a. Repression   b. Denial
   c. Adaptation   d. Projection
4. Mr. A hates Ms. B, but his superego tells him that such hatred is unacceptable. He "solved" the problem by believing that Ms. B hates him. What defense mechanism did Mr. A show?
   a. Regression   b. Projection
   c. Rationalization   d. Displacement
5. A 15-year boy after tonsillectomy has seen sucking thumb in between. What defense mechanism he exhibits?
   a. Regression   b. Repression
   c. Reaction formation d. Rationalization

15

Emotions in Health and Disease

Chapter Outline

- Emotion
- Polygraph
- Emotional Development
- Positive Emotions
- Emotional Quotient
- James–Lange Theory
- Cannon–Bard Theory
- Cognitive–Appraisal Theory

Learning Objectives

♦ Students will be introduced to types, characteristics and measurement of emotions.
♦ Orients students to different theories of emotion.

INTRODUCTION

"Anybody can become angry—that is easy; but to be angry with the right person, and to the right degree, and at the right time, and for the right purpose, and in the right way, that is not within everybody's power and is not easy."

—*Aristotle*

Emotion and motivation have the same Latin origin. The Latin word "emovere" means to be "stirred up". Anger, fear, surprise, joy, grief, love, affection, hope, anticipation, acceptance, disappointment, jealousy, and disgust are classified as emotions while hunger, thirst and fatigue are motives. Emotions are, usually, aroused by external stimuli and emotional expression is directed toward the stimuli in the environment that arouses it. Motives, on the other hand, are aroused by internal stimuli and are directed toward certain objects in the environment, e.g., food, water.

Chapter 15: Emotions in Health and Disease

We often think ourselves as rational beings that go about satisfying our motives in an intelligent way. To a certain extent we do that, but we are also emotional beings, more emotional than we often realize. Life would be drab without emotions. Emotions add color and spice to life.

Emotions and feelings are interchangeably used by many. Emotions are the outward expressions of feelings. Feelings persist for longer time than emotions. Feelings are simple and sensory. Emotions are more complex. Emotions are aroused not only by existing circumstances but also by a recollection of these circumstances.

Emotion is a strong feeling. It is a conscious stirred up state of the organism. Emotion is a disturbed glandular and muscular activity. It increases energy mobilization. Emotion is defined as a subjective response that is usually accompanied by a physiological change and is associated with a change in behavior.

Characteristics of Emotions

1. To a considerable extent, emotions are accompanied by the activation or an aroused state in the organism.
2. They are normally accompanied by physiological changes like gestures, muscular movements, changes in facial expression, and changes in physiological reactions like blood pressure, heart beat, pulse rate, and respiration.
3. Whenever an organism is experiencing an emotion, a lot of energy is released. Exception is grief, when the energy and activity level are reduced.

Psychological Changes in Emotions

1. During emotional experiences, other activities like perception, learning, consciousness, and memory are affected.
2. Along with bodily changes, there are psychological changes that also take place during the emotion. For example, confusion in perception, clouding of consciousness, and blocking of memory.

Parts of an Emotion

The four parts of an emotion are: (a) a subjective feeling, (b) an emotional expression, (c) a physiological expression, and (d) an interpretation.

1. Subjective means existing within one's own mind or thoughts. Subjective feelings are what you believe you are feeling. Others cannot directly see what you are feeling. Subjective feelings form a part of the emotion you experience before an exam.

2. The second part of an emotion is the emotional expression, e.g., you may express your feelings of fear in a number of ways, such as tensing your body, trembling, perspiring, urinating, and even vomiting.
3. The third part of an emotion is physiological change or arousal. Adrenaline is released in the body during most emotions through the action of autonomic nervous system.
4. The fourth part of an emotion is the interpretation of it by another person. A smiling person would be interpreted as a happy person and a frowning person would be interpreted as an unhappy person.

Primary and Mixed Emotions

In the primary emotional states, there is, generally, only one emotion, e.g., fear, surprise, sadness, disgust, anger, anticipation, joy, and acceptance.

Mixed emotions are those feelings which combine a number of primary emotions, e.g., love, submission, awe, disappointment, remorse, contempt, aggression, and optimism **(Fig. 1)**.

Internal Changes in Emotion (Physiological Changes)

The autonomic nervous system has two subdivisions—(a) Sympathetic division and (b) Parasympathetic division. The sympathetic division of the autonomic nervous system prepares the body for emergency action during aroused states. The sympathetic system causes discharge of hormones, epinephrine (adrenaline), and norepinephrine (noradrenaline). Adrenaline gets circulated to different parts of the body through blood and is responsible for the following physical changes **(Fig. 2)**:

- Increased blood pressure and heart rate.
- Changes in the rate of respiration. When excited, breath comes in short quick gasps. When depressed, breathing is slow.
- Dilation (widening) of pupils of the eyes.
- Sweating and decreased secretion of saliva.
- Increase in blood sugar.
- Production of more energy.

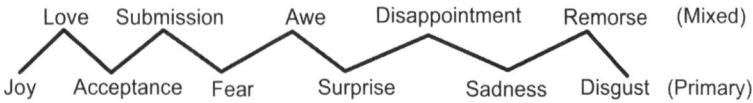

Fig. 1: Primary and mixed emotions.

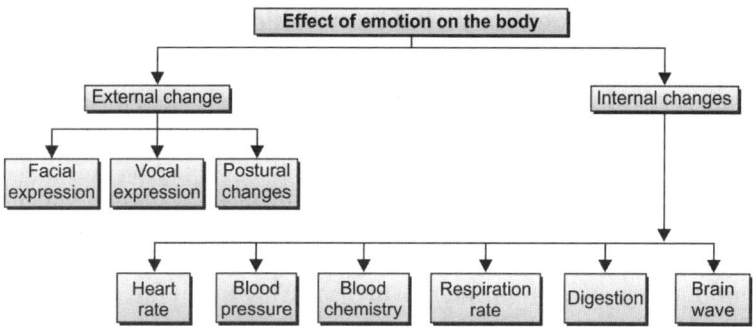

Fig. 2: Effect of emotion in the body.

- Increased mobility of the gastrointestinal tract.
- Erect hair on the skin (goose pimples).
- Changes in the frequency of the brain waves.
- Muscular tensions and tremors.

Tremors are, usually produced when opposing muscles are contracted simultaneously. They also occur when a person is experiencing severe conflicting desires.

Normally, emotions help us, so when there is danger they get into action altering the blood pressure increasing the flow of adrenaline and tensing up muscles. And once the fear ebbs, the emotions allow us to relax. But if there is no let up in danger, then the emotions keep flashing distress signals, which may manifest themselves in the form of a migraine, peptic ulcer, etc.

External Changes in Emotion

Change in the voice is experienced in many persons. Emotions like fear and excitement are expressed externally by a smile or laughter. A tremor in the voice, denotes sorrow and sharp high pitch indicates anger.

Changes in the facial expression are indicative of emotional responses. Primary emotions like interest, enjoyment, surprise, disgust, anger, shame, and fear are expressed externally by facial expressions.

Changes in the different parts of the body (body language) like stiffness of the body, the way the person holds his head and the way he folds his hands are non-verbal expressions of emotions.

Body Language: Nonverbal Communication

Body language means communication through body movement, such as facial expressions, postures, and gestures. It is called a language, because all of these movements send a message to another person along with anything that is said verbally.

Much body language is universal. Leaning toward another person or object means liking while drawing away means disliking. Smiling means pleasantness and frowning shows unpleasantness. Spitting at another person means contempt or disgust in any culture. Shaking or throwing one's shoe or sandal at another person is a sign of extreme disgust.

Fight or Flight Syndrome or Emergency Theory

Walter Cannon, the Harvard physiologist, has said that the internal changes in emotions are useful to people who must fight or flee. Cannon noted that the physical aspects of such emotions as anger or fear help the organism survive in case of danger. The adrenal glands pour out adrenaline into the blood stream and extra strength or power is available for quick action.

Measurement of Emotions

Emotions are difficult to be analyzed objectively but effects of emotions on behavior can be measured by:

1. **Introspective reports:** It is possible to identify and even quantify emotions by the introspective report of the individual. He may be able to identify the changes internal or external he undergoes on joy, fear, sorrow, etc., and also describes what he was feeling. Since, emotion is regarded as a highly subjective experience, self-reporting introspective reports play an important role in identification and measurement of emotions.
2. **Observations of facial expressions:** Face in the index of the mind. The nonverbal communications in the form of looks, gestures and bodily positions provide a clue to identify various emotional states. By looking at one's facial expressions, we can judge ones intended emotions and label it as anger, joy, fear, disgust, contempt, surprise, or love. The correlation between the facial expression and emotion is based on the sociocultural environment and one's inmate dispositions. The way of expressing emotions vary from culture to culture. For example, the Chinese put out their tongues when happy. These expressions may also

be innate responses to particular situations like jumping at the time of hearing a sudden noise and bearing teeth at the time of anger. But these expressions are not sufficiently objective, reliable and valid indications for identification and measurement of emotions as people can hide their feelings under the mask of false expressions.

3. **Measurement of physiological changes in emotion:** Emotions are always accompanied by physical and physiological changes in an organism. Some of these changes are easily observable some of this internal physiological changes need special instruments for their proper measurement. With technological progress today we have instruments which accurately measure physiological changes in terms of blood pressure, blood volume, respiration, pulse rate, muscle tension, temperature, skin resistance and sensitivity, brain waves (EEG), and pilometer reaction involving erection of body hair often associated with chilling of the skin. Under emotion the resistance of the skin to electric current is increased. This change is used in measuring emotions experimentally in psychogalvanoscope.

4. Emotions can be assessed using emotion quotient (EQ) test. It is a standardized test, which allows understanding oneself better. Nowadays, employers are using EQ test for recruitment of candidates. Awareness of your emotional intelligence allows you to improve your emotional intelligence and to live a happier and more balanced life style.

5. Emogram measures 11 basic emotions by presenting a series of photographs that precisely depict the emotions. Individuals respond to each photograph indicating a level of agreement with each photo. The eleven basic emotions that an emogram can measure include happiness, interest, surprise, contempt, disgust, anxiety, shame, fear, anger, and distress.

Polygraph-Lie Detector

The physiological changes accompanying intense emotions are the basis of the use of polygraph commonly known as the "lie detector" in checking the reliability of an individual's statement. The term "lie detector" is actually incorrect. The polygraph does not detect lies. It simply measures some of the physiological changes in emotion like alteration in heart rate, blood pressure, respiration, and the galvanic skin response (GSR), i.e., changes in the electrical conductivity of the skin.

IMPORTANCE OF EMOTIONS

Emotions occupy a very important position in a person's life as they motivate many in their job endeavors. A person in love makes sacrifices for the object of his love. The love of their offspring spurs the parents to great sacrifices.

Emotions have a stimulating effect. For example, a person who is in a happy state of mind invariably makes others also happy and sees happiness around him. Similarly, a person who is angry makes others angry. Thus, emotion is contagious. Emotions also play a crucial role in creative and artistic activities. A soldier lays down his life for the love of his country. The ability to understand and interpret the emotional states of others is very important in our social life. It is clear that emotions play a major role in our behavior and in understanding other's behavior. Sometimes, emotions are beneficial and at other times, they are harmful. It depends on the intensity and duration of emotion. When emotion becomes intense whether pleasant or unpleasant, they usually result in some disruption of thought or behavior. So also when emotions are prolonged or excessive they do harm because of the sustained physiological changes that accompany them.

EMOTIONS AND DISEASE

Good pleasant emotion constitutes a great power for good health and unpleasant emotion disturbs the whole organism.

Excess emotions not only have an inhibiting effect on the ability to think, but also have a permanent harmful effect on the body. Illness and excess emotions always go together. A branch of medical science has developed known as psychosomatic medicine.

Many physical complaints are related to the patient's psychological reactions to life. Peptic ulcer has its origin in emotional stresses. Colitis is caused psychosomatically. Many skin diseases, blood pressure, asthma, and migraine are caused by reactions to emotional stress. Emotion can interfere with the course of a disease even when it may not be a cause of the disease. Emotions work against the successful treatment of tuberculosis, diabetes, heart diseases, and epilepsy. Emotions need not be eliminated but should be controlled.

If the disease is entirely organic, the symptoms are likely to be definite and consistent. If it is chiefly emotional, there may be a variety of complaints—faintness, pounding of heart at night, sleeplessness—all involving unrelated systems of the body.

DEVELOPMENT OF EMOTIONS

In addition to genetic and environmental influences, maturation and growth play an important role in the appearance or nonappearance of particular patterns of behavior. While the basic developmental process is common in a general way for all individuals, this pattern is greatly influenced by social, cultural, and environmental factors.

The child has been described as a "big blooming buzzing confusion" as he reacts to a stimulus. The newborn child shows only general excitement as the only emotion. As the child grows older, an increasing number of emotions become apparent. Thus, in the 3-months-old child, distress and delight can be distinguished. During the next 3 months, distress is differentiated so that fear, disgust, and anger are also apparent. At about 12 months, delight is differentiated into elation and affection. Jealousy and affection for children, distinguished from affection for adults appear between 12 and 18 months. Between 18 and 24 months, delight develops into joy.

Maturation and Learning in Emotional Development

Both maturation and learning play important roles in emotional development. As the infant grows, even when no opportunity has been presented for learning them, such emotional responses as crying, weeping, smiling, and laughing begin to appear. These emotional reactions appear about the same age in all children, regardless of variations in stimulation provided by adults. This is due to maturation.

Many fears are learned. Children do not fear mice, rats, and other animals unless they are negatively conditioned to them.

AN EMOTION ACTS AS A MOTIVE

Emotion is a conscious stirred up state of organism, when there are marked physiological changes involving both visceral and peripheral areas.

An emotion acts as a motive. It implies a goal. In case of fear, for example, the motive is to avoid the situation that causes fear; in anger the motive is aggress against or harm the source of provocation. In pleasure, the motive is to seek or attain what gives pleasure.

Emotional states determine human behavior. Anger can cause a person to be rude and sarcastic. Disorders of emotion interfere with human efficiency, lack of appetite, increased risk of accidents, lack of sleep and palpitation. Emotional disorders in children may appear in the form of temper tantrums, abdominal pain, spasms and antisocial behavior like aggressiveness.

Emotions, generally, rise suddenly but die slowly. Sometimes, they persist in the form of a mood.

Emotional Quotient (EQ) and Emotional Intelligence

Our thinking, reasoning, perception, learning, memory, etc. are influenced by our emotional state. This shows the need to understand the dynamics of emotions to understand human behavior. Today one's success in any walk of life depends on Emotional Quotient (EQ) than on Intelligence Quotient (IQ).

Weightage should be more to EQ which also take into consideration the IQ. The ratio may be 70% EQ and 30% IQ. The reason is because IQ uses only aspects of brain, whereas EQ uses both the heart and the brain which are vital aspects of human psyche. It is the synthesis of two things—the heart of the Buddha, the enlightened and the brain of Einstein, the physicist, which constitute the Emotional Quotient (EQ).

Nurse must have high level of emotional intelligence as they come across many emotional situations in their duties, such as suffering and death of patients and the sorrow of their relatives.

THEORIES OF EMOTIONS (FIG. 3)

Peripheral Theories

James-Lange Theory: Felt Emotion is the Perception of Bodily Changes

One of the earliest theories of emotion was succinctly stated by the American Psychologist William James: "We feel sorry because we cry, angry because we strike, afraid because we tremble". This theory, presented in 1890 by James and the Danish physiologist Carl Lange, turns the common sense idea of emotions inside out. It proposes the following sequence of events in emotional states: (1) We perceive the situation will produce emotion; (2) We react to this situation; and (3) We notice our reaction.

James-Lange Theory (Fig. 4)

The emotional experience (the felt emotion) occurs after the bodily changes.

Our perception of the reaction is the basis for the emotion we experience. So the emotional experience (the felt emotion) occurs after the bodily changes; the bodily changes (internal changes in the

Chapter 15: Emotions in Health and Disease

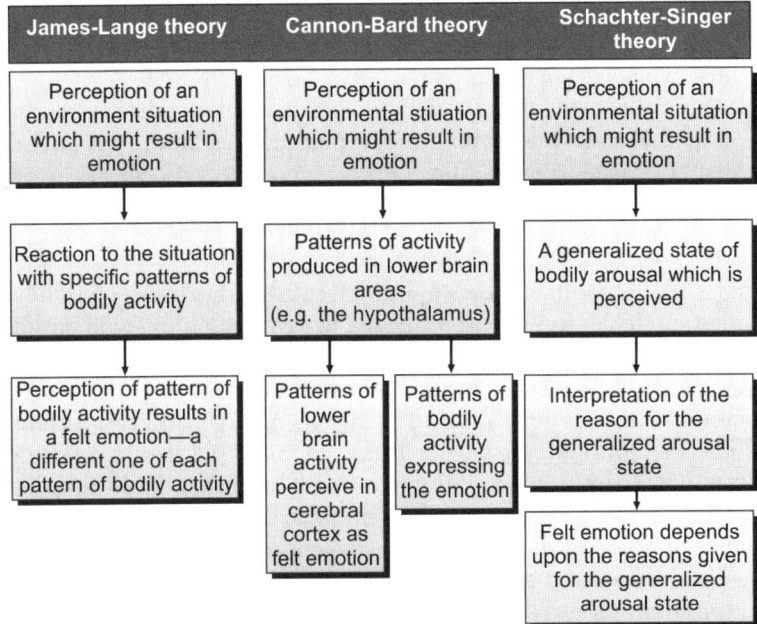

Fig. 3: Theories of emotions compared.

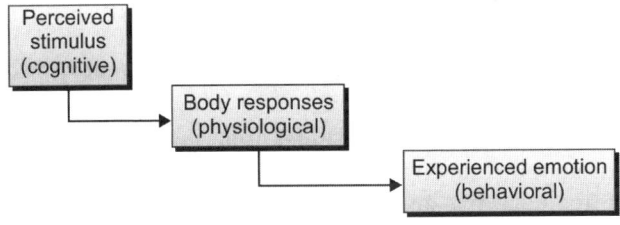

Fig. 4: James–Lange theory.

autonomic nervous system or movements of the body) precede the emotional experience.

The major objections to the James–Lange theory came from Walter Cannon (1871-1945), a physiologist at the University of Harvard who pointed out that:
a. Since, the internal organs are relatively insensitive, the bodily changes are very often too slow and appear only after the psychological experience of emotion.

b. The same bodily changes occur in different kinds of emotional experiences, e.g., our heart beats faster when we feel happy and also when we are unhappy.
c. Artificially inducing the bodily changes associated with an emotion (e.g. injecting a person with adrenaline) does not produce the experience of true emotion.

Cannon–Bard Theory: Felt Emotion and Bodily Responses are Independent Events

In the 1920s, another theory about the relationship between bodily states and felt emotion was proposed by Walter Cannon who based his approach to the emotions on the research done by Philip Bard. The Cannon–Bard theory says that felt emotion and the bodily reactions in emotions are independent of each other; both are triggered simultaneously. According to James-Lange theory, the body first responds physiologically to a stimulus, and then the cerebral cortex determines which emotion is being experienced. In the Cannon-Bard theory, impulses are sent simultaneously to the cerebral cortex and peripheral nervous system. Thus, the response to the stimulus and the stimulus are experienced at the same time, but independently.

Cannon-Bard Theory (Fig. 5)

An emotion arousing stimulus simultaneously triggers (1) Physiological responses, and (2) Subjective experience of emotion.

Schachter-Singer Theory (Cognitive Appraisal Theory) or Two Factor Theory

Stanley Schachter and Jerome Singer (1962) proposed a two factor theory of emotion known as cognitive appraisal theory. Observations suggest that cognitive appraisals are often sufficient to determine the quality of an emotional experience. This theory has incorporated elements of both James-Lange and Cannon-Bard theory. Like James

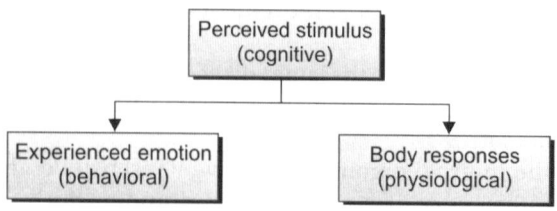

Fig. 5: Cannon–Bard theory.

and Lange, Schachter presumed that our experience of emotions grows from our awareness of our body's arousal. But he also believed like Cannon-Bard that emotions are physiologically similar. According to Schachter and Singer, the intensity of emotion depends upon the cognitive appraisal of the situation. Thus, people experience internal arousal, become aware of the arousal, seek an explanation for it, identify an external cue, and finally label the cue. Our physical arousal together with our perception and judgment of situation (cognition) jointly determines which emotions we feel. In other words, our emotional arousal depends on both physiological changes and method or cognition interpretation of those changes **(Fig. 6)**.

To experience emotion, we must be aroused and must cognitively label the arousal.

STATES OF EMOTION

There are ten different basic emotional states five positive and five negative as enumerated below:

Positive Emotions

1. **Love:** The power of love has a remarkable healing potential in major illnesses like cancer, colitis, etc. Babies who get a lot of love grow up healthier than children deprived of it. Forgiveness brings good health. Quality of mercy is doubly blessed.
2. **Laughter:** Some of the physical benefits of laughter are:
    * Increases muscular and respiratory activity
    * Stimulates cardio muscular system and sympathetic nervous system
    * Increases antibodies, the body's first line of defense
    * Decreases levels of stress hormones

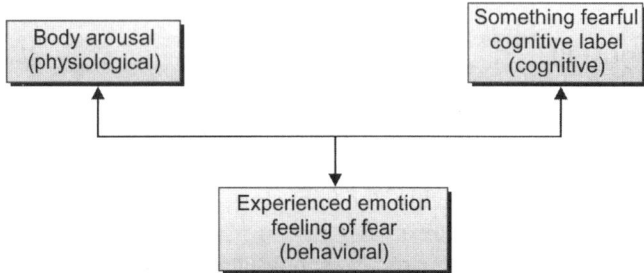

Fig. 6: Schachter-Singer theory.

- Decreases heart rate and breathing becomes easier
- Increases pain tolerance
- Even your relationships improve. Laughter is the best medicine.

3. **Hope:** If your life has hope, purpose, and meaning, you will be happier and healthier. Hope springs eternal in the human breast.
4. **Optimism:** Optimists put failures behind them, do their best to look at the bright side and generally have better health. There is a silver lining even in the darkest cloud.
5. **Self-confidence:** If you lack confidence and find it difficult to assert yourself, you may suffer from indigestion and headaches. Positive emotions can play wonders with your biology.

Negative Emotions

1. **Anger:** Suppressed anger causes high blood pressure, heart attacks, strokes, and stomach ulcers. Get rid of it with physical activity, chat with a friend or leave that irritating situation.
2. **Fear:** We worry about future, money, health, children, etc. To combat fear, learn as much as you can about it. If it is health related, meet a specialist doctor.
3. **Sadness:** It is our natural reaction to problems. Crying helps the body get rid of harmful wastes.
4. **Boredom:** Inactivity and boredom can damage your health like stress. Cultivate some hobby.
5. **Guilt:** It is the most damaging of emotions and very difficult to be distinguished from conscience. To counteract guilt build up your self-confidence. Think of your strengths and you will feel distinctly better.

THE NURSE AND CONTROL OF EMOTIONS

As a nurse, you should be concerned with the expression and control of emotions:

In Yourself

As a nurse, you are the central figure in health care. You will be much more poised and productive, if you are emotionally controlled and mature in your behavior. Emotional poise is also important for your physical and mental health. The following suggestions will help you to develop emotional poise:

- Try to understand yourself, your conflicts, and your physical and emotional limits.

- Learn as much as you can, about the causes and physical reactions. to emotions. The more you know better control over emotions.
- Control stress in your life. Plan your work to avoid emergencies.
- Balance your work with play, exercise, and social activities.
- Practice relaxation by meditation, listening to music, reading, dancing, or sports.
- Use your sense of humor. Laughter with others and laughing at yourself can relieve tensions in your body.
- Try to control unreasonable and excessive external expressions of emotions. These external expressions tend to increase the intensity of emotional experiences of the individual. They excite other people and cause further emotionality.
- A desirable philosophy of life will enable you to avoid mental conflicts and emotional tensions.

Control of Emotions in the Patients

When you first come into contact with a patient, he will respond to whatever message you give through the tone of your voice and body language.

Help the Patient Feel Welcome and at Ease

Give a warm welcome to the patient. Let him feel that he is an important guest. Let not the patient know your feelings, if any, of frustration due to the heavy work load or any negative feeling toward the patient. Your top priority at the beginning of a patient's relationship is to provide a pleasant, relaxed atmosphere.

Understand his Negative Emotions

Normally, the patients are less self-controlled than the nurses. They are tense, irritable, and unbalanced. Therefore, the nurse has to be very patient, mature, and balanced in her behavior toward the patients.

Promote Positive Feelings

The nurse has to substitute the negative emotions of the patient by positive thoughts. She should try to eliminate fear, anger, worry, anxiety, and resentment from her and her patients. This requires healthy interpersonal relationships.

Develop Empathy

It will be helpful, if the nurse develops empathy with the patient. Empathy means understanding the patient's situation, feelings, and motives. With proper understanding, you will be able to accept the patient as an individual.

Psychosomatic Illness

Patients with a psychosomatic illness may need more of your time, patience and attention. It is easy for the nurse to get impatient with such a patient. Such patients need help to relax and the nurse must arrange professional counseling for such patients when required.

Key Points ● ● ●

- Emotions are the outward expressions of feelings.
- Subjective feeling, an emotional expression, a physiological expression, and an interpretation are for parts of an emotion.
- Emotions can be measured in various ways.
- James–Lange theory proposes that the emotional experience (the felt emotion) occurs after the bodily changes.
- Cannon-Bard theory states that an emotion arousing stimulus simultaneously triggers physiological responses and subjective experience of emotion.
- According to Schachter and Singer theory, the intensity of emotion depends upon the cognitive appraisal of the situation.

STUDY QUESTIONS

Long Essays

1. Define emotion. Mention its states. Bring out the relevance of theories of emotion in understanding them.
2. Define emotions. Explain how emotions can be motives. What is the effect of emotions?
3. Discuss emotions and feelings and discuss their implications on behavior.
4. What are emotions? Discuss their influencing factors on health.
5. Elaborate the various theories of emotion and bring out the relationship between emotions and health.
6. Define emotion. Describe the various theories and states of emotion.

Short Essays

1. Discuss the different states of emotion.
2. Discuss the emotions that encourage health and list others that hamper the healthy functions of the body.
3. Explain the role of emotion in health and illness.
4. Elaborate the theories of emotion.
5. What emotions do patients usually experience? What experiences usually provoke these emotions?

Chapter 15: Emotions in Health and Disease

Short Answers

1. Discuss emotion as a motive.
2. James-Lange theory.
3. Psychosomatic disorders.
4. Emotions during illness.
5. Discuss the development of emotions.

Multiple Choice Questions

1. During most emotions _____ is released in the body.
   - a. Oxytocin
   - b. Adrenaline
   - c. Insulin
   - d. Tyroxine
2. Emogram measures emotions by presenting a series of _____ _____.
   - a. Statements
   - b. Ink blots
   - c. Photographs
   - d. Stories
3. According to _____ theory of emotions body changes precede emotions.
   - a. James-Lange
   - b. Cannon-Bard
   - c. Schachter-Singer
   - d. Both a and d
4. The seat of emotion is found to be in the _____.
   - a. Reticular formation
   - b. Hind brain
   - c. Limbic system
   - d. Cerebellum
5. The word "emovere" means:
   - a. Relax
   - b. Stirred up
   - c. Goal directed
   - d. Act out

16

Attitude: The Way We See Things

Chapter Outline

- Attitude
- Balance Theory
- Favorable Attitude
- Social Distance
- Rank Order
- Paired Comparison
- Sentiments
- Attitude Change

Learning Objectives

♦ Students will be familiarized with the concept, characteristics, components, and factors influencing attitude.
♦ Students will be oriented to types, development, and measurement of attitudes.

INTRODUCTION

An attitude is a predisposition to react in a persistent and characteristic manner to some situation, idea, material object, or person. Our set ways of reacting to religious rituals, to our parents and teachers, to our profession and other professions are examples of attitudes. Attitudes can be positive or negative. An attitude of respect toward elders is a positive attitude. An attitude of hatred toward a certain community is a negative attitude. Attitudes accompanied by strong feelings are called sentiments.

We often remark that certain person has a great attitude or bad attitude or should change his or her attitude. The media regularly reports on people's attitude toward a wide range of topics like drugs, smoking, marriage, dowry, divorce, sexual harassment, assisted suicides, capital punishment, fast food, etc.

Chapter 16: Attitude: The Way We See Things

An attitude is any belief or opinion that includes an evaluation of some object, person, or event along a continuum from negative to positive. It predisposes us to act in a certain way toward that object, person, or event.

Our attitudes have a great effect on our behavior and have many other functions. Attitude research has become a big business. Large sums of money are spent each year on measuring or trying to change buyers' attitude toward consumer products and in measuring and trying to change attitude of voters toward candidates.

Terri—A Case History

In 1991, a certain Terri employed in the US "Continental Airlines" as an airport sales agent was dismissed from her job as she refused to wear makeup (lipstick and eyeliner), which was compulsory as per their dress code manual. Terri had not worn makeup in her 2 years in airline industry and no one had ever complained before. Her attitude was that she was doing a fine job without wearing makeup, so why should she start now. After a few weeks, she was reinstated in her job without having to wear makeup.

Characteristics or Functions of Attitude

Three general features of attitudes are given below:
1. **Evaluation:** An attitude is evaluation. It involves likes and dislikes. An attitude is like a point in the thermometer that ranges from very negative to very positive, e.g., Terri makes negative evaluation of using makeup which means she has developed a negative attitude toward makeup.
2. **Targeting:** The evaluation is targeted toward same object, person, or event. Terri's negative attitude is targeted against a specific event that is wearing makeup.
3. **Predisposition:** An attitude predisposes us to behave in a certain way. This means we approach some objects, people, and events and avoid others because of corresponding positive or negative attitudes. Terri's attitude toward wearing makeup predisposed her to fight against it, even to the point of losing her job.

Components of Attitude

An attitude has three components.
1. **Affective:** How one feels about it (feeling really shows concern)?
2. **Conative or behavioral:** Behavioral tendency of both verbal and nonverbal, toward the objects (psychomotor aspects) how one acts?

3. **Cognitive:** What a person knows of it and their belief about it (awareness, knowledge), how one perceives events and how one thinks about them?

If one could predict this, it should be useful to know what a person feels and thinks and now one is likely to act.

Examples
1. **Terri's case:**
   a. *Cognitive component:* One reason Terri does not wear makeup is that some cosmetics are tested on animals, which she believes is a cruel practice.
   b. *Affective component:* Another reason, Terri does not approve of using makeup is that when she does, she feels uncomfortable, because she does not like what she sees in the mirror. Terri's strong negative feeling about how she looks in makeup is an example of affective component of attitudes.
   c. *Behavioral component:* Terri's negative attitude toward cosmetics predisposed or influenced her behavior. Her refusals to wear makeup and fight to save her job are examples of behavioral component of attitudes.
2. **Cruelty to patients:** A nurse may have definite attitudes about the way patients should be treated. Cruelty to patients may make her feel angry (affective component); because she feels strongly about it, she may be on the lookout for cruelty and detect the slightest sign of any fellow nurse's impatience and irritability with a patient (cognitive component). The nurse's own behavior could never include any act of cruelty toward any patient (behavioral component).
3. **Attitude to health:** Some people have very strong positive feeling about healthy life styles (affective component). They will pay attention to what is said and written about healthy eating (cognitive component). One would expect such people to choose, for example, brown bread when they go shopping (behavioral component).

Factors that Determine Our Attitude

There are primarily three factors that determine our attitude. They are as follows:
1. Environment,
2. Experiences, and
3. Education.

Environment

Environment consists of the following:
- **Home:** Positive or negative influences,
- **School:** Peer pressure,
- **Work:** Supportive or over-critical supervisor,
- **Media:** Television, newspapers, magazines, radio, movies, etc.
- Cultural background,
- Religious background,
- Traditions and beliefs,
- Social environment, and
- Political environment.

All of these environments create a culture. Every place—be it a home, organization, or a country—has a culture.

Experiences

Our behavior changes according to our experiences with people and events in our life. If we have a positive experience with a person, our attitude toward him becomes positive and vice-versa.

Education

Knowledge strategically applied translates into wisdom, ensuring success. A teacher affects eternity. The ripple effect is immeasurable.

We are drowning in information but starving for knowledge and wisdom. Education ought to teach us not only how to make a living but also how to live.

Development of Attitudes

Our attitudes are acquired by us, and in acquiring them, we are influenced by our social environment, by our own thinking, our own motives, our schooling, and cultural norms, our early training and the factual knowledge we have about things and situations.

Heredity plays only a very small part in the development of attitudes, through differences in physical characteristics and intelligence. It is mainly the environmental factors that are responsible for development of attitudes.

Early in life a child's attitudes are shaped primarily by parents. During the period between the age 12 and 30 years, the critical period, a person's attitude takes the final form. The major influences during this period are a person's peers, the information received through various media and education. After 30 years, attitudes change very little except that there is a tendency to become more conservative. We can however modify the established attitudes by changing our

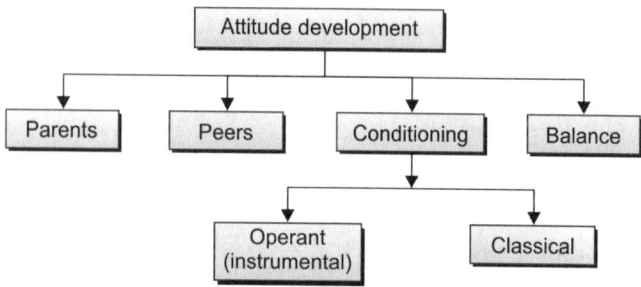

Fig. 1: Classification of attitude development.

perceptions, by controlling our motivational factors through efforts of home and school (**Fig. 1**).

Family is the first place for formation of attitudes. Parents begin the information flow that forms beliefs and attitudes about things. Information provided by the parents in the earliest stages of life is very difficult to undo. Erroneous and nonadaptive attitudes molded from parental feedback have tremendous implications for further personality development. Motives, emotions, parent-child relationships, and the ways of perceiving things—all influence our attitude formation.

Attitudes originated in the family are further strengthened when they are appreciated by peers, playmates, neighbors, etc. A child is likely to internalize the attitudes of people whom he likes or whom he wishes to please. Similarly, a child tends to reject attitudes of people whom he dislikes.

Classical Conditioning

Griffitt (1970) had people interact in small groups either in a comfortable room or one which were hot and uncomfortable. When asked to rate how much they liked the other people present in the room, individuals in the hot room reported liking the others less than individuals in the comfortable room. In this manner, attitudes can be formed simply by association.

Instrument Conditioning

If you express an attitude to a friend who then provides positive reinforcement by smiling or nodding, your attitude is likely to be strengthened. But if your friend provides punishment by showing or expressing disapproval, your attitude is likely to be weakened.

Balance Theory

Balance theory states that people prefer consistency or harmony in relationship with others. Since balance is preferred by everyone, people develop attitudes that are harmonious with other sentimental relationships. Unbalanced structures will produce tensions and discomfort.

Measurements of Attitudes

The scientific study of attitudes requires that they be measured. In order to measure attitudes, evaluations must be translated into some number system. For some purpose, it is adequate to measure attitudes with only two categories ("favorable" and "unfavorable"). By far the most common method of measuring attitudes is the self-report method, in which people are asked to respond to questions by expressing their personal evaluations.

An attitude involves beliefs or disbeliefs, acceptance or rejection, favoring or disfavoring some aspects of the physical or social environment. In order to measure attitudes, many scales have been constructed. These scales have small statements referring to various aspects of the issue under study. Each statement involves acceptance or rejection of the idea implied in the statement. These statements serve as the units of a yardstick. These statements are equally spaced throughout the entire range of attitude continuum from complete acceptance to rejection. Some of the important attitude scales are as follows:

1. Thurston's scale of equal appearing interval, developed to measure attitudes toward war, Blacks, etc.,
2. Rammers and Sitanee master scale suitable to measure a variety of issues,
3. Likert's method of summated rating scales,
4. Paired comparison method,
5. Rank order method, and
6. Social distance scales.

Public opinion (attitude) polling: Opinion polls are used either to predict something or to provide information. They are used to predict the outcome of elections, the likelihood of buying a product, or the degree of public support for implementing new policies of the Government.

POSITIVE AND NEGATIVE ATTITUDES

People with positive attitudes are caring, confident, patient, and humble. Positive attitudes foster teamwork, solve problems, reduce stress, and make the person an asset to his society. Negative attitudes lead to bitterness, resentment, a purposeless life, ill health, and high level of stress to themselves and others.

To develop a positive attitude the following suggestions will be helpful:

1. **Look for the positive:** Look for what is right in a person or situation instead of what is wrong.
2. **Avoid procrastination:** Procrastination causes fatigue and leads to a negative attitude. A completed task is fulfilling and energizing.
3. **Develop an attitude of gratitude:** Count your blessings and not your troubles. There is a lot to be thankful for. "I complained about my bad shoes, till I met a person with no feet".

Change of attitudes: The attitudes once originated and developed in the family environment are changed by school and other world experiences. A teacher, a friend, a specific event content of school curriculum, etc., can make attitudinal changes in children.

Communication is the strongest means by which attitudinal changes can be effected in adults. Through effective communications people can be persuaded to the extent that their attitudes may even make a shift from positive to negative. To make communication effective, three variables are to function proportionately as below:

1. Source of the communication (who says it),
2. Nature of the communication (how he says it), and
3. Characteristics of the audience (to whom does he say it).

Allport (1935) has defined attitude as a mental and neural state of readiness, organized through experience, exerting a directive or dynamic influence upon the individual's response to all objects and situations, with which it is related. Attitudes are formed toward social as well as nonsocial aspects of the environment. Attitudes play a very significant role in our social life. Our success and failure depend on our attitudes toward our work and abilities.

Our attitudes are acquired from our family and peer group during early childhood and later periods of life. So most of our attitudes are formed within the group to which we belong. Second source is the personal experience gained during the course of interactions with the society. The third source is traumatic experience which compels us to form attitudes about others. Attitudes once formed become stable and try to resist any change. However, attitudes can be changed in a variety of ways.

Some of the ways of changing the attitudes are given below:
1. Obtaining new information coming from others and through mass media. This information produces changes in the cognitive component; affective and behavioral components also change.
2. Attitudes change through direct experience.
3. Changes in attitude can be brought about by legislations.

The external situation around the person also has some effect on the attitude change.

Attitudes and the nurse: The nurse who carries out an assessment of a new patient may be prevented from giving an adequate history by his attitude to his illness. The nurse who attempts to assess the patient's attitudes in order to plan appropriate care, herself brings into the situation her own complex attitude system. Her studies and her knowledge will affect her attitude to the patient's illness; her previous nursing experience influences her attitude to hospital, treatment, staff, and patients.

The nurse should try to understand her patients' attitudes. Some of them enter the hospital ready and willing to cooperate others enters hospital afraid or resentful to the ideas of receiving treatment and to the rigidity of the ward routine. Favorable or unfavorable attitudes may be the result of their own previous experience in the hospital or of the experience of their friends and relatives. These may be the result of also insufficient knowledge of what is going to happen to them when they are in the hospital.

The nurses should try to find out the causes of unfavorable attitudes and should change them into favorable ones, because favorable attitudes help in treatment and recovery. She can do this by providing better experience, by adequate explanations, by giving them a feeling of security and self-confidence, by means of efficient and skillful care, assurances and giving them a sense of being at peace by exercising patience and not being rushed. The nurse needs to develop and cultivate professional attitude, which will contribute to her success in her work.

Key Points

+ Attitudes can be favorable, unfavorable, positive, and negative.
+ A child's attitudes are shaped primarily by parents.
+ Attitudes can be formed simply by association.
+ Attitudes can be measured.

STUDY QUESTIONS

Long Essays

1. Define attitudes. Describe the characteristics, components, and functions of attitudes.
2. How can attitudes be changed? Describe the role of a nurse is changing the negative attitude of one of her patients into a positive one.

Short Essays

1. Discuss the development and modification of attitudes.
2. Attitudes during health and illness.
3. How does study of attitudes help nurses?
4. Describe the development and identification of attitudes.

Short Answers

1. Attitudes.
2. Characteristics of attitudes.
3. Measurement of attitudes.

Multiple Choice Questions

1. Which is the most common method of measuring attitude?
    a. Observational field study method
    b. Physiological measurements method
    c. Self-report method
    d. History taking method
2. A phobia may be based on which components of attitudes?
    a. Only affective
    b. Only cognitive
    c. Only behavioral
    d. Cognitive, affective, and behavioral
3. The defining characteristics of which of the following is that they express an evaluation of some object?
    a. Beliefs
    b. Attitudes
    c. Interaction
    d. Perception

4. Which people tend to have the strongest attitudes?
    a. Children
    b. Young adults
    c. Middle-aged adults
    d. Older adults
5. The emotional component of attitude is also called_____ component.
    a. Cognitive
    b. Affective
    c. Psycho motor
    d. None of the above

Personality
(Is What the Man is)

Chapter Outline

- Temperament
- Personality
- Psychoanalytical Theory
- Type and Trait Theories
- Humanistic Theory
- Personality Development
- Personality Assessment
- Projective Tests
- Personality Inventories

Learning Objectives

♦ Enables students to understand the various approaches to personality theories.
♦ Helps students understand how personality is assessed.

INTRODUCTION

❖ *"Personality may be defined as the most characteristic integration of an individual's structure, modes of behavior, interests, attitudes, capacities, abilities, and aptitudes."*
—**Munn NL (Psychology)**

❖ *"Personality is the dynamic organization within the individual of those psychosocial systems that determine his unique adjustment to his environment."*
—**Gordon Allport**

The word "personality" is derived from Greek word "Persona", the mask used by actors in Greek drama.

Personality is the total quality of an individual's behavior as it is shown in habits of thinking, in attitude, interests, manner of acting, and personal philosophy of life. It is the totality of ones being.

Personality is more than the sum total of an individual's traits and characteristics. It is expressed through behavior. The characteristic combinations of behavior distinguish one individual from another giving each a unique personality and identity.

Personality is often confused with character and temperament. Character means a judgment of the individual based upon certain qualities. A person has a good or bad character depending on whether or not he/she is honest and dependable. Character reflects the part of the personality related to one's value system.

Temperament is the hereditary emotional aspects of personality. We refer to a person's temperament as "irritable and fuzzy", "moody", or "sensitive".

CLASSIFICATIONS OF PERSONALITY

1. By types, and
2. By traits or factors.

Type Approach

The theory approached human personality and behavior characteristics using somatic structure, blood type, and secretions.

Types Based on Temperament

Hippocrates (about 400 BC), the father of medicine, classified people into four types as per temperament depending on which one of one's bodily humors or fluids they believe to predominate.
1. Sanguine—cheerful, vigorous, confident, optimistic (blood).
2. Phlegmatic—calm, slow moving, unexcitable, unemotional (mucus).
3. Choleric—irritable, hot tempered (yellow bile).
4. Melancholic—depressed, morose (black bile).

This is similar to dividing people into Vatha, Pitha, and Kabham in Ayurveda.

Types Based on Body Build (Physiological Types)

a. Kretschmer (physic and character), and
b. William Sheldon (based on body build).

Kretschmer (1925) divided people into three types based on body structure:
1. Asthenic—introvert, tall, thin, sensitive.
2. Athletic—active, aggressive, well-developed muscular body.
3. Pyknic—extrovert, round and fat.

William Sheldon (1954) divided people into three types according to body build and behavior.
1. Endomorph—plumb, soft, fat and round—sociable even tempered and relaxed.
2. Mesomorph—heavy set and muscular—physically active and noisy.
3. Ectomorph—tall, thin and flat-chested—self-conscious, shy, fond of solitude, and reserved (introverts).

On the same basis, temperament too is classified into the following three classes:
1. **Viscerotonic (endomorphic) eating predominates:** They love comforts and food also seek love of others. They also sleep deeply. They like others help them when they are in trouble.
2. **Semantotonic (mesomorphic):** They have a brittle, clear, competitive nature and generally powerful, daring, authoritative, and loud talkers. In troubles, they are more active.
3. **Cerebrotonic (ectomorphic):** They are habituated in suppressing their emotions. They are self-controlled and withdrawing. They love solitude. Instead of seeking assistance in trouble, they keep to themselves. They speak slowly and their sleep is often disturbed.

Although a person's physique may have some influence on personality, the relationship is much more subtle. Research has shown little correlation between body build and specific personality characteristics.

Type A and B based on emotions and stress as classified by health psychologists.

Classification by Psychological Types

On the basis of sociability, Dr Karl G Jung classified people into two main groups namely: (a) Extroverts, and (b) Introverts.
1. **Extroverts** are people who are sociable and take interest in others and like to move with people and are skilled in etiquette. They are friendly and sociable and not easily upset by difficulties. They are dominated by emotions, whereby they take decisions quickly and act on them without delay. They are realistic and face the problems of life objectively.
2. **Introverts** are those who are interested in themselves, their own feelings, emotions, and reactions. They are busy in their own thoughts and are self-centered. They are reserved and like to work alone. They are very sensitive and are unable to adjust easily to social situations. They are inclined to worry and easily get embarrassed. Many poets, philosophers, scientists, and artists belong to this group.

There are very few people who are pure extroverts or introverts. Majority of the people are ambiverts having the qualities of extroverts and introverts in different proportions.

Trait Approach

Personality Traits

Allport (1961) used different traits to describe the uniqueness of each individual. The most common way to describe people, say a nurse, is to list a number of qualities she should possess, e.g., patience, honesty, perseverance, thoroughness, and initiative. These qualities are called personality traits. Groups of personality traits are known as personality factors or dimensions of personality. When traits are analyzed and results are put on a graph, it is called personality profile.

Personality traits of a nurse
- Discipline,
- Responsibility,
- Patience,
- Commitment,
- Dedication,
- Punctuality,
- Hard work,
- Good physical stamina,
- Alertness of mind,
- Adaptability to follow difficult time schedules,
- Ability to think in crisis to take a quick decision,
- Calm, pleasant, compassionate, and understanding,
- Good team spirit, and
- Ability to help and serve needy people without getting sentimentally attached.

Factors of personality
- The physical factors include the physique of the individual—his size, strength, looks, and constitution.
- The environmental or social factor.
- Mental or psychological factors including motives, interests, attitudes, will and character, intellectual capacities as intelligence, reasoning, attention, perception, and imagination. These traits and factors are assessed by psychological tests. Trait theory is an

approach for analyzing the structure of personality by measuring, identifying and classifying similarities, and differences in personality characteristics or traits.

THEORIES OF PERSONALITY DEVELOPMENT

Personality refers to a combination of long-lasting and distinctive behaviors, thoughts, motives, and emotions that typify how we react and adapt to other peoples and situations.

A theory of personality is an organized attempt to describe and explain how personalities develop and how personalities differ.

There are a number of approaches for studying human development. There are several theories or set of principles of personality development which have been developed to explain personality differences. Some focus upon the internal growth of personality, others are based on the effect of one's external environment and still others emphasize personal experience and growth of self-image.

Personality has been considered from the point of view of types, on one hand and traits, on the other. The more popular and reasonable view is a compromise with traits organized type wise. Kretschmer, Jung, and Sheldon have classified personality based on types. Bhagavad Gita speaks of three types— (a) Tamasik, (b) Rajasik, and (c) Satwik, which are similar to Sheldon's classification correlating temperament with body types as described below:

Indian Approach

1. **Rajasik** have rajaguna, kind, optimistic, light hearted, sociable, easy going, noble, honest, and sincere, will do anything for their loved ones. Kings possessed rajaguna.
2. **Satvik** have satvaguna; reserved, pessimistic, frustrated, gets angry fast, difficult to understand, depressed easily.
3. **Tamosik** possess tamoguna; pleasure seeking, not punctual, lazy, do not want to be active even while expecting pleasure. The major personality theories are tabulated **(Box 1)** below:

Psychoanalytical Theory (Internal Growth)

Sigmund Freud (1856–1939) developed the best known theory of personality focused upon internal growth or psychodynamics.

Freud's theory stresses the influence of unconscious fears, desires and motivation on thoughts and behavior. The theory has three parts:

> **Box 1:** Major personality theories.
>
> - **Theories adopting type approach:** Hippocrates, Kretschmer, Sheldon, and Jung.
> - **Theories adopting trait approaches:** Allport, Cattell, the Five Factor Model.
> - **Theories adopting type-cum-trait approach:** Eysenck's theory of personality.
> - **Theories adopting developmental approach:** Psychosexual theory of Sigmund Freud, Psychosocial theory of Erik H Erikson.
> - **Humanistic theory of personality:** Carl Roger's self-theory, Abraham Maslow.

Structure of Personality (Anatomy of Personality or Subsystems of Personality)

Freud thought of personality as being based upon a structure of three parts: (a) Id, (b) Ego, and (c) Superego.

The id is composed of biological instincts including the drives of sex and aggression. Id is self-centered, impulsive but unconscious. All the drives of a person toward pleasure and self-satisfaction are coming from id. This uninhibited demand for self-satisfaction is called the pleasure principle. Id does not bother about the environment, the needs of others or reality but demands complete self-satisfaction. An infant is all id as it demands immediate satisfaction of its basic needs like hunger, thirst, relief from discomfort, or pain without concern for how it will be done immediately.

The ego called self, gets energy from the id but serves as a control for the id through its contact with reality. Ego directs the behavior of personality through the reality principle. Many demands of id are not realistic and hence will be controlled by the ego. The ego is primarily determined by the experience of reality and is, therefore, guided by reality principle. It is predominantly conscious though some parts (like ego-defense mechanisms) are unconscious. Ego maintains a balance between the id and superego, on one hand and the reality, on the other.

For example, an individual observes a pleasurable object surrounded by a barrier. Id wants immediate gratification by obtaining the object without seeing the reality of a barrier around it. The superego, on the other hand, proclaims that it is sinful to derive pleasure from an object surrounded by a barrier. The ego strokes and balance between the two as well as real world and decides to

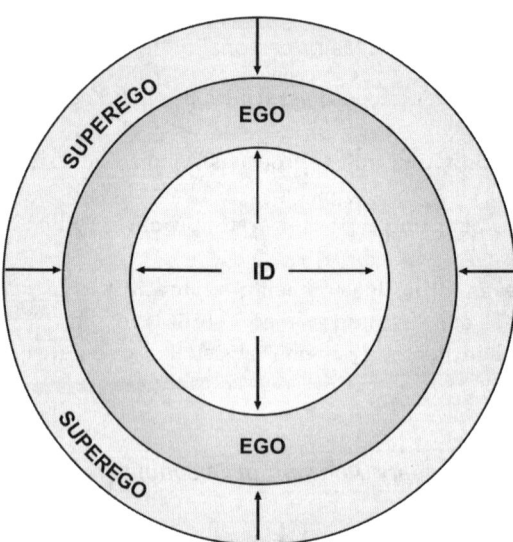

Fig. 1: Structure of personality.

wait and find a way to climb the barrier and derive pleasure. Ego delays gratification in view of the reality. Ego is the seat of conscious, intellectual, self-preservative and defensive functions of the mental apparatus (**Fig. 1**).

The superego is predominantly unconscious subdivision of mental apparatus that develops from ego.

The superego is made up of the conscience and the ego ideal. It is developed through the cultural environment and learning from social contacts, such as parents, family members, and authority figures. It judges the thoughts and actions of the ego. When a person behaves against the standards of his superego (= conscience) he will feel guilty.

Freud believed that the id, ego, and superego were in constant conflict with one another, the ego controlling the demands of the id and the superego checking the behavior of the ego.

Psychosexual Stages

According to Freud, all human beings pass through a series of five psychosexual stages:
1. The oral stage from birth to 1.5 years; pleasure is obtained through stimulation of the mouth as in nursing or thumb sucking.
2. The anal stage occurring during 1½ to 3 years of life when toilet training is attempted—gratification is obtained through holding or expelling feces.

3. The phallic or oedipal stage from about age 3 to 6-pleasure is obtained by fondling the genitals.
4. A latency stage 6–12 years (onset of puberty) called latency, because sexual interests are repressed and lie dormant till puberty. Period of gang formation and fierce gang loyalties. Boys cling together and shun girls and girls despise boys.
5. The genital stage (adolescence) begins with puberty. Young people begin experiencing romantic infatuation and emotional upheavals. Problems encountered, at any one stage, either of deprivation or overindulgence, may produce fixation at that stage. A person fixated, at the oral stage, when the infant is totally dependent upon others for satisfaction of needs may, as an adult, be excessively dependent and overly fond of such oral pleasures as eating, drinkin, or smoking. A person fixated, at the anal stage, may be abnormally concerned with cleanliness and orderliness [obsessive compulsive disorder (OCD)].

Freud's theory paints a picture of humans filled with irrational and unconscious forces that control our behavior without any free choice.

For Freud, the first 6 years of childhood are most critical for personality development. What happens to the individual in later life is fashioned during the child's first 6 years.

Personality Dynamics (Structure of the Mind or Division of the Mind)

Topographical description of psyche or mind or levels of consciousness: Mind is a function of the body; it does not exist apart from the body. It is the sum total of the various mental processes or activities. Mental processes can be conscious, unconscious, or preconscious.

Conscious: As per Freud, the conscious part of the mind consists of those mental activities of which we are aware, such as thoughts, feelings, and sensations. It functions only when the individual is awake. It directs the individual as he behaves in a rational way.

Unconscious: The unconscious is by far the largest part of the mind. It includes our repressed desires, our fears, and phobias for which we do not know the reasons and many others. Material stored in the unconscious has a powerful influence on our thoughts, or feelings (unconscious motivation).

Preconscious or subconscious: It is that part of the mind, in which ideas and reactions are stored and partially forgotten. The preconscious also prevents certain unacceptable, disturbing unconscious memories from reaching the conscious mind. Materials from the subconscious can be brought to the conscious, if the individual concentrates on recall.

Mind and body interact on each other. Our nervous system and glands are responsible for our ways of thinking, feeling, and wishing. Our feelings or our emotions can cause bodily illnesses.

Freud's theory has been criticized for its (a) Excessive emphasis on the unconscious, (b) Too much emphasis on sex impulse, and (c) The interpretation of normal through abnormal.

Psychosocial Theory of Emotional Development

This theory was developed by Eric H Erikson (1902-1994). He challenges Freud's theory that personality is primarily established during the first 6 years and says that the personality continues to develop over the entire life cycle. Individuals develop a healthy personality by mastering inner and outer dangers with positive solutions to life's social problems **(Table 1)**. The individual is in a state of progress, but at the same time also faced with constant threat of decay.

Table 1: Erikson's eight life stages (1959).

Age (stage)	Developmental task	Central issue	Significant relations	Favorable outcome
0–18 months (Infancy)	Trust vs. Mistrust	Testing of the trustworthiness of the infant's significant others	Mother	Hope, trust optimism
18 months–3 years (Early childhood)	Autonomy vs. doubt	Testing of the individual capabilities in relation to significant others	Parents	Self-control, adequacy
3–5 years (Middle childhood)	Initiative vs. Guilt	Testing out abilities to compete in the outside world	Basic Family	Purpose, initiates own activities
5–12 years (Late childhood)	Industry vs. Inferiority	Gaining mastery of cultural tools	School	Competence Developing intellectual social physical skills
13–19 years (Adolescence)	Identity vs. Role confusions	Developing a sense of personal identity	Peer Groups	Awareness of self as a unique individual

Contd...

Contd...

Age (stage)	Developmental task	Central issue	Significant relations	Favorable outcome
20–40 years (Early adulthood)	Intimacy vs. Isolation	Merging of identity with another to achieve intimacy	Friends	Forming close relationships, making career commitment
40–65 years (Mature adulthood or middle age)	Generativity vs. Stagnation	Investing creative energies in promoting the social welfare	Household	Care concern for family and society
65 years–Death (old age)	Ego integrity vs. Despair	Acceptance of the life one has lived as worthwhile	Mankind	Satisfaction with life

The concept of stages is controversial, stages overemphasize the rapidity of changes ignoring the continuity of human development. Stages should be considered only as convenient points for identification related to age but not determined by age per se.

These are called psychosocial changes because many aspects of psychosocial and social functioning are interrelated. At each stage, the focus is on a specific crisis in our relationships with other people.

Relevance of Psychosocial Development Theory to Nursing Practice

Erikson's theory is particularly relevant to nursing practice in that it incorporates sociocultural concepts into the development of personality. Erikson provides a systematic stepwise approach and outlines specific tasks that should be completed during each stage. This information can be used in psychiatric nursing. Many individuals with mental health problems are still struggling to achieve tasks from a number of developmental stages. Nurses can plan care to assist such individuals to fulfil these tasks and move onto a high developmental level.

Humanistic Theory (Self-theory, Growth of Self-image)

When personality development focusses upon the development of self, it is called humanism. Humanists like Carl Rogers and Abraham Maslow reject the internal conflicts of Freud's view and the mechanistic nature of behaviorism. They believe that each person is creative and responsible, free to choose, and each strives for fulfilment or self-actualization. Human beings want to grow and develop to their greatest potential.

Abraham Maslow

Maslow broke away from the reward/punishment/observable behavior mentality of behaviorism and developed his humanistic theory. His theory emphasized two things: (i) Our capacity for growth or self-actualization, and (ii) Our desire to satisfy a variety of needs. Maslow's need hierarchy arranges needs in an ascending order, with biological needs at the bottom and social and personal needs at the top. As needs at one level are met, we advance to the next level.

Carl Rogers' Self-theory

Carl Rogers (1902–1987) rejected the psychodynamic approach, because it placed too much emphasis on unconscious, irrational forces. Instead Rogers developed a new humanitarian theory called "Self-theory" (1980). Self-theory has two primary assumptions:
a. Personality development is guided by each person's unique self-actualization tendency.
b. Each of us has a personal need for positive regard.

Rogers said that the self is made up of many self-perceptions, abilities, personality characteristics, and behaviors that are organized and consistent with one another. People have a basic need to be loved and respected. If you have an unconditioned positive regard from others, you will develop more realistic self-concepts/self-actualization but if the response is conditional, if may lead to anxiety and frustration.

Social Cognitive Theory

Freud's psychodynamic theory, developed in the early 1900s, grew out of his work with patients. Humanistic theories were developed in the 1960s by an ex-Freudian (Rogers) and an ex-behaviorist (Maslow) who believed that the previous theories had neglected the positive side of human potential and fulfilment.

In comparison, the social cognitive theory, developed in the 1960s and 1970s, grew out of a strong research background that emphasized a more experimental approach to developing and testing concepts that could be used to understand and explain personality development **(Fig. 2)**.

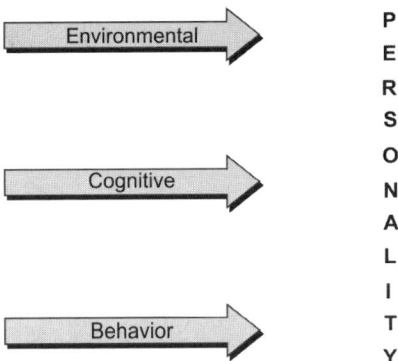

Fig. 2: Social cognitive theory.

Social cognitive theory says that personality development is primarily shaped by three factors:
a. Environmental conditions,
b. Cognitive—personal factors, and
c. Behavior.

Behavior includes a variety of actions, such as what we do and say. Environmental influences include our social, political, and cultural influences as well as our particular learning experiences. Just as our cognitive factors influence how we perceive and interpret our environment, in turn, affects our beliefs, values, and social roles. Cognitive-personal factors include our beliefs, expectations, values, intentions, and social roles as well as biological and genetic influences. Thus, what we think, believe, and feel affect how we act and behave.

Bandura's social cognitive theory developed in 1970s says that personality development, growth and change are influenced by four distinctively human cognitive processes:
a. Highly developed language ability,
b. Observational learning,
c. Purposeful behavior, and
d. Self-analysis.

Reciprocal interaction between the behavior and environment. Society and individual are interdependent. Bandura's theory emphasizes cognitive factors, such as personal values, goals, and beliefs.

Three particular beliefs have been shown to influence personality development.
a. **Locus of control** which refers to how much control we think we have over our environment.

b. **Delay of gratification,** which involves voluntary postponing an immediate reward for the promise of a future reward.
c. **Self-efficacy,** which refers to our personal beliefs of how capable we are in performing specific tasks and behaviors.

Trait Theories

In trait approach, the personality is reviewed in terms of traits like honest, shy, lazy, dull, dependent, etc. Traits are defined as relatively permanent and constant behavior patterns that the individual exhibits in many situations. These behavior patterns are considered as the basic units of personality. If a person behaves honestly on several situations, he is called honest. Honesty or laziness becomes a behavior trait of his personality.

GB Allport (1887–1967) was the first personality theorist who adopted trait approach. According to him, an individual develops a unique set of stable tendencies or traits organized around a few primary traits.

RB Cattell, the British born American research worker, defined trait as a structure of the personality inferred from behavior in different situations. He described four types of traits:

a. Common traits, widely distributed in general population.
b. Unique traits, unique for a person, e.g., temperamental traits, emotional traits.
c. Surface traits, able to be recognized as a manifestation of behavior like curiosity, dependability, tactfulness, honesty. For example, a student showing proficiency in both mathematics and literature has a surface trait, because two different factors influence him to achieve success in these subjects.
d. The inner qualities of human being, which find behaviors and act as sources of surface traits and called source traits underline sources or structures that determine ones behavior, such as dominance, submission, emotion, and motivation.

The theory of Cattell intends to give certain specific dimensions to personality, so that human behavior related to a particular situation can be predicted. Cattell has adopted factor analysis as a technique for his work (The 16 factor personality theory).

Assumptions made:
1. Traits are common to all individuals.
2. Traits are relatively stable.
3. Traits are quantifiable. Human personality development is influenced by some active and forceful traits.

THE FIVE FACTOR MODEL OR THE FIVE TRAITS THEORY

For over 50 years, a major goal of personality researchers was to find a way to define the structure of personality with the fewest possible traits. The search for a list of traits that could describe personality differences among everyone began in 1930s with a list of about 4,500 traits and ended in 1990s with a list of only five traits.

The five (traits) factor model traits theory organizes personality traits under five categories: (1) Openness, (2) Conscientiousness, (3) Extraversion, (4) Agreeableness, and (5) Neuroticism (OCEAN). These traits which are referred to as the big five traits raise three major issues.

Firstly, although traits are stable tendencies to behave in certain ways, this ability does not apply across all different situations.

Secondly, personality traits are both changeable and stable. Most change occurs before age 30 years, because adolescents and young adults are more willing to adopt new values and attitudes or revise old ones. Most stability occurs after age 30, but adult do continue to grow in their ideas, beliefs, and attitudes.

Thirdly, genetic features have a considerable influence on personality traits and behaviors. Genetic factors push and pull the development of certain traits whose development may be helped or hindered by environmental factors.

Traits are useful in that they provide shorthand descriptions of people and predict certain behaviors.

Trait theory says relatively little about the development or growth of personality but instead emphasizes measuring and identifying differences among personalities.

METHODS/TECHNIQUES OF PERSONALITY ASSESSMENT

Personality testing is done for various reasons. A personnel psychologist may want to identify people for a salesman's job. A clinical psychologist often uses personality tests to evaluate psychological disorders. Personality tests do not have "right" and "wrong" answers. Instead they seek answers that will reveal people's characteristic tendencies or behavior.

The techniques of personality assessment can be divided into five categories:
1. Where one can see how the individual behaves in actual life situations.
    a. Observation technique, and
    b. Situation technique.

2. Where one can find out what an individual says about himself: Subjective
   a. Autobiography,
   b. Questionnaire/personality inventory, and
   c. Interview.
3. Techniques by which one can find out what others say about the individual whose personality is under assessment. Objective
   a. Case history taking, i.e., extracting information,
   b. Biography,
   c. Rating scales, and
   d. Sociometry.
4. Techniques by which one can find how an individual reacts to an imaginative situation involving fantasy. For example, projective methods.
5. Techniques by which one can indirectly determine some personality variables in terms of physiological responses by measuring (technical) instruments.

ASSESSMENT OF PERSONALITY

The following are some of the methods used for evaluation and measurement of personality traits:
1. Observational methods (the interview),
2. Personality inventories (based on trait theories), and
3. Projective techniques (based on psychoanalytical theory).

Interviews: Interview is the most popular method of observation. Appearance, bearing, and speech can be noticed. Questions can be asked about attitudes and interests. Interviews are used to evaluate a person's personality for the purpose of employment and for education as well as for identifying personality traits. An interview may be informal or unstructured. It can be formal or structured, where specific topics are selected by the interviewer before and the flow of conversation is controlled.

Body language of the client can be observed, during an interview. The body language may be posture, movement of the hands, facial expressions, or voice. However, interviews take place under stress and great skill is needed to put the interviewee at ease.

Questionnaires: This is the most common written method of measuring personality. A personality inventory is a questionnaire in which the person reports his or her feeling in certain situations.

Table 2: Examples of questions used in questionnaires.

Questions	Answers	
a. Would you rate yourself as a quiet person	Yes	No
b. Do you prefer to work alone rather than with others	Yes	No
c. Do you frequently feel sad	Yes	No

They are very easily checked and scored. More often the answers are scored by machines which eliminate the prejudice of the tester, making the test more objective **(Table 2)**.

Minnesota Multiple Personality Inventory (MMPI): One of the most commonly used personality tests is the MMPI. This test asks for answers of "True", "False", or "Cannot Say" to 567 statements (one for men and another for women) about different personality traits, such as attitudes, emotional reactions, physical and psychological symptoms, and past experiences. The answers are quantitatively measured and personality assessment is done based on the norm scores. Dr HN Murthy of NIMHANS, Bangalore has reduced it to 100 items called Multiphasic Questionnaire (MQ).

Personality questionnaires are used in psychology for counseling and research. They are used for selection for employment or promotion.

Projective Tests

Projective tests focus upon what is inside a person rather than what can be seen in a person's behavior. These tests try to find out more about a person's feelings, unconscious desires, and inner thoughts.

The Rorschach ink blot test was the first projective test and is still widely used. It was developed by the Swiss Psychologist Hermann Rorschach in 1920. Another projective test is the Thematic apperception test (TAT) developed by Henry Murray of Harvard University in 1943. The Rorschach test uses ten different kinds of ink blots, which must be described by the person taking the test. The TAT uses twenty sketches about which the person is asked to make up a story.

These tests make use of people's tendencies to makeup stories about things they see. When shown an ink blots, for example, people see butterflies, dancing girls, pictures of skeletons, or many other images. When a vague picture is shown depicting two people, a story can be made about their relationship to each other, their difficulties and troubles. The stories people make up about pictures reveal something about their own personality. They project into the picture, feelings, and thoughts of their own.

Projective Tests Based on the Phenomenon of Projection
- RIBT—Rorschach's Ink Blot Test developed by Hermann Rorschach.
- TAT—Thematic Apperception Test developed by Henry Murray.
- CAT—Children's Apperception Test developed by Leopard Bellarck consisting of ten cards.
- Word Association Test.
- Sentence Completion Test.

Rorschach's Ink blot test
The responses differ from person to person based on the individual's personal experiences. For example, teen aged college students saw ink blot no 1 as:
- A bat,
- Two ladies standing back-to-back,
- Face of an owl, and
- A patch of cloud.

Rorschach responses can reveal the following information:
- Degree of intellectual control of the subject on his actions,
- Emotional aspects,
- Mental approach to given problems,
- Creative and imaginative capacities,
- Security and anxiety,
- Personality growth and development, and
- Phobias, sex disturbances and severe psychological disorders can be detected which serve as a guide for treatment program.

Thematic apperception test (TAT) developed by Henry Murray
Thematic apperception test consists of three sets of pictures, one set is used with both men and women, and a second set only for men, and a third set for women. The pictures are shown in a definite sequence and the subject is asked to makeup a story based on what he sees in these pictures. It is believed that he would project his own experience, biographical data, major conflicts, interests, and problems into his description of pictures: Findings of TAT are compared with case history. TAT is more structured unlike the ink blot test, which however is more popular. TAT is also less standardized.

TAT throws light in the following areas of life:
- Family relationships,
- Motivation of the subject,
- Inner fantasies,
- Level of aspiration,
- Social relationships,

- Functioning of sex urge,
- Emotional conflicts,
- Attitude to work,
- Outlook toward future, and
- Frustrations, if any.

Sentence completion test

When the subject is asked to complete the sentence without giving time to deliberate on it, it is assumed that his unconscious process will direct his response. The test will give an insight to his desires, hopes, conflicts, frustrations, fears and annoyances, e.g.,

1. I feel happy when ....
2. I tell lies only when ....
3. On rainy days, I ....
4. Other people think I ....

Word association test (WAT)

The word association test popularized by Jung, consists of 50 or more words, which are presented to the subject one at a time. Mixed in the list are words related to conflicts of the patient or words producing emotional reaction, which is related to a hidden complex.

When the subject gives a quick response word, he is taken unaware of and his unconscious process directs his association. Here the subject has to answer as quick as possible with the first word which comes to his mind when he is given a stimulus word.

Projective tests are often used in clinical practice. They are helpful in showing a person's inner areas of conflict, anxieties or any problems in relationships because the person is free to describe anything.

A man who interprets a woman's smile as a sexual come on, may be projecting his own sexual feelings on to the woman and thus revealing a good deal about himself.

In nursing, suitable pictures can be devised to test attitudes to patients, work, or hospital.

PERSONALITY DEVELOPMENT

Domains of Development

Development refers to a progressive series of changes that occur in an orderly predictable pattern as a result of maturation and experience. The human being is never static. From conception to death, change is constantly taking place in his physical and psychological capacities. Abilities, interests and personality of the individual change with age.

His ability to think, speak, and problem-solving—all develop with growing years.

A study of personality is important, because it provides a means of predicting human behavior. People behave, normally, in a way consistent with their personalities. A person who is warm and outgoing will not remain withdrawn for long. Under no circumstances, will a shy person behave aggressively.

Physical Development

It involves all those changes occurring in a person's body like changes in height, weight, in the brain, heart, and other structures and processes, and in skeletal, muscular, and neurological features that affect motor skills. At puberty boys and girls undergo growth and development very fast.

Cognitive Development

It involves all those changes that occur in the mental activity including sensation, perception, memory, thought, reasoning, and language.

Psychological Development

It includes all those changes that concern a person's personality, emotions, and relationship with others. Society distinguishes between children, adolescents, and adults.

Process of Development

Growth

The increase in size that occurs with changing age is called growth. Most organisms become larger as they become older. Growth takes place through metabolic processes from within. The organism takes in a variety of substances, breaks them down into their chemical components and then reassemble them into new materials.

Maturation

Maturation is the unfolding of genetically prescribed patterns of behavior or biological potential. Such changes are relatively independent of the environment. For example, an infant's motor development after birth, i.e., grasping, sitting, crawling, standing, and walking follows a regular sequence. Both growth and maturation involve biological change. While growth refers to the increase in the individual's cells and tissue, maturation concerns the development of organs and limbs to become functional.

Chapter 17: Personality (Is What the Man is)

Learning

It is more or less a permanent modification in behavior that results from the individual's experience in the environment. It differs from maturation which occurs without any specific experience or practice.

Factors Influencing Personality Development

Personality is a dynamic growing thing different in each person and influenced by the following three factors:
1. Environmental or social factors
   a. Heredity
   b. Influence of home
   c. Order of birth—the first born child may be dominating
   d. Only child—may become a problem child
   e. School and peer group
   f. Community and social roles
   g. TV, cinema, radio, and newspaper
2. Biological factors
   a. Endocrinal glands and personality
      – Thyroid glands
      – Adrenal glands
      – Sex glands
   b. Blood glucose level
   c. Externally imposed biological conditions
      – Drugs and alcoholism
      – Diseases
      – Diet.
3. Mental or psychological factors.
   These include our motives, acquired interests, our attitudes, our will, and character, intellectual capacities, such as intelligence, reasoning, attention, perception, and imagination. These determine our reactions in various situation and thus affect the growth and direction of our personality. An individual with a lot of will power will make decisions more quickly than others. Intelligence will enable him to make adequate adjustment and in collecting facts and understanding relationships.

Personality and the Nurse

An understanding of personality will help the nurse to predict her behavior as well as the behavior of others. Major decisions of life depend upon this knowledge, e.g., selection of a career, spouse, and colleagues. Her relationships with friends and relatives depend upon her expectations of their behavior from an understanding of their personalities.

A successful nurse will have a strong and pleasing personality. Besides possessing such professional qualities as integrity, dignity, mental abilities, poise, self-confidence and dependability, she must have personal qualities like sympathy, understanding, friendliness, and adaptability. Patients appreciate a nurse who brings physical comfort to them with her skills and who understands their emotional difficulties, caused by illness. The nurse must also have good health, fresh, and neat appearance, will power, high standard of moral values, sense of humor, teaching, and managerial capabilities, self-control, and friendly interpersonal relationships.

PRACTICAL EXPERIMENT

Personality Assessment

Eysenck Personality Inventory

Hans J Eysenck, a German psychologist, proposed that personality consists of four dimensions. They are introversion, extraversion, psychoticism, and normal mental deficiency. Personality inventories ask people about a sample range of their behavior. Eysenck's personality involuntary is brief, having only 57 questions, out of which 24 questions measure introversion—extroversion, 24 questions measure stability-instability and 9 questions measure the tendency to lie. An extroverted person is carefree, easy going, and optimistic. An introverted person is quiet, retiring sort of person, who keeps his feelings under control. A stable person in even tempered, calm, and lively, whereas an unstable person is anxious, moody, touchy, and restless.

Problem

To study the personality of the subject using Eysenck personality inventory.

Materials Required

1. Eysenck's personality inventory
2. Key and norms
3. Writing materials

Procedure

The subject is seated comfortably. An atmosphere is created where the subject gives honest answers. The subject is given a copy of Eysenck personality inventory and he is asked to go through the instructions. After the subject has understood what he has to do, he is allowed to answer the inventory. At the end, the answers are checked with the help of the key. The place of subject on introversion-extroversion and instability—stability is identified.

Result: In the introversion-extroversion dimension, if the score is more than 17, the subject is an extrovert. If he gets less than 17 he is an introvert. In the instability—stability dimension, if he gets more than 14 he is unstable and if he gets less than 4, he is stable. If the score is between 5 and 12 he is normal. If he gets 5 and more on the scale, it indicates a tendency to lie.

He observed that the person, who suffers from psychoticism is not fluent in speaking and cannot adjust well to a new situation. His intention is not bold and his learning and memory power are not developed. His level of aspiration is also low. Psychotics suffer from mental disorders. They are quite different from introverts and extroverts. Persons suffering from mental deficiency are different from introverts and extroverts. They show different symptoms. In their case, psychological factors are main and hereditary factors along with nerve diseases are subsidiary. On the other hand, the man suffering from mental deficiency is dominatingly influenced by heredity and newer sensations. After getting three dimensions of personality, Eysenck accepted intelligence as the fourth dimension **(Fig. 3)**.

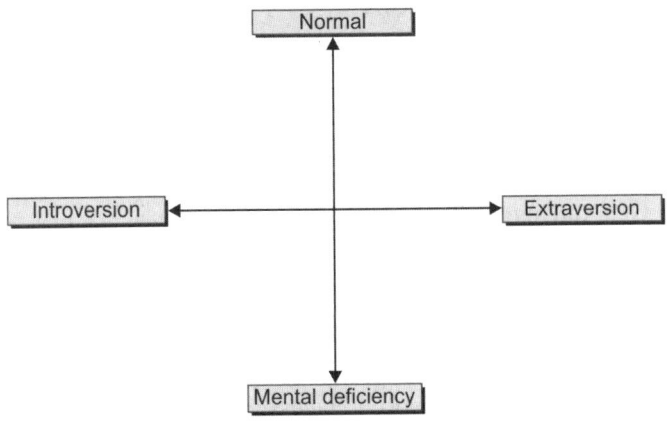

Fig. 3: Eysenck personality inventory.

Key Points

- Personality is more than the sum total of an individual's traits and characteristics. It is expressed through behavior.
- Freud proposed the psychoanalytic theory of personality.
- Carl Rogers and Maslow–humanistic theory of Personality.
- Allport, Catell, Eysenck–Trait theories of Personality.
- Personality can be assessed using different methods/techniques.

STUDY QUESTIONS

Long Essays

1. What is personality? Discuss the various trait compositions to have effective nurse-patient relationship.
2. Write an essay on different types of personality and methods of assessment of personality.
3. Discuss the role of projection tests in assessment of personality.
4. Explain the principles on which id, ego, and superego function.
5. Write an essay on different types of personality.

Short Essays

1. Define personality. Discuss the determinants of personality.
2. Explain the trait theory of personality. Discuss the various trait compositions necessary to have effective nurse-patient relationship.

Multiple Choice Questions

1. According to the psychosocial stages, what is the conflict that occurs during adulthood?
   a. Ego integrity vs. Despair
   b. Identity vs. Identity diffusion
   c. Intimacy vs. Isolation
   d. Generativity vs. Stagnation
2. TAT is an example of:
   a. Objective personality test
   b. Intelligence test
   c. Projective personality test
   d. Objective attitude test
3. According to the psychosexual stages of development, between the ages of 6 and 12 years, the child is said to go through the _____ stage.
   a. Phallic

b. Latency
   c. Anal
   d. Genital
4. The extent to which people believe that they can bring about an outcome is referred to as_____.
   a. Extraversion
   b. Neuroticism
   c. Self-efficacy
   d. Self-regulation
5. The social cognitive theory was put forth by_____.
   a. BF Skinner
   b. Abraham Maslow
   c. Albert Bandhura
   d. Cattell

18. Developmental Psychology

Chapter Outline

- Development
- Nature–Nurture Controversy
- Moral Development
- Emotional Development
- Cognitive Development
- Gender Identity
- Stages of Development
- Early Childhood
- Late Childhood
- Adolescence
- Adulthood
- Old Age
- Grief
- Death

Learning Objectives

- Students will be introduced to various developmental theories.
- Students get oriented to the impact of nature and nurture on development.

INTRODUCTION

Development means a progressive series of changes that occur in an orderly, predictable pattern as a result of maturation and experience. The human being is never static. From conception to death, change is taking place constantly in his physical and psychological capacities. Abilities, interests and problem solving skills—all develop with growing years.

There are three issues, sometimes called controversies in life-span development. They are as follows:

1. **Nature-Nurture debate:** Is your development the result of your genetic structure (nature) or your experience (nurture)?
2. **Whether the development occurs continuously or in stages:** Is your development a gradual and continuous process or does it pass through stages which have to be negotiated one after the other?

3. **Stability or change issue:** Is your personality stable over your life span or does it change as you develop?

NATURE–NURTURE DEBATE

Nature view: What aspect of your behavior is controlled and what happens when we grow?

Nurture view: What aspect of your behavior can we attribute to the way in which we are brought up—what are the environmental, social and human influences on us? As present, there is universal agreement that both nature and nurture are involved.

DEVELOPMENT: CONTINUOUS OR IN STAGES

Behaviorists like Watson, believe that our development is a steady continuous process based on the rate at which we learn new behaviors.

But stage theorists, such as Freud, Erikson, and Piaget believe that development or maturation is an uneven process, with periods of little development followed by dramatic changes in a relatively short time. They argue that however good or enriched the environment, however keen the parents are that their children should speak or walk—until the child is ready or has matured enough for the next stage, it will not happen. In other words, until the child has matured biologically, the next stage will not occur. Biological change precedes or prepares us for psychological change.

At present, the stage theorists appear to have the upper hand. Nature theorists tend to be stage theorists while nurture theorists tend to hold to the continuous view.

STABILITY OR CHANGE ISSUE

Finally with respect to the question of personality: Is it stable or does it change with development? The answer is a mixture of both. There is a list of evidence supporting the view that children and young people often change as they mature, but also that some aspects of personality continue through life.

Theoretical Perspectives

The four major theoretical perspectives that have shaped our understanding of human development are:
a. Psychoanalytic approach (Freud, Erikson)
b. Behaviorist approach (Watson, Bandura, Skinner)

c. Cognitive approach (Piaget) and
d. The ethological approach (Gessel).

EMOTIONAL DEVELOPMENT IN CHILDREN

According to Izard (1982), primary emotions emerge between 3 and 6 months, typical of these is distress, happiness and other extreme emotions. Izard believes that these emotions are more biologically than socially prompted. Secondary or complex emotions start to occur from about 12 months, these include embarrassment, pride and similar emotions. There is a connection between the appearance of these emotions and the child's cognitive development.

Another stage is reached when the child can recognize itself as an individual. This normally taken place at about 18 months and when the child can evaluate a situation where an emotion requires both an awareness of rules and a self-awareness.

Coming up to 24 months, the child's emotional development is such that, in many instances, the child has learned to deliberately manipulate its own emotions, to control others.

Socialization

Socialization can be defined as, the process by which we learn the things we need to know to enable us to fit into the society to which we belong. Early socialization refers to those things which occur first in this process. The connection between the developing emotions and early socialization is fairly obvious. As the baby expresses its emotions, it is clearly communicating with its parent or care giver that the socialization process has begun.

Development of Self

Development of a child's self-concept is closely related to the child's social development Lewis and Brooks-Gun (1979) developed a technique of placing the child in front of a mirror and observing the child's reactions. They concluded that self-recognition started to occur at about 16 months; but they believed that it was not until 18–24 months that the child was fully able to recognize itself as an individual. These data were confirmed when photographs of the child were shown to the child. This is the same age in Piaget's scheme that the child is able to form mental images. **Table 1** shows Piaget's stages of cognitive development.

Table 1: Piaget's stages of cognitive development.

Age	Stages	Major developmental tasks
Birth to 2 years	Sensorimotor	With increased mobility and awareness, development of a sense of self as separate from the external environment; the concept of object permanence emerges as the ability to form mental images evolves
2–6 years	Preoperational	Learning to express self with language; development of understanding of symbolic gestures; achievement of object permanence
6–12 years	Concrete operations	Learning to apply logic to thinking; development of understanding of reversibility and spatiality; learning to differentiate and classify; increased socialization and application of rules
12–15 + years	Formal operations	Learning to think and reason in abstract terms; making and testing hypotheses; capability of logical thinking and reasoning expand and are refined; cognitive maturity achieved

Gender Identity

Immediately from birth, parents and others will treat the child based on its biological sex, and this social input begins the process of gender identity. The acquisition of sexual identity—the child knowing his/her own sex—starts at about 24 months. This learning continues over a period. During this time, the child also learns certain behaviors that are associated with boys, other behaviors with girls, so as well as learning about his/her sex, he/she learns a gender role as well.

Deprivation Effects

Maternal deprivation is one of the worst forms of deprivation. Children living in an institution—an orphanage or children's home showed less concern for other people than a control group of children who had been brought up in a normal family situation with mother as the primary care giver. The institutionalized children also demonstrated more delinquency than control group. The early years of life are critical but research with severely deprived children has shown that these children, given an improved, enriched and loving environment are capable of almost complete recovery.

DEVELOPMENT IN THE LIFE CYCLE

The understanding of the principles of heredity and environment as well as physical, social and cognition development, gives the foundation for human development throughout the life cycle. Earlier the emphasis in developmental psychology was on child development but more recently, there has been a shift toward the view that development continues through the whole of life.

Havighurst in 1953 prepared a development model for the American population giving developmental test for adolescence, early adulthood, middle age, and old age **(Box 1)**.

Box 1: Developmental task model.

Havighurst's Developmental Tasks Model
Havighurst, writing in America in the 1950s, developed what he called developmental tasks. He proposed a series of tasks that stretched from birth to death. He defined a developmental task as:
"a task which arises at or about a certain period in the life of the individual, successful achievement of which leads to his happiness and to success with later tasks, while failure leads to unhappiness and difficulty with later tasks."
Havighurst (1953), cited in Hurlock (1959), Developmental Psychology.

Developmental tasks—Havighurst (1953)
Havighurst prepared a development model in which he has presented the list of developmental tasks from early childhood to old age. Every cultural group expects its members to master certain essential skills and acquire certain approved patterns of behavior at various stages during life span.
Although most people master these tasks at the appropriate time, some are unable to do so while others are ahead of the schedule. The developmental tasks are as described here:

1. *Infancy (first 2 weeks of life): The newborn infant must make four major adjustments to postnatal life viz.*
   a. To temperature changes
   b. To sucking and swallowing
   c. To breathing
   d. To elimination
2. *Babyhood and early childhood:*
   ➤ Learning to take solid foods
   ➤ Learning to walk and talk
   ➤ Learning control of elimination of body wastes
   ➤ Learning sex differences and sex modesty
   ➤ Getting ready to read

Contd...

Contd...

- ➢ Beginning to develop conscience. Learning to distinguish right and wrong
3. *Late childhood:*
   - ➢ Learning physical skills necessary for ordinary games
   - ➢ Building a wholesome attitude toward oneself as a growing organism
   - ➢ Learning to get along with age-mates
   - ➢ Beginning to develop appropriate masculine or feminine social roles
   - ➢ Developing fundamental skills in reading, writing, and calculating
   - ➢ Developing concepts necessary for everyday living.
   - ➢ Developing a conscience, a sense of morality and a scale of values
4. *Developmental tasks of adolescence:*
   - ➢ Accepting one's physique and accepting a masculine or feminine role
   - ➢ New relations with age-mates of both sexes
   - ➢ Emotional independence of parents and other adults
   - ➢ Achieving assurance of economic independence
   - ➢ Selecting and preparing for an occupation
   - ➢ Developing intellectual skills and concepts necessary for civic competence
   - ➢ Desiring and achieving socially responsible behavior
   - ➢ Preparing for marriage and family life
   - ➢ Building conscious values in harmony with an adequate scientific world picture
5. *Developmental tasks of early adulthood:*
   - ➢ Selecting a mate
   - ➢ Learning to live with a marriage partner
   - ➢ Starting a family
   - ➢ Rearing children
   - ➢ Managing a home
   - ➢ Getting started in an occupation
   - ➢ Taking on civic responsibility
   - ➢ Finding a congenial social group
6. *Developmental tasks of middle age:*
   - ➢ Achieving adult civic and social responsibility
   - ➢ Establishing and maintaining an economic standard of living
   - ➢ Assisting teenage children to become responsible and happy adults
   - ➢ Developing adult leisure-time activities
   - ➢ Relating oneself to one's spouse as a person
   - ➢ Accepting and adjusting to the physiological changes of middle age
   - ➢ Adjusting to aging parents
7. *Developmental tasks of old age:*
   - ➢ Adjusting to decreasing physical strength and health
   - ➢ Adjusting to retirement and reduced income
   - ➢ Adjusting to death of spouse
   - ➢ Establishing an explicit affiliation with age group
   - ➢ Meeting social and civic obligations
   - ➢ Establishing satisfactory physical living arrangements

Role of Nurse: Nurses working in hospitals will come across patients of all the above stages of life. Some of them might have failed to resolve their developmental tasks enumerated for each stage. Their personalities are not sound and they are disturbed and unhappy. Knowledge of their problems and developmental psychology will help nurses to understand the patients' psychology better and extend proper nursing care with warmth and empathy. Such behavior of nurses will soothe the feelings and attitudes of the patients necessary for early cure.

EIGHT PSYCHOSOCIAL STAGES OF ERIKSON

Erikson's concept differs from that of Havinghurst in that he divides the lifespan into eight psychological stages. These are called psychosocial stages, because many aspects of psychological and social functioning are interrelated and show consistent changes at certain times in the life cycle. A psychological crisis has to be resolved as each stage for healthy development.

Infancy: Oral Stage Infant Trust versus Mistrust

In infancy, the development is in the direction of complexity and variety. The baby responds as a whole to feeding, to noise and other stimuli. Gradually the tissues, the organs and the interacting systems make possible a wide variety of responses. The various parts and systems grow or mature at various rates at different times **(Table 2)**.

There are individual variations and all the newborn babies will not fit into any one time-table. Growth and development of the baby is called maturation. The rate at which an infant matures may vary but the order in which development takes place is the same anywhere in the world. For example, an infant will sit before it stands and stand before it walks.

Readiness is an important principle in maturation. The readiness principle means that a child will not be able to learn a particular skill until the physical structures needed for the skill are ready or mature.

Table 2: Motor development sequence.

Development (in months)	Action
2–4 months	Head and back can be raised with support
4–6 months	Can sit with support
8–10 months	Can stand with support
10–12 months	Can walk with support
12–14 months	Can walk alone

Thus, a child cannot learn to walk or be toilet-trained until the muscles needed for those skills are mature.

As per Erikson, trust is fostered by consistency, continuity, and sameness of experience. If the child is given affection, he will trust the adult members (parents) who give the affection. Child will think that the world is safe and dependable. The child identifies its mother and other members of the family. On the other hand, if the child is ill-treated and not given affection and the treatment given by the adults is inconsistent, the result is mistrust. The child forms emotional attachment with the caretaking person.

When an infant does not receive warm and loving care or is isolated from others or from a natural environment, it is called need deprivation. Deprivation has far reaching effects upon the emotional and intellectual development of the child. An infant develops language as the nervous system develops.

The Nurse and the Infant

An infant is in the need of tender loving care at home or in the hospital. Many hospitals have nurse care for the infant for the duration of its stay. Touching the infant is the first communication from the nurse. The nurse should plan to give as much personal attention as possible, such as handling, cuddling, holding and loving the infant under her care.

An accurate observation of the infant is very important as it cannot speak. The nurse must be able to interpret the infant's needs through its crying and body language. The nurse should observe the physical abnormalities and unusual growth and development.

Assisting, teaching, and advising the mother is the responsibility of the nurse. New mothers need emotional support and encouragement. Maturation and normal development as the infant matures should be explained to the mother with the help of available literature. Mothers of infants with physical abnormalities need special sympathy.

Early Childhood: Anal or Habit Training Stage (Toddlers)— Autonomy versus Shame and Doubt (18–36 Months)

By the second year of life, the muscular and nervous systems have developed well, and the child, eager to acquire new skills, is no longer content to sit and watch. The infant moves around and examines its environment, but judgment develops more slowly. What the child wants is not necessarily what the parents want as they are anxious about the child's health and safety.

The child learns to control elimination of waste or do things himself or fails at this task. The child derives much pleasure from the anus and the urethra by evacuating the bowels and evacuating the bladder. If the toilet training is too rigid, the child may express anal aggression in the form of retention of feces, soiling and scattering. The habit training stage is extremely important because self-control and autonomy are initiated in this stage. The child learns that he cannot depend entirely on the mother and that he has to take some degree of care himself.

The child needs guidance and the caretaker's decisions about how much freedom to allow are very important. In case of autonomy versus doubt, the critical issue is the child's feeling of independence. In an extremely permissive environment, the infant encounters difficulties that it cannot yet handle, and the child can become overwhelmed, doubling itself but developing a sense of independence. Similarly, if the control is too severe, the child feels worthless and shameful of being capable of so little. The appropriate middle position, respecting the child's needs and environmental factors, requires the caretaker's careful and constant attention. If the child is respected as an individual, the child will develop a sense of autonomy; otherwise feelings of shame and doubt about oneself are developed.

Keeping a good relationship with the younger child will be challenging to the nurse. The child will be self-centered and may not cooperate. The nurse needs a good relationship with the child's family. The parents may need reassurance if the child is very ill. They will also need explanation and information to help them understand and plan for the future.

Middle Childhood (Preschool): Phallic Stage or the Period of Family Triangle—Initiative versus Guilt (3–6 Years)

The pleasurable sensations have now shifted from the mouth and excretory organs to the genitals. The child will now begin to identify with parent of the same sex and unconsciously wish to replace that parent in the family.

The child learns to plan and carry out a task. His initiative should be encouraged otherwise, the child feels guilty.

During this period, the little boy who always had a great deal of attention and love from his mother, begins to feel very possessive toward the mother. He wants her for himself and resents the close tie that he feels exists between his father and mother. He develops competitive feelings toward his father and tries to be rival with him for his mother's love. The father, however, is such a large and formidable opponent that the little boy develops resentment and fear of him. This is Oedipus complex.

Eventually, the little boy concludes that being like his father is more effective way of obtaining his mother's love and attention. Thus, he begins to take on the masculine behavior of his father. This is identification. Similarly, the little girl identifies herself with the mother. Thus, the basic future relationship with men and women is initiated, during this period. If for any reason, parents are people with whom the child cannot identify, future adjustment may be seriously affected. Do not get upset by questions by children. Nonsense is nothing but creativity.

Latency or Later Childhood (School Child)—Industry versus Inferiority (6–12 Years)

It is called latency, because the sexual interests are repressed and lie dormant till puberty. This is a period of gang formation and fierce gang loyalties. Boys cling together and shun girls. Similarly, groups of girls come together and declare that they despise boys.

During this period, the child becomes somewhat independent of the family and finds a place for himself among his peer groups. At school and playgrounds, he develops his skills that help him to compete, cooperate and get along successfully with others. Playing games in groups is very popular in the later years of later childhood. Group games with rules which have to be followed help teach moral rules to the child. The child learns how to compete with others, how to play for the benefit of a team, how to be a good loser and why it is wrong to cheat.

During this stage, the child develops a sense of industry and learns perseverance and diligence. The difficulty of this stage is that the child may develop a sense of inferiority if it is unable to master the tasks set by teachers and parents.

Fixation refers to the point in the individual's development at which certain aspects of the emotional development cease to advance. Further development seems to be blocked. The result is a complex, e.g., Oedipus complex and inferiority complex.

The Nurse and the Older Child

The older child is gaining more independence but continues to need guidance and special care. He needs direction to understand what behavior is expected of him or what are the *do's and don'ts* when hospitalized. The child needs frequent praise and encouragement especially in loneliness, pain, and discomfort.

Puberty and Adolescence—Identity versus Role Confusion (12–18 Years)

The transition period from childhood to adulthood is known as adolescence. Through physical, social, and mental changes, the child must develop into an adult.

Physical change: Toward the end of later childhood, sexual changes or puberty begins. Secondary sexual characteristics develop—enlarged hips and breasts develop in girls and muscular development and voice changes in boys. Both sexes begin to grow pubic hair. Puberty is completed when primary sexual functioning occurs.

Social changes during adolescence: Life is in a state of disequilibrium. Every aspect of life is likely to be characterized by stress, storm, and turmoil as the young individual attempts to become completely free from his family. Because of this conflict over dependency-independency needs, the adolescent may be hostile toward adults, particularly parents and teachers and rebellious toward authority. He craves for love, recognition and encouragement.

Developmental task, at this stage is to develop a sense of identity regarding occupational, familial and social roles as opposed to the development of role confusion. This requires a stable, loving home life and wise, mature parents who understand the needs of their children and treat them as individuals. The adolescent, during the stage of identity formation is likely to suffer from a confusion of roles or identity confusion. This state causes one to feel isolated, empty, anxious and indecisive. Helping adolescents feel good about themselves will promote a good nurse-patient relationship.

Young Adulthood—Intimacy versus Isolation (20–40 Years)

The major developmental tasks of early adulthood include choosing a mate, establishing a home and accepting the responsibility of parent. Children cannot be effectively nurtured unless the family has a reasonable degree of security. A successful parent must also be a good citizen and a participating member of a social group.

Mature Adulthood or Middle Age—Generativity versus Stagnation (40–65 Years)

People find themselves in a crisis leading to increased rate of divorces and major shift in career plans, e.g., a woman who has been satisfied as a housewife for the past 15 or 20 years may feel that she had been left out of the mainstream of life and so may take up a job. A father and husband may think that he has made a mistake not only in the choice of the job but also in the marriage partner and place of residence. The mid-thirties usher in the "deadline decade (35–45)", the crossroads of life.

At the mid-forties, the equilibrium is regained. Children take up a job away from home or are married. Parents have to redefine their roles in relationship to one another, to their family and to the larger world outside the family. They become involved in work outside the family. For example, a nurse who has been both a mother and nurse, may become increasingly involved in giving leadership in professional nursing. She may become involved in a group that is deciding whether nurses should strike, her attention moving from merely doing her job to broader issues of social justice.

Changes that occur during adulthood have given rise to various expressions, such as "middle age crisis", "mid-career crisis", "middle age slump"—referring to recognition of losing youth and coming of old age. Individuals become aware of ageing process and realize that time is moving on.

The conflict within this period is between generativity and stagnation. We begin to look at what we have generated-products and ideas, the legacy we leave to future generations. When generativity is weak and not given expression, the personality regresses or stagnates.

Individuals unable to make the transitions of this period, will be frightened of growing old, rather than enjoying a new type of fulfillment as they grow old. Energies are invested in holding back the tide of time, e.g., the middle-aged woman dressing like a young girl.

Old Age or Senescent–Ego Integrity versus Despair (65 Years to Death)

Old age is subject to stresses and strains.
a. Retirement and reduced income which may create a feeling that one's usefulness is essentially over and activities are restricted.
b. With the passage of years, the old people become weaker and weaker.
c. Even though the old people become weaker physically, they want to tighten their grip over the younger ones in the family and also over family matters and business issues. The younger ones in the family instead of developing a sympathetic outlook toward the old, start asserting their rights and power leading to tension in the family.
d. Reduction in physical attractiveness
e. Failing health and invalidism
f. Isolation and loneliness
g. The problem of meaning of life and death

This period is characterized by integrity. According to Erikson, integrity sums up our ability to live the later portion of life with dignity and a sense of order and meaning to life. It involves a continued joy in living, a sense of accomplishment, of things well done. Integrity is the acceptance of one's life cycle. Despair expresses the feeling that what has been done is not of much value and that not much time is left to do anything. While looking back, if he feels that his life was successful, then he has integrity; otherwise despair, which causes depression.

It is necessary to adjust to the reduced income and deteriorating health. Frequently friends or husband/wife die leading to loneliness.

Nurse and the Adult Patients

Listening to the worries and concerns about family and work responsibility in both the young and middle adulthood is most helpful. Physical signs of stress should be noted. The adult should be assisted to become independent until able to assume responsibility for his or her own health.

Older adults will be hospitalized more than any other group. The elderly need warmth and personal touch of others and should be helped to prevent social isolation. They have a special need to be respected and valued as a person. They should be helped to take food, dressed and protected from cold by covering with blankets. The nurse should help the elderly hear and see more easily. Also they should be physically protected especially if disoriented.

Generally, old people become impatient and show irritability and willfulness. The nurse should realize that these are due to the normal deteriorating process. It is necessary to keep old people interested in life and make them feel important and useful.

Life and then Death

There are five stages in the reactions of dying patients:
1. **Denial:** Patient insists that it was a mistake. The diagnosis is wrong or something has been overlooked.
2. **Anger:** Patient then asks "Why me" and becomes annoyed with God.
3. **Bargaining:** Patient makes promises in exchange for longer life. He promises to give up addictions or promises to God that he will lead a better life.
4. **Depression:** There is a loss of interest and sense of despair.
5. **Acceptance:** Patient becomes void of feelings. He develops an inner peace and accepts death.

The nurse has the responsibility to help families to face and accept death. Patients should be encouraged to share their memories and feelings and talk about death. Most people prefer to die at home. This concept has been accepted by the hospice movement, committed to making the end of life as free from pain, anxiety and depression as possible.

Effective treatment of the older people suffering from mental and other problems requires a comprehensive use of medical and psychological procedures. Administration of group therapy to older patients would mean the creating of a social environment in which the person can function successfully. Scientists in many areas of the biological and social sciences are investigating the pathological and normal aspects of aging including ways to minimize the aging process. **Table 3** shows the Erikson stage of psychosocial development and Freud analytical theory. **Table 4** shows the difference between Piaget's intellectual stages and Kohlberg's Moral level. **Table 5** shows the stage of Mahler's theory of development. **Table 6** shows the Kohlberg's stages of moral development. **Table 7** shows the stages of development in Peplau's interpersonal theory.

Table 3: Stages of Erikson psychosocial development and Freud Analytical theory.

Stages	Erikson's Psychosocial Stages			Freud's psycho-sexual stages	Significant persons
	Approximate age	Tasks	Negative counterpart		
Infancy	0–1	Sense of trust	Mistrust	Oral	Maternal person or substitute
Toddler	1–3	Sense of autonomy	Shame and doubt	Anal	Parental persons
Preschool	3–6	Sense of initiative	Guilt	Phallic	Basic family
School	6–12	Sense of industry	Inferiority	Latency	Neighborhood, school
Early adolescence	12–18	Sense of identity	Identity diffusion	Puberty	Peer groups and out groups models of leadership
Late adolescence and young adult	18–40	Sense of intimacy and solidarity	Isolation	Genitality	Partners in friendship, sex competition, cooperation

Table 4: Difference between Piaget's intellectual stages and Kohlberg's moral level.

Tasks	Lasting virtues	Piaget's intellectual stages	Kohlberg's moral levels
• Getting • Tolerating frustration in small doses • Recognizing mother as distinct from others and self	Drive and hope	Sensorimotor (0–2 years)—Differentiates self from objects	Preconventional morality Stage 0 (0–2 years)—The good is what I like and want
• Trying out own powers of speech • Beginning acceptance of reality	Self-control and will power	Preoperational (2–7 years)—Functions symbolically using language as major tool Preconceptual phase (2–4 years)—Uses representational thought	Stage I (2 and 3 years) Punishment-obedience orientation

Contd...

Contd...

Tasks	Lasting virtues	Piaget's intellectual stages	Kohlberg's moral levels
versus pleasure principle		to recall past, represent present, and anticipate future, transductive reasoning	
• Questioning Exploring own body and environment • Differentiation of sexes	Purpose and direction	Intuitive phase (4–7 years)— Increased symbolic functioning: transductive reasoning	Stage 2 (4–7 years)—Instrumental hedonism and concrete reciprocity
• Learning to win recognition by producing things • Exploring, collecting • Learning to relate to own sex	Competence and method	Concrete operational (7–11 years)—Inductive reasoning and beginning logic, ability to order and relate experiences to an organized whole	Conventional morality Stage 3 (7 to 8 or 9 years) Orientation to interpersonal relations of mutuality Stage 4 (10–12 years) Maintenance of social order, fixed rules, and authority
• Moving toward heterosexuality • Selecting vocation • Beginning separation from family • Integrating personality (altruism, etc.)	Devotion and fidelity	Formal operational (11–15 years)—Abstract and deductive reasoning: can plan and implement scientific approach to problem solving	Postconventional morality (adolescence and adulthood) Stage 5A—Social contract, utilitarian lawmaking perspective Stage 5B—Higher law and conscience orientation Stage 6—Universal ethical principle orientation

Contd...

Contd...

Tasks	Lasting virtues	Piaget's intellectual stages	Kohlberg's moral levels
• Becoming capable of establishing a lasting relationship with a member of the opposite sex • Learning to be creative and productive	Affiliation and love		

Table 5: Stages of development in Mahler's theory of object relations.

Age	Phase/subphase	Major developmental tasks
Birth to 1 month	I. Normal autism	Fulfillment of basic needs for survival comfort
1–5 months	II. Symbiosis	Development of awareness of external source need fulfillment
	III. Separation-Individuation	
5–10 months	a. Differentiation	Commencement of a primary recognition of separateness from the mothering figure
10–16 months	b. Practicing	Increased independence through locomotor functioning, increase sense of separateness of self
16–24 months	c. Rapprochement	Acute awareness of separateness of self; learning to seek "emotional refueling" from mothering figure to maintain feeling of security
24–36 months	d. Consolidation	Sense of separateness established; on the way to object constancy (i.e., able to internalize a sustained image of loved object/person when it is out of sight); resolution of separation anxiety

Contd...

Table 6: Kohlberg's stages of moral development.

Level/age*	Stages	Developmental focus
I. Preconventional (common from age 4–10 years)	1. Punishment and obedience orientation	Behavior motivated by fear of punishment
	2. Instrumental relativist orientation	Behavior motivated by egocentrism and concern for self
II. Conventional (common from age 10 to 13 years, and into adulthood)	3. Interpersonal concordance orientation	Behavior motivated by expectations of others. Strong desire for approval and acceptance
	4. Law and order orientation	Behavior motivated by respect for authority
III. Postconventional (can occur from adolescence on)	5. Social contract legalistic orientation	Behavior motivated by respect for universal laws and moral principles; guided by internal set of values
	6. Universal ethical principle orientation	Behavior motivated by internalized principles of honor, justice, and respect for human dignity, guided by the conscience

*Ages in Kohlberg's theory are not well-defined. The stage of development is determined by the motivation behind the individual's behavior.

Table 7: Stages of development in Peplau's interpersonal theory.

Age	Stages	Major developmental tasks
Infancy	Learning to count on others	Learning to communicate in various ways with the primary caregiver in order to have comfort needs fulfilled
Toddlerhood	Learning to delay satisfaction	Learning the satisfaction of pleasing others by delaying self-gratification in small ways
Early childhood	Identifying oneself	Learning appropriate roles and behaviors by acquiring the ability to perceive the expectations of others
Late childhood	Developing skills in participation	Learning the skills of compromise, competition, and cooperation with others; establishment of a more realistic view of the world and a feeling of one's place in it

Key Points ● ● ● ●

- Readiness is an important principle in maturation.
- Deprivation has far reaching effects upon the emotional and intellectual development of the child.
- Late childhood child becomes independent of the family.
- The transition period from childhood to adulthood is known as adolescence.
- Elizabeth Kubler-Ross proposed the five stages of grief.
- Piaget's theory is the theory of cognitive development.
- The theory of moral development is given by Kohlberg.
- Psychosocial development theory is proposed by Erikson.

STUDY QUESTIONS

Long Essays

1. Elucidate factors influencing the development of personality and its characteristics.
2. Describe the life cycle of human development.
3. Describe Kohlberg's theory of moral development.

Short Essays

1. Elaborate the various stages of human development.
2. What are the personality changes due to illness?
3. Discuss the role of personality in health and illness.

Short Answers

1. Adolescence.
2. Middle age crisis.
3. Integrity versus despair.
4. Preconventional stage.
5. Preoperational stage.

Multiple Choice Questions

1. According to the psychosocial stages what is the conflict that occurs during puberty?
    a. Ego integrity vs. despair
    b. Identity vs. identity diffusion
    c. Intimacy vs. isolation
    d. Generativity vs. stagnation

Chapter 18: Developmental Psychology

2. According to the psychosexual stages of development, between the ages of 3 and 6 years, the child is said to go through the _____ stage.
   a. Phallic
   b. Latency
   c. Anal
   d. Genital

3. A child who failed to learn multiplication and division in grade school did not successfully complete which of Erikson's stages of personality development?
   a. Autonomy vs. shame and doubt
   b. Integrity vs. despair
   c. Industry vs. inferiority
   d. Initiative vs. guilt

4. According to Freud, fixation at which psychosexual stage of development is associated with sarcasm, and criticalness, in adults?
   a. Oral
   b. Anal
   c. Phallic
   d. Genital

5. Theoretically, the correct order of the stages of dying are:
   a. Depression - Anger - Bargaining - Denial - Acceptance
   b. Denial - Acceptance - Bargaining - Depression - Anger
   c. Denial - Anger - Bargaining - Depression - Acceptance
   d. Denial - Anger - Begging - Depression - Acceptance

6. According to Piaget, during the _____ stage, children typically master the principle of _____.
   a. Concrete operational; Conservation
   b. Preoperational; Abstract reasoning
   c. Concrete operational; Object permanence
   d. Sensorimotor; Conservation

7. According to Piaget's theory, what term is given to the flexible mental patterns that can be combined with one another to solve problems?
   a. Operations
   b. Simulations
   c. Symbolism
   d. Mentalism

8. Jack studying in 5th standard, visits church because his family is going regularly to church and his parents think he should also do the same. According to Kohlberg, which stage of moral reasoning, Jack is in?
   a. Preconventional
   b. Conventional
   c. Postconventional
   d. Generative morality
9. Which among the following is the sequential order of Piaget's cognitive development theory?
   a. Preoperational, Sensory motor, Concrete operational, Formal Operational stage
   b. Sensory motor, Concrete Operational, Preoperational, Formal Operational stage
   c. Formal operational, Preoperational, Concrete Operational, Sensory motor stage
   d. Sensory motor, Preoperational, Concrete Operational, Formal Operational stage
10. In the DABDA stages of Elizabeth Kubler-Ross's theory, the first and third "D" stands for _____.
    a. Depression, Denial
    b. Denial, Death
    c. Denial, Depression
    d. Depression, Death

19. Mental Health and Mental Illness

Chapter Outline

- Mental Health
- Mental Illness
- Mental Hygiene Movement
- Personal Adjustment
- Counseling
- Psychotherapy
- Empathy
- Genuineness
- Unconditional Acceptance
- Guidance

Learning Objectives

♦ Students will be familiarized with mental health and characteristics of mentally healthy individual.
♦ Students will be oriented to ways of promoting mental health.
♦ Students will be able to differentiate guidance, counseling and psychotherapy.

INTRODUCTION

In older days, emotionally disturbed people were thought to be possessed by the devil or by evil spirits, and they were treated accordingly. They were beaten, whipped, or dipped in hot liquids in the hope of "driving the devil" out of them.

The return to reason and scientific method was witnessed due to great changes generated by the *renaissance*. Emphasis was placed on anatomy and physiology and physical treatment of mental disorders was stressed by physicians. A new social and political philosophy to the problems of mental illness was applied by the French physician, Philippe Pinel (1745-1826) who is called the Father of Modern Psychiatry. In 1793, he removed the chains from mentally ill patients confined in Bicêtre, a hospital outside Paris, thus bringing about the first revolution in psychiatry. He emphasized the need to treat asylum inmates as human beings rather than as dangerous animals. His human and progressive ideas had considerably influenced the care and treatment of mentally disturbed people throughout the civilized world.

MENTAL HYGIENE MOVEMENT

This movement spread in the United States with the efforts of Dorothea Lynde Dix (1802–1887), a school teacher of Massachusetts. She launched a 40-year crusade to improve the plight of the mentally ill. Having achieved success in her program in the US, she took steps to spread the movement to England and Scotland. In 1908, Clifford W Beers published his autobiography. "A mind that found itself" which exposed existing evils. The book was widely read and quoted extensively as he suggested ways in which these unfortunate conditions could be corrected. Today the work of the mental hygiene movement is taken up in different parts of the world by the World Federation of Mental Health and the World Health Organization (WHO).

Mental health and mental illness are relative terms. They are closely related to one another. Imagine healthy and unhealthy behavior as part of a continuum or scale. Mental health or very definite healthy behavior is at one end of the scale and mental illness or very definite unhealthy behavior is at the other end of the scale. Borderline behavior is in the middle of the scale or approximately halfway between the two ends as shown here.

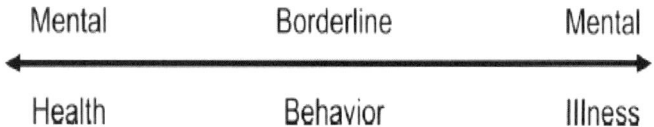

Unhealthy behavior can be identified when it becomes extreme for prolonged periods of time and prevent adjustment in society. Solitude is a healthy withdrawal but paranoia is unhealthy; a minor annoyance which is quickly forgotten is healthy anger but rage is unhealthy. Anxiety before an interview, is healthy behavior but euphoria is unhealthy. Being excited about a promotion is a healthy behavior but panic is unhealthy. Other unhealthy behavior includes delusions, hallucinations, flight of ideas, compulsive actions or ideas and phobias.

MEDICAL CLASSIFICATION OF MENTAL ILLNESS (WORLD HEALTH ORGANIZATION)

1. **Organic mental disorders** are caused by physical damage to the brain, e.g., diseases of the brain, senility, and injury.
2. **Substance use disorders** caused by dependency upon drugs and substances, such as alcohol, and tobacco.
3. **Psychotic disorders** are most severe and require hospitalization. Patients lose touch with reality and are unable to control their thought and behavior. Examples are schizophrenia and paranoid disorders.
4. **Affective disorders** are those involving abnormal moods and emotions, such as euphoria, agitation, depression, and hyperactivity. Affect means emotions, or strong feelings.
5. **Anxiety disorders** involving chronic and extreme fears which cannot be explained, e.g., phobias.
6. **Somatoform disorders** (psychosomatic) show physical symptoms for which there is no cause, e.g., blindness or pain due to psychological factors.
7. **Dissociative disorders:** When individual separates themselves from their real personalities to avoid stress and responsibility, e.g., amnesia, multiple personality.
8. **Personality disorders** are when individuals develop abnormal behavior patterns, e.g., very suspicious of others, extremely dependent, very self-centered, compulsive, aggressive and antisocial.
9. **Psychosexual disorders:** Abnormal sexual behavior.

MENTAL HEALTH—ITS MEANING AND NATURE

A healthy individual is not only physically healthy but also mentally healthy. A healthy mind in a healthy body. The modern concept of health extends beyond the proper functioning of the body. It includes a sound, efficient mind, and controlled emotions. Health is a state of being hale, sound or whole in body and mind. It means that both body and mind are working efficiently and harmoniously.

Mental health is an important aspect of one's total health status and it is a basic factor that contributes to the maintenance of physical health and social effectiveness. It means the ability to balance feelings, desires, ambitions and ideals in one's daily life. It means the ability to face and accept the realities of life. Mental hygiene is the ability to withstand stress.

Personal Adjustment

Mental health has two important aspects. It is both individual and social. Social forces are in constant flux. They are constantly moving and changing. Similarly, our mental adjustment is affected by various stresses. Mental health is a process of adjustment, which involves compromise and adaptation, growth and continuity. Because of the significance of individual and social aspects, some psychologists have defined mental health as the ability of the individual to make personal and social adjustments.

The word "adjustment" needs some explanation. If one can establish a satisfactory relationship between himself and his environment, his needs and desires and those of other people, or if one can meet the demands of a situation, he has achieved adjustment. Adjustment results in happiness because emotional conflicts and tensions have been resolved and relieved.

Characteristics of a Mentally Healthy Individual

From the earlier discussion, we can deduce certain characteristics that a mentally healthy individual or a well-adjusted person possesses or develops in his daily life. These characteristics can serve as criteria for optimum mental health.

1. A well-adjusted person has some awareness of his/her motives, desires, ambition, and feelings. He/she knows himself/herself and accepts his/her strength and weakness gracefully. He/she chooses a task of moderate difficulty to achieve.
2. He/she has a high degree of self-esteem and confidence. Unlike a maladjusted person, he/she feels adequate and equal to others in facing the challenges and responsibilities of daily life.
3. He/she is able and willing to assume responsibilities appropriate to his/her age. Participates with pleasure in experiences belonging to each successive age level.
4. He/she attacks problems that require solutions. Makes decisions with a minimum of worry, conflict and advice seeking. Abides by the choice he/she makes until convinced it is a wrong choice. Accepts the fact that life is an endless struggle.
5. He/she can use thinking before action and not as a device for delaying or escaping action.
6. He/she learns from defeats instead of finding excuses for them, can endure pain and emotional frustration when necessary; can compromise when encounters difficulties. Can concentrate his/her energy on a goal considered important for him.

Chapter 19: Mental Health and Mental Illness

7. He/she can say "no" to situation harmful to his/her best interest; can say "yes" to situations that will ultimately aid him/her.
8. He/she can show anger directly when injured or when rights are violated. Can show affection directly and appropriately in kind and amount.
9. As he/she is mentally healthy, he/she will express his/her emotions in a desirable and controlled manner.
10. He/she has the capacity to socially adjust with others and get along well with them in different situations.
11. His/her intellectual powers are well-developed. He/she thinks independently and takes appropriate decisions as and when required.
12. He/she lives in a world of reality and not in a world of fantasy. He/she does not run away from harsh realities of life.
13. He/she has the courage for facing failures in his/her life. He/she learns from his/her mistakes and improves in his/her functioning.
14. He/she conforms to the norms of his/her group and has a sense of belongingness to his/her group.
15. He/she sorts out his/her problems appropriately and so does not suffer from anxiety, frustration, or conflicts.
16. He/she is always punctual for his/her duties and does not suffer from forgetfulness.
17. He/she is self-confident and optimistic.
18. He/she has an adequate sex adjustment and does not suffer from sex abnormalities.
19. He/she is well-adjusted and happy with his/her profession.
20. He/she leads a balanced life of work, rest, and recreation.

FOUNDATIONS OF MENTAL HEALTH

Basic factors:
1. Heredity
2. Physical factors
3. Social factors
   a. Home
   b. School
   c. Community
4. Satisfaction of basic needs in childhood

Heredity (refer Chapter 4 for more details)

It gives the raw material or the potentialities of the individual. It sets the limits for his mental health. What the individual inherits is the potentialities in relation to growth, appearance, intelligence, and health. The development and utilization of these potentialities are determined mainly by the environmental opportunities. Heredity may also predispose a person for some mental diseases.

Physical Factors

Physical health factors make a significant ground for mental health. People with greater strength, better looks, and health enjoy a social advantage in the development of personality characteristics.

He/she has a desire to live, to achieve, and be happy. Physical health improves mental vitality, motivation, and drive. Continued hunger, overwork or sleeplessness produce fatigue affecting mental health adversely. Vitamin deficiencies also can cause many personality disorders.

Social Factors

Every individual is born into a society which influences his behavior. The social factors which affect mental health, among them the most important are the home, school, and community.

Home: Broken homes or unstable homes where parents are in constant conflict produce children usually with adjustment problems. There should be sympathetic understanding from both the parents. Both the parents should have interest in their children, pride in their achievements and sympathy for their problems. Discipline is through patience, affection, understanding, and reasoning. Child is respected as a person and is given freedom to develop. His early mistakes are recognized as part of "growing up". Children will have respect for parents, respect based on love and not on fear.

School: Parents and teachers should note the individual differences of children and respect these differences. Physical needs of the child should be properly looked into including his need for exercise.

A good school provides an environment in which each pupil is respected as an individual. Extracurricular activities, such as dramatics, athletics and debates promote the physical and emotional development of pupils. Such a school is a positive factor in the development of sound mental health.

Community: The community provides the framework and climate within which each family lives and develops. The community should provide a healthy atmosphere and a well-organized network of public utility services of high standard.

Satisfaction of Basic Needs

Mental health is also determined by the way our basic needs are satisfied especially in our childhood. These needs include besides physiological needs, safety and security needs, belongingness and love and esteem needs. Thus, the home and school should provide satisfaction for these needs—the need for security through love and affection of the parents, the need for recognition as a person of worth and importance, the need to grow independently, the need to play, and the need to belong to a group. This will be another positive factor in the development of sound mental health.

ROLE OF NURSES IN PSYCHOTHERAPY

The main responsibility of the nurse is to instill confidence in the patient and to make him like the company of others. The hesitant, shy patient should be encouraged by the nurse to mix with people. Her feelings expressed or unexpressed toward her patients are vital for any psychotherapeutic attempt.

Nurse-Patient Relationship

It is important to focus upon the person with respect and concern rather than upon behavior alone. Most patients will need extra time and special attention, acceptance of their behavior without criticism or punishment, sincere praise and encouragement, protection from self-injury or injury to others and an environment which will ease their most disruptive behavior.

Promoting Mental Health

As a nurse, your responsibilities are four fold:
1. You should live in a life style which would promote your own mental health,
    a. *Accept your personal feelings:* Like home sickness, fear, or anger. It is healthier to recognize them and find ways of releasing the tensions they cause.
    b. *Know your weaknesses:* Know your fears, what upsets you or hurts you under stress and protect yourself from these situations. Avoid people or situations which upset you. If you cannot avoid these situations, work out a way of dealing with them.
    c. Develop talents and interests.
    d. Share yourself with other people.
    e. Get help when you need.

f. Follow the suggestions already given in this book for emotion control and stress reduction in your life.
2. You should recognize unhealthy behavior in yourself and others, so that the need for help can be identified. This is very necessary for effective client relationship.
3. **Knowing and using sources of professional help in your geographical location:** You should know the details of the nearest psychiatric institutions, clinics and counseling services, both private and government sponsored. You should also know the sources of funds to pay the bills of patients who cannot pay.
4. **Promoting education and positive attitudes towards mental health in the community:** It is your duty to know more about the national programs of mental health. Your role as a professional nurse can be used in a very positive way in your personal relationships, within the institution of your employment, professional organizations and in the community. You can teach others through planned programs of education and your example and positive attitudes toward mental health and mental illness.

Health-For-All by AD 2025

On September 12, 1978, at Alma-Ata in Kazakhstan, representatives of 134 nations agreed to the terms of a solemn declaration pledging urgent action by all governments, all health and development workers and the world community to project and promote health for all people of the world.

Through the implementation of primary health care as a part of "Health-for-all by AD 2000", major health gains have been realized throughout the world. Life expectancy has increased, infant mortality rates decreased and access to health services has also improved. Despite these gains, the world faces significant political, economic, environmental, social and demographic challenges as well as technological opportunities in future.

In the inter-regional meeting held in Geneva from 26th to 30th August, 1996, the progress of Health-for-all was reviewed and the target date was renewed from AD 2000 to AD 2025. Sharp inequalities in health and wealth remain, even within many countries and these together with changes in other determinants of health, will affect future health status.

In the consultative document for the above Geneva meet **(Table 1)** major depression was considered as the top disease of the developing countries including India by AD 2025.

Chapter 19: Mental Health and Mental Illness

Table 1: The top five causes of burden of disability in developing countries (Projection for AD 2025).

Causes	Rank	Percentage of burden in developing countries	Change between AD 1990 (%)
Major depression	1	88	92
Road traffic accidents	2	90	161
Ischemic heart disease	3	78	168
Chronic obstructive pulmonary disease	4	91	123
Cerebrovascular disease	5	84	111

National Mental Health Program for India

For the implementations of Alma-Ata Declaration of Health-for-all by AD 2000, the Central Council of Health Program in its meeting held from 18th to 20th August, 1982 recommended:

a. Mental health must form an integral part of the total health program of India.
b. In all training courses for medical professionals, mental health education will be an integral part.

The program will have three components: (a) Treatment, (b) Rehabilitation, and (c) Promotion of positive mental health.

The mental hospitals, medical colleges, and mental health institutions shall be linked together into the national grid for mental health care. Specific psychiatric services will be provided at district level.

Role of Nurses

In the implementation of the above program, the role of the nurses especially trained in mental health is very important. The nurses working in primary health centers have the responsibility of educating the rural masses by making them understand the importance of preventing mental illness and also considering mental illness as something to be cured by medical treatment and not to go for traditional methods.

Nurses will also give counseling services for problems, such as alcoholism, and drug abuse.

SHARED RESPONSIBILITY

Reaching the Health-for-all in the 21st century is the shared responsibility of everyone. World Health Organization has the unique responsibility as the international organization whose mandate is solely concerned with human health, to mobilize and promote global support for this to be universally achieved. Action in support of this vision will move us toward a world in which human rights are respected, global health equity is achieved, and all people are able to enjoy the highest attainable state of health.

COUNSELING

Counseling is a helping service. The essential nature of counseling consists in helping individuals to help themselves.

It is, therefore, different from advising when the individual becomes dependent on the advisor and not self-directed.

Some adolescents and youth develop a feeling of inadequacy, inferiority and lack of self-confidence as they grow up. Some young men and women show these deficiencies openly and may overreact. They may cover up their feeling of inferiority and lack of self-esteem by acting aggressively or withdrawing and showing no interest in things that should concern them the most.

Counseling is the psychotherapy to help such individuals suffering from mild mental difficulties. The counselor plays a dynamic role in not only sympathetically understanding the problem himself but in making the individual understand the problem clearly. More often than not, individuals who experience problems or who report problems do not really understand them fully. We cannot see ourselves as others see us. This is the greatest weakness of individuals. They do not have the necessary patience and maturity for such a calm and collected examination of the problem. They cannot be dispassionate, because they are involved in the problem. The counselor, on the other hand, can take a more dispassionate and objective view of the problem as he is not directly involved in the situation.

The individual is helped to help himself through counseling. It means that the solution for the problem should be one discovered by the subject himself. This makes the problem of implementation easy. When a solution is suggested by an outsider, it is not one's own solution and therefore remains something outside one's own personality. But when the solution is found from one's own personality resources as in counseling, the solution is very much one's own and not foreign or alien.

Characteristics of a Counselor

a. Empathy,
b. Genuineness, and
c. Unconditional acceptance.

By providing an atmosphere of trust and confidence, the counselor can patiently listen to the young men/women who dissent and protest and exhibit aggressive behavior. By talking with them the counselor helps them to examine their own concept of themselves and makes them feel the need for building a positive self-concept. Even the worst criminals would not like to think of themselves as dirty, ugly, or evil individuals. Everyone would like to consider himself/herself as good. They would like to have a positive self-concept. The counselor can take advantage of this aspect of human nature, invite the youth (or anyone needing counseling-services) to look into themselves without the fear of criticism or being ridiculed, bring out their true self and encourage them to do something to change the picture of their personality.

Counseling, thus, helps the individual to understand himself both in terms of his strengths and weaknesses and gives understanding of the world and act on them. Through this verbal communication, the patient's mind becomes lightened of its load of various painful thoughts with guilt feeling. This technique involves the counselor's patient hearing of the patient's outpourings, without any comment of his own. From the point of view of mental hygiene, if we have indulged in some shameful activities, it is best for us to understand them rather than pretend that we have never done them.

Every patient mental or otherwise must be helped by the counselor to face facts.

Characteristics of Guidance and Counseling in Educational Institutions

Guidance is not direction. It is not the imposition of one's point of view upon another. It is not making decisions for an individual which he should make for himself. It is not carrying the burden of another's life. Rather guidance is assistance made available by competent counselors to an individual of any age to help him direct his own life, develop his own point of view, make his own decisions and carry his own burdens.

An analysis of the above viewpoints shows that guidance has the following main characteristics:

1. **It is a process:** It helps every individual to help himself to recognize and use his inner resources, to set goals, to make plans, to work out his own problems of development.
2. **It is a continuous process:** It is needed right from childhood, adolescence, adulthood, and in old age.
3. **Choice and problem points are the distinctive concerns of guidance:** The individual's unique world of perception interacts with the external order of wants in his life.
4. **It is assistance to the individual in the process of development rather than a direction of that development:** The aim is to develop the capacity for self-direction, self-guidance, and self-improvement through an increasing understanding of his problems and his resources as well as limitations to solve the problem.
5. **Guidance is a service meant for all:** It is a regular service which is required at every stage for all students; not only for awkward situations and abnormal students. It is a positive program geared to meet the needs of all students.
6. **It is both a generalized and a specialized service:** It is generalized service because every one—teachers, tutors, advisors, deans, parents—play a part in the program. It is a specialized service because specially qualified personnel as counselors, psychiatrists, and psychologists join hands to help the individual to get out of his problem.

Difference between Guidance and Counseling

Very few terms have been more loosely or interchangeably used than the terms "guidance" and "counseling".

Guidance is the total program or all the activities and services engaged in by an educational institution that is primarily aimed at assisting an individual to make and carry out adequate plans or to achieve satisfactory adjustment in all aspects of his daily life. Guidance is not teaching, but it may be done by teachers. It is not separate from education but is an essential part of total educational program. Guidance is a term which is broader than counseling and which includes counseling as one of its services.

In another logical separation, counseling is defined as having two phases—one "adjustive" and the other "distributive". In the adjustive phase, the emphasis is on the social, personal and emotional problems of the individual, whereas in the distributive phase, the focus is upon his educational, vocational, and occupational problems. In that case, distributive phase can be called "guidance" and adjustive phase as "counseling".

Key Points

+ A healthy individual is not only physically healthy but also mentally healthy.
+ Mental health is also determined by the way our basic needs are satisfied especially in our childhood.
+ Guidance is the distributive phase and counseling is the adjustive phase.

STUDY QUESTIONS

Long Essays

1. Characteristics of a mentally healthy person.
2. Foundations of mental health.

Short Essays

1. National mental health program for India.
2. Role of nurses in promoting mental health.
3. Counseling and guidance for nurses.

Short Answers

1. Guidance.
2. Counseling.
3. Skills required for a counselor.

Multiple Choice Questions

1. Who is called the Father of Modern Psychiatry?
   a. Beers			b. Pinel
   c. Lyndae			d. Gall
2. _____ started the mental hygiene movement.
   a. Dorothea Lyndae		b. Clifford Beers
   c. Paul Beatrice		d. Jack Springer
3. When individual separates themselves from their real personalities to avoid stress and responsibility, it is referred to as _____ disorder.
   a. Somatoform		b. Personality
   c. Affective			d. Dissociative

4. A specialized service whose primary concern is with the individual and to help them to solve their problems.
   a. Teaching
   b. Learning
   c. Advice
   d. Guidance
5. What is/are useful in a therapist/client relationship?
   a. Trust
   b. Warmth
   c. Acceptance
   d. All of the above

20. Psychological Tests: Measurement of Individual Differences

Chapter Outline

- Psychological Tests
- Individual Differences
- Rating Scales
- Intelligence Tests
- Aptitude Tests
- Personality Tests
- Achievement Tests
- Halo Effect
- Reliability
- Validity

Learning Objective

Students will be familiarized about the types and psychometric properties of psychological tests

INTRODUCTION

The purpose of psychological tests is to get the right persons for right jobs. Some of the most interesting things about people cannot be seen by a casual observer. Attitudes, personality characteristics, and abilities cannot be viewed directly. Psychological tests help us to observe people's behavior in a systematic way. A psychological test is a structured technique used to generate a carefully selected sample of behavior. This behavior sample is used in turn to make inferences about the psychological attributes of the people who have been tested—attributes, such as intelligence, aptitudes, attitudes and many abilities and personality traits. The purpose of psychological tests is to get the right people to the right place.

KINDS OF PSYCHOLOGICAL TESTS

1. Speed test versus power test (task oriented, no time limit), e.g., assignments,

2. Group test versus individual test,
3. Verbal test versus nonverbal test (minimum language), and
4. Paper-pencil (written) test versus performance test.

Classification of Tests as per Functions they Measure

1. **Intelligence tests:**
   a. Stanford-Binet test
   b. Raven's progressive matrices (used in selecting nurses)
   c. Bhatia's battery of performance tests of intelligence
2. **Aptitude tests:** Aptitude is innate potential or capacity or ability, e.g., Differential aptitude test (DAT) for counseling high school students and non-college adults.
3. **Achievement tests:** Term ending examinations
4. **Personality tests (for assessment of personality):**
   a. Self-reported or open reports
   b. Rating Scales
   c. Questionnaires
      – The Bell adjustment inventory
      – Minnesota Multiphasic Personality Inventory (MMPI)
      – RB Cattell's 16 personal factors test (1965) (measures 16 personality factors)
      – Eysenck's personality questionnaires (1970) (measures the personality scales psychoticism, extraversion and neuroticism)
   d. Projective tests
      – Rorschach ink blot test
      – Thematic apperception test (TAT) by HA Murray
      – Sentence completion test
      – Word association test
   e. Performance tests (accuracy, speed, perseverance, manual dexterity are some of the personality characteristics for which performance tests have been designed)
   f. Situational tests
   g. Interviews

Personality description of a student nurse is usually by open reports and rating by ward sisters. Open reports are widely relied on as it is assumed that ward sisters know their student nurses well. One method is using blank paper and writing whatever appears important to the reporter. The method will highlight the student's faults and merits. Its overall tone gives an indication of the students' general ability. Examples and episodes may also be mentioned. There are three serious drawbacks, in this method. It is possible for a ward sister to leave out statements about large areas of students' personality. Another drawback is the emphasis each sister places on those aspects which to her appear to be of particular importance. One ward sister may always comment on tidiness and punctuality; another ward sister may only write about ability to teach others or to cooperate. This bias makes comparison of successive reports difficult.

"Halo effect" is another drawback. Any one outstanding characteristic may influence the opinion of the reporter to such an extent that the whole report is colored by it, e.g., he is kind, so he must be honest!

Rating scale: The above difficulties are overcome by making the report in the form of a rating scale.

The reporter is given a number of headings and asked to state the degree to which the characteristic is present in the student.

The question of punctuality must always be filled in because the heading already appears on the paper. The ward sister has to rate each item on the report on a five-point rating scale, meaning that the student nurse is:
1. Always punctual,
2. Usually punctual,
3. Average in punctuality,
4. Frequently unpunctual, and
5. Always unpunctual.

On some report forms the questions are all set out and the ward sister ticks the answer which applies. This makes it possible to give detailed examples of what is meant by rating. For example:
- Her work is always accurately done without any need to supervise.
- She usually works accurately; occasionally asks for guidance.
- She works well with only cursory supervision.
- She works well only when supervised.
- She does nothing at all unless closely supervised.

Rating scale can be used for assessing the work of any subordinate in any organization. It is particularly useful in reporting a patient's progress and particularly on the behavior, attitudes, and interests of mentally ill patients.

Interviewing: Appearance, bearing, and speech of the candidate can be noticed, during an interview. Questions can be asked about attitudes and interests. Answers may even reveal the interviewee's emotional approach. Interviewing can be very effective, provided it is well-prepared and questions asked cover a wide area in order to make possible an assessment of all aspects of personality.

There are some drawbacks. Interviews take place in stressful circumstances and great skill is needed to put the person who is interviewed at ease. Interviewer's gestures, eye contact, facial expression, attitude of approval or disapproval may influence the answers. People often try to give the answer they think may be the expected one. In business, the interviews are conducted over lunch and a more relaxed atmosphere.

The seven-point plan (Roger, 1974) is the most widely used plan for job interview to select a candidate for a job:
1. Physical characteristics or abilities which are important to the job, e.g., good health, vision, hearing, and speech.
2. Attainments include education, professional background.
3. Overall general ability—general intelligence.
4. Special aptitudes, e.g., social skills. Though at an interview for student-nurse selection, this is difficult, as a young person needs time to develop social attitudes.
5. Interests which are occupationally significant and how they are pursued, e.g., intellectual, physical and social pursuits.
6. Personality attributes, such as self-perception, reliability, and sociability.
7. Financial circumstances—not important for a nursing student if the training is free.

PREREQUISITES OF A TEST: RELIABILITY AND VALIDITY

Reliability is the internal self-consistency of a test. It means that repeated administration of a test will give the same result. This is like a thermometer which would show the same reading on successive occasions if the temperature had not changed.

Validity indicates truth. The test must in fact measure something which it is intended to measure. A thermometer may always read 100°C but it would not be valid because it would not have taken notice of the temperature changes outside. A question paper in psychology should contain questions from topics given in the syllabus only and should not have questions say from sociology or any other subject. A reliable test need not always valid but a valid test is always reliable.

Chapter 20: Psychological Tests: Measurement of Individual...

Key Points ● ● ● ●

- A psychological test is a structured technique used to generate a carefully selected sample of behavior.
- Psychological tests can be classified based on nature and as per the functions they measure.
- Reliability is the internal self-consistency of a test.
- Validity means the test is to measure what it is intended to measure.

STUDY QUESTIONS

Short Essays

1. Classification of tests as per function they measure.
2. Prerequisites of a test.

Short Answers

1. Rating scale.
2. Halo effect.
3. Kinds of psychological tests.

Multiple Choice Questions

1. Which of the following is not a projective test?
    a. Word association test
    b. Rorschach's inkblot test
    c. Thematic Apperception test
    d. Sentence completion test

2. What is the correct meaning of psychological test?
    a. Psychological test measure traits/abilities
    b. Psychological test is a standardized measure of sample of behavior
    c. Psychological test is only a qualitative measure of behavior
    d. Psychological test is only a quantitative measure of behavior

3. A test in which there is generous time limit so that most examinees are able to attempt it is known as:
    a. Speed test
    b. Power test
    c. Verbal test
    d. Nonverbal test

4. The major feature of nonverbal test is that:
    a. It contains pictorial items
    b. It has manipulative items

c. It contains only verbal items
d. It contains both pictorial and manipulative items

5. _____ measures what the test purports to measure.
   a. Reliability   b. Standardization
   c. Validity   d. Objectivity

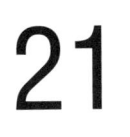

21 Attributions: Our Explanations of Behavior

Chapter Outline

- Attributions
- Internal Attributions
- External Attributions
- Attributional Analysis
- Fundamental Attribution Error
- Self-serving Bias

Learning Objective

Students will be introduced to the concept, types and errors of attribution.

INTRODUCTION

Why do people do the things they do? To answer this question, we make attributions, that is, we assign or attribute causes to explain the behavior of others as well as to explain our own behavior. We are particularly interested in the causes when behaviors are unexpected, when goals are not attained and when actions are not socially desirable.

Although, we can actually observe behavior, we can only infer its causes. Whenever we try to determine why we or someone else behaved in a certain way, we can attribute or assign internal or external reasons.

Attributions are things we point to as the causes of events, other people's behaviors or our own behavior. Attributes are characteristic traits, intentions, and abilities inferred on the basis of observed behavior, an aspect of social perception.

A famous social psychologist, Fritz Heider believed that we all function to some extent like social psychologists as we try to explain everyday behaviors. Heider was the first to distinguish between internal and external causes or attributions of behavior.

PAN POSTHEMA'S CASE

After 13 seasons and 200 games in minor leagues, Pan Posthema was not promoted to be umpire in major baseball leagues. She filed a discrimination suit against professional baseball in America because she felt that baseball was not ready for a woman umpire, however efficient. If you had to explain why there is no female umpires, you would assign internal and external attributions to their behavior.

External (situational) attributions are explanation of behavior based on external circumstances or situations. They are sometimes called situational attributions.

If you used external attributions to explain why Posthema was not promoted, you would point to external circumstances such as saying that major baseball leagues are run by men and they do not want a woman umpire. Internal (dispositional) attributions are explanations of behavior based on the internal characteristics or disposition of the person performing the behavior. They are sometimes called dispositional attributions.

For example, if you used internal characteristics (attributions) to explain why Posthema was not made a major league umpire, you would point to her personal characteristics or dispositions, such as saying that she was not a good judge of balls and strikes.

Using internal or dispositional attributions to explain Posthema's lack of promotion results in very different reason compared with external or situational attribution.

Although, we can actually observe behavior, we usually can only infer its causes. Whenever we try to determine why we or someone else behaved in a certain way, we can make situational attribution (an external attribution) and attribute the behavior to some external cause or factor operating within the situation.

Thus, after failing in an examination one might say "the test was unfair", or "the professor did not teach the material well" or we might make a dispositional attribution (an internal attribution) and attribute the behavior to some internal cause, such as personal trait, motive, or attitude. We might attribute a poor performance to our own lack of ability or to a poor memory.

ATTRIBUTIONAL BIASES: DIFFERENT ATTRIBUTION FOR OURSELVES AND OTHERS

There are basic differences in the way we make attributions about our own behavior and that of others. We tend to make situational attributions to express our own behavior, because we are aware of the factors in the situation that influenced us to act as we did. Also being aware of our past behavior, we know whether our reactions are typical or atypical.

When we try to explain the behavior of other people however, we focus more on them personally than the facts operating within the situation. Not knowing how they have behaved in different situations in the past, we assume a consistency in the behavior. Thus, we are likely to attribute the behavior to some personal quality. The tendency to overemphasize internal factors and underemphasize situational factors is so common and fundamental that it has been named the fundamental attribution error.

In the USA, the plight of the homeless and people on welfare is often attributed to laziness, an internal attribution, rather than to factors in their situation that might explain their condition. However, the fundamental attribution error is not universal. In India, for example, middle class adults tend to make situational attributions for deviant behavior, attributing it to "role, status or caste and kin structures", rather than to internal dispositional causes and blame our failures on external or situational causes. If we interview for a job and get, it is because we have the right qualifications. If someone else gets the job, it is because he or she knows the right people. Self-serving bias allows us to take credit for our successes and shift the blame for our failure to the situation.

CHANGING ATTRIBUTIONS

Research was conducted in the USA on freshmen who had academic problems, such as scoring poorly in examinations, not submitting assignment as per schedule, and considering dropping out of the course. These students were divided into two equally talented and similar groups, (a) Experimental group, and (b) Control group.

The experimental group (attributions group) were given a number of procedures that changed their attributions about their poor performance from a permanent cause to only a temporary condition.

For example, students in the experimental group read a booklet about previous freshmen who had similar academic problems but showed improvement later in the college. The experimental group watched videotapes of senior students who described very convincingly how their grade point averages had risen after their freshman year. Next the experimental group were asked to write down all the reasons they could think of why grade point averages might increase after the freshmen year. The other group who also had academic problems, did not receive any of this information and served as the control group.

RESULTS AND CONCLUSION

Experimenters found that by changing students' attributions for poor academic performance from permanent to temporary had two significant effects:
1. Freshmen who were told how to attribute their academic problems to temporary conditions had a significant improvement in grade point averages 1 year after completion of this program.
2. Only 5% of the freshmen who changed their attribution for poor academic performance from permanent to temporary dropped out of the college while 20% of those in the control group dropped out.

FACTORS INFLUENCING ATTRIBUTIONS

1. **Distinctiveness:** The extent to which the person behaves in the same way in similar situations. For example, if Alison only smokes when she is out with friends, her behavior is high in distinctiveness. If she smokes at any time or place, distinctiveness is low.
2. **Consistency**: The extent to which the person behaves like every time the situation occurs. For example, if Alison only smokes when she is out with friends, consistency is high. If she only smokes on one special occasion, consistency is low.
3. **Consensus**: The extent to which other people behave in the same way in a similar situation. For example, Alison smokes a cigarette when she goes out for a meal with her friend. If her friend smokes, her behavior is high in consensus. If only Alison smokes it is low.

High consistency, low distinctiveness and low consensus—internal attribution.

High distinctiveness and consensus, low consistency—external attribution.

MODIFYING OUR ATTRIBUTES

To avoid the common errors in attributing others behavior, we should modify our attributes for accurate judgment. The following points may be remembered in this connection:
a. We should process the information in a logical way.
b. Think that to err is human. We may be wrong and others right.
c. All of us have many positive and negative characteristics.
d. Consider both dispositional and situational causes to explain our behavior.
e. Try to collect as much information as possible. Avoid overemphasizing others behavior with dispositional causes. Examine the environmental causes also.

ATTRIBUTIONS AND THE NURSE

The nurse who attempts to assess the patients attributes in order to plan appropriate care, herself brings into the situation her own complex attributes system. Her studies and her knowledge will affect her attributes to the patient's illness, her previous nursing experience influences her attitude to hospital, treatment, staff, and patients.

When nurse and patient meet, the behavior of each is the result of his own and other person's attributes.

Attributional analysis: One interesting way of analyzing situation is "attributional analysis". Whenever we interact with another person, our behavior to him depends on the kind of person we think he is and how we think he will behave toward us. At the same time, his behavior depends upon the expectations that he has, of our behavior. Both parties to an interpersonal encounter are constrained by the extent to which they attribute to the other abilities, intentions, attitudes, power, and responsibility.

When a nurse describes a patient, she may be trying to keep herself out of the picture, but it is unlikely that, interviewed by any other nurse, the picture of the patient would have emerged the same. The nurse makes an "internal" attribution if she believes that the patient would have behaved the same way, had the situation been different. She makes an "external" attribution, if she considered how much her own behavior has affected the patient. It is important that nurses learn to observe themselves in their interactions with the patient. To see oneself on videotape can be very revealing.

Key Points ● ● ● ●

+ Attribution refers to the process by which the individual assign causes to the behavior he/she conceives.
+ Attribution theory was developed by Fritz Heider 1958 extended by Kelly.
+ Attribution is influenced by factors of distinctiveness, consensus, and consistency.
+ Internal attribution is assigning the cause of behavior to some internal characteristic, rather than to outside forces.
+ External attribution is assigning the cause of behavior to some situation or event outside a person's control rather than to some internal characteristic.
+ Fundamental error and self-serving bias are common attribution errors.

STUDY QUESTIONS

Short Answers

1. Attribution factors.
2. Errors in attribution.

Multiple Choice Questions

1. The process of assigning causes of behavior, both your own and that of others is called_____.
   a. Perception
   b. Attribution
   c. Attitude
   d. Motivation

2. According to Kelley's Attribution Theory, if a person's behavior varies across different situations, his behavior is said to have _____.
   a. Low distinctiveness
   b. High consensus
   c. Low consensus
   d. High distinctiveness

3. Which of the following is correct regarding situational attribution?
   a. Situational attribution occurs when there is high consensus, high consistency, and high distinctiveness
   b. Situational attribution occurs when there is low consensus, high consistency, and high distinctiveness
   c. Situational attribution occurs when there is high consensus, low consistency, and high distinctiveness
   d. Situational attribution occurs when there is low consensus, low consistency and low distinctiveness

4. When are people relatively less likely to exhibit the fundamental attribution error (or correspondence bias)?
   a. When forming attributions about people they know well
   b. When forming attributions about the self
   c. Both a and b
   d. Neither a nor b
5. A teacher making the fundamental attribution error would attribute a student's poor test grade to:
   a. Her failure to teach the material clearly
   b. Personal conflict in the student's home
   c. The students lack of motivation
   d. The difficulty of the test material

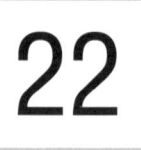

22. Educational Psychology: Scope and Methods

"Education is something which makes an individual self-reliant and selfless"
—**Rig Veda**

"By education, I mean an all-round drawing out of the best in the child and man—body, mind and spirit"
—**Mahatma Gandhi**

"Education is the manifestation of divine perfection already existing in man"
—**Swami Vivekananda**

"Education means enabling the mind to find out the ultimate truth, making truth its own and giving expression to it."
—**Tagore**

Chapter Outline

- Educational Psychology
- Education Goals
- Learner
- Learning Process
- Sociometry
- Observation
- Case Study
- Questionnaire
- Inventory
- Remedial Education

Learning Objectives

♦ Students will be introduced to the field of educational psychology.
♦ Students will be aware of methods in educational psychology.

EDUCATION

Education is a social process by which the innate capacities of an individual are drawn out and he/she is adjusted to the society in which he/she lives. Thus, it is a two-fold process of growth of personality and enhancement of the degree of adjustability to the surroundings. The basic aim of education is to modify behavior.

PSYCHOLOGY

Psychology is the science of human behavior. It attempts to analyze and interpret human behavior in diverse situations in life. It bases itself on a keen examination of human experience and arrives at conclusions on human behavior. It studies the physical, mental, emotional, and social traits of an individual.

Pestalozzi, the great Swiss educationalist, was the first to point out that the mind of the pupil is the primary concern of the teacher. Since then, other educationalists have stressed the importance of the knowledge of child development, principles of learning and principles of mental hygiene for improving one's work as a teacher.

Education is normative in its outlook, since it is concerned with aims, ideals, values, and standards. On the other hand, psychology is a positive science, trying to ascertain the facts of behavior, how it is developed and how it is modified. Two general aims of education are social and the individual.

Long ago Whitehead distinguished between a craft and a profession. A craft is based on customary activities and it is modified by trial and error with course of practice. On the other hand, a profession is one when the activities are subjected to theoretical analysis. Psychology helps in educational research.

The three ways in which the study of educational psychology benefits the teacher, are as follows:
1. It will enable him to understand the students for whose benefit he/she has been employed and for whom the college organization is existing.
2. This realization will give him/her greater power to mold the students in the definite direction of their educational goals.
3. Educational psychology will help him/her to understand himself/herself, his/her strength and weakness and make him/her adjust to the college environment completely.

Psychology has contributed a great deal toward the improvement of the processes and products of education. Theories of learning, motivation, personality development, etc. have been always helpful to shape and design educational systems to meet the needs of students. Educational psychologists have contributed a lot for improving teaching methods, preparation of curriculum, lesson plans, time tables, and training aids.

EDUCATIONAL PSYCHOLOGY

Educational psychology is an applied branch of general psychology dealing with the application of psychological principles in the field of education. It deals with the learning process of an individual, in the light of his physical, mental, emotional, and social traits. It is a combination of the study of the individual and the study of the environment that affect the learning process. It helps the teacher to foster harmonious overall development of the learner.

Objectives of Educational Psychology

The general objectives of educational psychology are:
a. To provide a body of facts and methods which can be used in solving teaching/learning problems.
b. To develop a scientific and problem solving attitude.
c. To train in thinking psychologically about educational problems.

Teaching Objectives of Educational Psychology

a. To develop an understanding and appreciation of the hereditary and environmental factors which underline learning ability.
b. To provide a base for understanding the nature and principle of learning and to supply the techniques for its improvement.
c. To understand and appreciate factors influencing individual ability to learn.
d. To provide understanding of the external factors, such as training aids, libraries, class rooms which are largely within the control of the teacher and the institution.
e. To evaluate teaching efficiency.
f. To develop an appreciation of the individual (importance of the individuals with their individual differences).

Scope of Educational Psychology

Educational psychology has important applications in the following three areas:
1. Learner,
2. Learning process, and
3. Evaluation of learning process.

Learner: Educational psychology helps in understanding the developmental characteristics of the students, their individual differences in intelligence and personalities, their adjustment abilities and their attitudes toward learning. With the help of educational psychology a teacher is able to understand individual differences and can adjust teaching to the needs and requirements of the class. He/she may also study the factors which are responsible for individual differences. He/she may create conducive environment in the schools where the students can develop their inherent potentialities to the maximum.

Good mental health is very important for efficient learning. The teacher, from the study of psychology can know the various factors which are responsible for the mental ill health and maladjustments. The teacher will also understand the causes of the problems which occur at different age levels and can successfully solve them.

Personality needs of the individual are of major importance to learning readiness. The individual's value system and the controlling influence of intrinsic motivation are very important in learning. Motivation includes achievements motivation, anxiety, self-concepts, and locus of control. The learner must be made self-directed in the pursuit of achievement of knowledge and skills.

Learning process: The knowledge of educational psychology provides the knowledge of learning process in general and the problems of classroom learning in particular.

a. To instruct effectively in the class, the teacher must understand the principles of learning and the various approaches to the learning process, problems of learning and their remedial measures.

   Educational psychology provides us with the knowledge of different approaches and theories to organize classroom teaching to different age groups, with scientifically developed curriculum.

b. The curriculum incorporates the needs of the students, their development characteristics, learning patterns and needs of the society.

   Another important contribution of educational psychology is the organization of special education for the handicapped (exceptional) children.

Evaluation of learning process: With the help of psychological tests, learning outcomes or evaluation of the curriculum are conducted. Measurements of aptitudes and any innovation introduced by the teacher should also be evaluated without delay as immediate feedback and knowledge of results enhance learner's motivation. Evaluation is also important for research studies.

Methods of Educational Psychology

Generally, educational psychology uses similar methods as that of general psychology namely—introspection, observation, experiment, case history, and clinical methods.

Observation

In natural observation, we observe the behavior characteristics of children or adults in natural settings. The subjects do not know that they are being observed, e.g., observation in the ward or in the playground.

Clinical/Case History Method

Some students are not able to perform satisfactorily during their course. Their problems can be studied with clinical methods. The reasons may be emotional problems, such as conflict at home, over anxiety, poor coping skills, or less intelligence. With case history, interview, and psychological tests, problems can be identified and modified to help the students.

Experimental Method

The experimental method is most useful in certain areas of educational psychology, e.g., to study the role of motivation in learning. You will arrange for two groups A and B comparable in age, intellectual level, social economic status and educational background. Both the groups would be given similar learning task but incentive on learning will be given to the experimental group (A) while the control group (B) gets no incentive. Learning outcomes of the two groups are compared to see which group has done better.

Merits of the experimental method are the following:
a. It is most systematic, provides objective, and reliable information.
b. Observations can be made under strictly controlled conditions.
c. Findings are verifiable by other investigators under identical conditions in which original experiment was conducted.
d. Cause-effect relationship can be studied and provides guidelines to solve teaching and learning problems.

Limitations: Experimental methods are mainly centered around controlled conditions in which it is conducted. It is often not feasible to strictly study human beings under controlled conditions. It is not only undesirable but legally and ethically not permissible to control human beings in certain ways or tamper with their psychological functioning or subject them to certain social, physiological and psychological conditions of deprivation. Another problem is cost-effectiveness in terms of time and money.

Inventory or Questionnaire Method

Different kinds of questionnaires or inventories are developed and standardized. The most important of them used in the fields of education are the interest, aptitude, attitude, and personality tests. Strong's Vocational Interest Blank (SVIB) for men and women is a very useful device to assess the interests of pupils and young people. The information can be used in vocational guidance and career planning. Aptitude tests are used in helping the young people to discover their potentialities and promises in different areas and activities of work, e.g., Differential Aptitude Tests (DAT) and the General Aptitude Test Battery (GATB). For educational guidance, the Scholastic Aptitude Tests (SAT) are widely used.

Sociometry

This method, introduced by the American Psychologist Moreno, has very large application and use in classroom and out of the classroom situations in the school. The method consists of asking the pupils in the class to choose three pupils from their class whom they like the best and with whom they like to work in the order of preference. Similarly, they are also asked to give names of three classmates whom they dislike and with whom they do not like to work. Individual preferences and dislikes are thus obtained and a sociogram prepared.

With the help of the sociogram, the teacher can effectively organize group work and other team activities. Sociogram is a good index of classroom climate. It will indicate whether there are any major cliques or divisions in the class. It will help the teacher to take necessary steps to remedy the situation, before it leads to serious rivalries and problem of discipline.

Special education: There are many children with handicaps, such as vision, hearing, speech and language, mental retardation, and emotional problems. Special education provides appropriate educational assistance to handicapped children. It offers a continuous form of special teaching for children who need either special environment, special medical treatment, special methods of teaching, or special curriculum. For handicapped children, special education is needed for most of their school life. For some others, it may be required, only during the period of months or years when their illness is being treated.

Remedial education: It is normally part time, relatively short-term and limited to learning some school subjects in which the child is weak.

Compensatory education: It involves modification of curriculum, methods of teaching, educational social work required by pupils whose development has been retarded by cultural and social limitations.

Significance of Educational Psychology to Nursing

The study of educational psychology will help the student nurse to study more effectively, improve her memory and understand the individual differences between students. With understanding of her capacity she can plan her academic achievements. If aspirations are set too high without matching capabilities, the result will be frustration due to failure. If the goals are lower than the capacity, then the motivation will be lowered and there would be no challenges to meet.

It will also help her understand and to develop positive attitudes toward patients and nursing care, problems of other people and in accepting newer technology.

It would prepare the nursing students to be future teachers, understanding the students and their problems and teach more effectively with a better understanding of the advancements in educational technology.

Key Points

- Educational psychology deals with the application of psychological principles in the field of education.
- Educational psychology has various methods to do research.
- Sociometry was introduced by Moreno.
- Special education provides appropriate educational assistance to handicapped children.

STUDY QUESTIONS

Short Essays

1. Teaching objectives of educational psychology.
2. Scope of educational psychology.
3. Methods of educational psychology.
4. Significance of educational psychology for nurses.

Short Answers

1. Education.
2. Psychology.
3. Sociometry.
4. Differentiate between educational psychology and developmental psychology.
5. Educational psychology.

Chapter 22: Educational Psychology: Scope and Methods

Multiple Choice Questions

1. Educational psychology applies knowledge of psychology in the field of:
   a. Psychology
   b. Industrial
   c. Social sciences
   d. Education

2. The primary aim of educational psychology is:
   a. To contribute to an understanding of sound educational practices
   b. To provide the academic background essential for effective teaching
   c. To provide a theoretical framework for educational research
   d. To provide the teacher with great appreciation of their role in the child's education

3. What is a case study?
   a. Study of historic movement
   b. In depth investigation of a single person, group or community
   c. Addition of knowledge
   d. Studies the events in planned manner

4. The observer becomes a part of the group, which type of observation is this?
   a. Artificial
   b. Naturalistic
   c. Participant
   d. Non-participant

5. Teacher should study education psychology so that:
   a. Easily impress the student
   b. Understand oneself
   c. Make teaching more effective
   d. To create learning materials

23

Effective Teaching

Chapter Outline

- Education Process
- Teacher
- Learner
- Lesson Plan
- Curriculum Appraisal

Learning Objectives

♦ Students will be introduced to different effective teaching methods
♦ Students will be oriented to teacher-student communication process

EDUCATION AS A PROCESS OF COMMUNICATION

Introduction

Communication in simple words implies communication of ideas. It is a process in which the students and the teacher act and interact between themselves and with one another. It is, therefore, evident that three elements are required for any communication to take place. These are as follows:
1. Source also called the *Encoder*,
2. Message also called the *Signal*, and
3. Destination also called the *Decoder*.

For effective communication, the teacher and students must know what to impart, why and what to receive. The teacher must have the correct information and transmit accurately and at the optimum speed. The receiver must understand it and add the knowledge as a meaningful addition to his/her communication skill. It is essentially a sharing process or an interaction of minds.

Ingredients in Education Process

Why, what and how are the three ingredients of communications:
- Why connotes the *motive,*
- What indicates the *matter,* and
- How implies the *method.*

Motive

The teacher must be clear in his/her mind what his/her motive is or he/she should know what exactly he/she wishes to teach during the lesson. Otherwise he/she will develop a tendency to digress. The student should also be told what he/she is going to learn and why. The fact why the things he/she is going to learn would be important to him/her should also be explained.

Matter

Before facing the class, the teacher must prepare his/her lessons, fully prepared material to be taught to the class should be available with the teacher. If the teacher has the material with him/her, he/she builds up confidence in himself/herself and enhances the confidence of the class. This plays an important role in imparting instruction effectively.

Method

A particular lesson can be taught by different methods. If the proper method is used, the students' interest will be maintained and they will be all set to receive the communication from the teacher. Let us take, for example, a lesson on "X-ray". If the lesson is taught with the help of an X-ray machine and X-ray film and other teaching aids, the impression formed by the students will be clear. Otherwise the lesson will not be learned effectively by the student. A good teacher should always prefer the best method suited to a given topic.

Barriers of Communication in Education

- Referent confusion,
- Day dreaming,
- Time and space,
- Individual differences,
- Physical discomfort,
- Atmosphere,
- Lack of interest in studies,
- Verbalism,
- Increasing population in schools,
- Changing curricula, and
- Radio, TV, and cinema.

Teaching and Internal Factors Influencing Behavior

Teacher's Problems

In the process of teaching problems faced by teachers fall into two main parts:
1. Presentation of the matter to make the greatest impression on student's mind
2. Follow-up measures to retain these impressions

How to Make Impressions?

Before going about attempting to make the impressions, the teacher has to ensure the preparedness of the mind of the learner to receive the information by assessing the following:
- The internal needs of the learner
- The external stimuli required

Needs of Learner

The internal needs of the taught, as of any human being, in the order of importance from the point of view of the individual are given below:
- **Physical:** The most compelling of all needs, such as food, sleep, air, water, bodily comforts, clothing, protection, etc.
- **Security and safety:** The desire to avoid danger or hurt to the body and mind.
- **Belongingness:** The need for affection—which in simple words means the desire to be petted or fondled, but also includes the love that is generated by belonging to a group.
- **Self-esteem or self-regard:** The desire to be recognized.
- **Self-realization:** The urge to be creative and express oneself.

It is no use trying to teach a person anything if some of these needs within him/her are so strong that he/she cannot think of anything else but satisfying them. If he/she is hungry, thirsty, cold, wet or extremely tired, or if he/she is frightened, nervous or worried, or lacks a feeling of belongingness, he/she will not be in a state to learn. Hence, it is paramount that these needs are reasonably satisfied.

After the internal needs are satisfied, external stimuli; by the way of motivation, are provided by impressing on the learner the need to learn.

External Factors Influencing Behavior and Strengthening of Impressions

Having thus satisfied the internal needs of the learner to the extent he/she is prepared to receive what is taught, the next task of the teacher is to present the matter to the learner so as to make the greatest possible and right impression on the learner's mind. "Stimuli" caused in the brain by what is seen, heard, felt, smelt or tasted set up "traces" leading to the formation, ultimately, of patterns and "forms". The factors affecting the strength of an impression are as follows:

- **Attention:** It governs the depth of the impression or the strength of the traces.
- **Vividness:** Clarity is the second factor on which the strength of a trace depends.
- **Mental imagery:** That dominant sensory faculty which is most appealing to the mind. Depending on the individual, the mental imagery may be visual, auditory or sense of touch, etc. It should be the endeavor of the teacher to appeal to as many senses as possible. Another cardinal rule is that matter must be presented in the form in which it is going to be used.
- **Heterogeneity, homogeneity, and variety:** Heterogeneity of material as well as presentation relieves the class of monotony, speeding up the learning process.
- **Maximum sense appeal:** We must aim at appealing to as many of the senses as possible. We must also make sure that the knowledge or skill is made available in the form in which it will be, by teaching mainly through the sense appeal.

Preparation (Matter)

In preparing the matter, teacher should have:
- Mastery of the subject.
- Adequate background of the subject to give him enough confidence, enable him to answer any question and make his teaching interesting.

After the matter is collected, the teacher has to decide:
- How much is to be taught.
- How much can the class take in.
- How much is absolutely necessary.
- Job analysis of what exactly a man must know to fit himself for his type of job.
- Classification of matter into "Must Know", "Should Know", and "Could Know" points, according to the teacher's target and keeping in mind, the intelligence and capacity to learn of the learners.
- The type of training aids required.
- The method of transmission.
- The manner of testing the assimilation.
- Home assignment.

TRANSMISSION

Steps Involved

Communication involves transmission or presentation and reception. It includes all those activities undertaken by the teacher during the time of his interaction with the learners. It involves the following steps:
a. A good introduction designed to capture interest.
b. A logical development having a series of connected ideas built up into an integral whole. There are five distinct stages in the presentation of a single idea:
 1. *Problem:* Pose a problem and make the learners think.
 2. *Suggestion:* If the problem is put across clearly, the learners will soon be waiting to make suggestions.
 3. *Amplification:* At the right moment amplify the suggestions that are suitable, and build up the lesson.
 4. *Illustration:* By way of training aids.
 5. *Consolidation:* It is necessary to consolidate what has been taught. It is generally done by writing on the wall board, brief statement of essential facts, special terms or definitions, etc.

Methods of Transmission

The primary consideration affecting the selection of the method of transmission is whether the teacher wants the students to acquire:
a. Facts,
b. Skills, and
c. Technique, i.e., application of facts and skills.

The methods of transmission and their characteristics are given below:
a. Lecture
 - It cannot be used for teaching skills.
 - It can be used only for teaching knowledge or facts.
 - Appeals to only one sense, the sense of hearing.
 - No class activity, and no contribution, therefore, toward individual development.
 - Useful for motivating a class by giving an interesting general background to a subject before starting teaching it.
b. Lesson
 - A much more intimate form of instruction than lecture, where the teacher deals with a small number of learners, not >10–15.
 - Greater individual attention is possible.
 - There is scope for individual development.
 - It can be used to teach both knowledge and skills.
 - Both visual and auditory senses can be appealed to.

c. Discussion
   - It cannot normally be satisfactorily used when the learners are in their early stages of learning.
   - In teaching knowledge of facts, once the learners learn certain amount, it is often an excellent way of strengthening or broadening their knowledge, or, of teaching the uses to which the knowledge can be put.
   - Skills cannot be taught.
   - Class is kept mentally active.
   - Not suited to classes larger than 10 or 15 unless the class is divided into syndicates.
d. Demonstration
   - It involves considerable difficulty in putting a demonstration.
   - Normally, follows a lesson or lecture or other form of instruction.

Manner of Transmission

Personal Characteristics: Teacher's Personal Qualities

a. **Bearing:** Has effect even before teaching starts.
   - Dress and carriage have to be clean and tidy, smart and spruce. Carriage has to be scholarly, bright and cheerful.
   - Overenthusiasm is to be avoided to avoid wrong perspective of the subject leading to loss of confidence in the teacher when the learners realize this later.
b. **Voice and manner of speech:** Though a natural gift, can still be improved.
c. **Delivery:**
   - Slow. To enable the thinking of the students to go along with what is spoken.
   - Pause. Raises the expectancy and eagerness of the class and gives the teacher as well as the class time to think. However, too long pauses make the talk monotonous.
   - Emphasis breaks the monotony of speech by repetition of words.
   - Simplicity of language.
   - Meaningless expressions, such as "I see", etc., to be avoided.
   - Provincial accent: To be overcome.
d. **Gestures and mannerisms:** These are to be avoided since more often, than not, they are distracting.

Attitude toward the Class

- **Sarcasm:** To be avoided since it leads to loss of mutual confidence.

- **Favoritism:** Brooks resentment and jealousy, results in loss of respect for the teacher.
- **Unfriendly attitude:** A student should never feel that his/her teacher is hostile toward him/her. The attitude of teacher has to be friendly and firm avoiding familiarity, since familiarity breeds contempt.
- **Bluffing:** Never to be done. In case of more information, the teacher can promise to find out the answer and give it at the earliest opportunity later.
- **Humor:** Of cheap and obscene nature is to be avoided. No special effort should be made to introduce humor.
- **Know the learners:** By name since it evokes greater response.
- **Chasing red herring:** The habit of being diverted from topics by some students. Results in the teacher being led rather than leading the students. The objects of the lesson are to be kept in mind and the teacher has to be firm. Adhere to lesson plan as far as possible.
- **Shooting a line:** To be avoided
- Avoid familiarity
- Loyalty

Assimilation-Questions

Good questioning technique can be used not only to check assimilation but also as a stimulus. Types of question are as follows:
- The rote questions are used to find out the extent of factual knowledge of the learners, e.g., what is the conventional sign of a Church? Which of these antibiotics has the broadest range?
- **Reasoning questions:** Those designed to make the learners reason out for themselves some logical process and understand. These are also meant to arouse curiosity, e.g., what happens when the piston moves? Why is discipline necessary?
- **Rote plus reasoning:** It is combination of the first two types. Learners have to use the knowledge of facts, and in addition, reason out things, e.g., wind is blowing from left to right; a man is walking from right to left 300 m away; where do you aim?

Questions should be:
- **Suitable:** Answers reasonably expected, within the scope and depth of learning by the class, as to test knowledge or skills. They should also be realistic and arouse the curiosity of the class.
- **Clear:** In meaning without ambiguity and asked from the point of view of the students' thinking ability.
- **Simple:** In vocabulary without high-flown jargon.
- **Heard by the whole class:** Both questions and answers, whether from the teacher or from the learners, for the benefit of the whole class.

Chapter 23: Effective Teaching

- **To the class and then the person:** To set the whole mental machinery of the class working.
- **Evenly distributed:** To cover the whole class, with no set pattern of rotation to prevent expectation of turn of questions.

Questions should not be:
- **Fifty-fifty:** Questions which can be answered by a "yes" or "no" or having only two alternatives. This encourages guessing, e.g., is the high-tension switch red or blue? (Correct questioning would be—what is the color of the high-tension switch?).
- **100 to 1 Question** an unfair trap, e.g., the high-tension switch is not red, is it?
- **To test expression or language ability:** Example asking a learner to explain taking the blood pressure when it can be shown practically or drawn.

TRAINING AIDS: VALUE AND CHARACTERISTIC

Introduction

The sophistication and modernity of the equipment being introduced in the medical sciences warrant a quick grasp of subjects starting from fundamentals. This means the need for a better system of imparting a vast amount of knowledge in a short time. The limitations imposed on the teacher in quickening the pace of instruction can be set off with the aid of modern training aids. A training aid is a device or means employed to focus a trainee's attention on a subject or help him in understanding a subject. A training aid helps to stimulate the interest and curiosity, makes a more vivid impression on the learner's mind and saves time.

Value of Training Aids

Training aids are invaluable for teaching because:
- **They sell:** Training aids help us to stimulate interest and curiosity and to maintain the interest and attention of a class. They produce a sense of realism.
- **They stick:** Training aids help to make a more vivid impression, make it remain longer and easy to recall.
- **They simplify:** Training aids help to explain things to a learner and give him that understanding which is vital to learning.
- **They save time:** Training aids save time.
- **They give variety to classroom techniques:** They generally represent a rest from the traditional activities of the school.

- They create an informal atmosphere in the classroom. While using sensory aids, the trainees may move about, talk, laugh, question, comment upon, and in other ways act in a natural manner. The attitude of the teacher is also very friendly and cooperative.
- **They provide with opportunities to handle and manipulate:** An opportunity to touch, feel, handle or operate a model, specimen, picture, map, press a button or turn a crank, gives an added appeal, because it satisfies temporarily at least the natural desire for mastery and ownership.
- They supply the context for sound and skillful generalization. Books lack the specificity, the "warmth" and the clarity of concrete audiovisual experiences, which are provided by training aids.

Essential Characteristics of Training Aids

A visual aid, in particular, must have the following characteristics:
a. **Simple:** It should be quite simple because unnecessary material tends to confuse the issue.
b. **Brief:** It must directly pertain to the subject in view.
c. **Big enough:** So that all can see it in detail.
d. **Interesting:** It must have the capacity to produce a desire to correlate learning and retention.
e. **Realistic:** It must be meaningful and purposeful.
f. **Cost-effective:** It should not be very costly.

CURRICULUM APPRAISAL

What is a *curriculum*? A curriculum is said to be the activities between a teacher and students. The curriculum is the sum total of all the experiences which the student undergoes in a school or college. These are planned activities and experiences which are available to students under the direction of the school and college. A good curriculum is the cooperative effort of students and teacher and it helps to solve the problems which the students face.

To develop curriculum, following important principles should be borne in mind:
- It must base on present need and circumstances of the students (student-centered).
- Curriculum should be dynamic than static.
- Curriculum must provide a rich and concrete experience to the students.
- It should be related to everyday life.

❖ The curriculum should bridge the understanding between teacher and student.
❖ The curriculum should be elastic and flexible and should emphasize attitudes more than skill.
❖ The curriculum should lay emphasis on learning to live rather than on living to learn.
❖ The curriculum should be integrated; continuity of the whole program, uniformity and variety maintained.

The teacher must play an important part in the planning of objectives—the attitudes, skills, and intellectual abilities to be developed. As a teacher, he must select suitable materials and tools and create curriculum so that teaching becomes effective.

LESSON PLAN

A lesson plan is a plan of action of the teacher for his students/learners. It points out what has been already done and in what way pupils should be guided and helped and immediate work to be taken up.

"Careful planning is the foundation of all good teaching."

It enables the teachers to conduct the lesson efficiently by covering the entire subject within the specific time. It guides the teacher to make use of various training aids, such as charts, boards, OHP and models at appropriate time **(Fig. 1)**. The standardization of teaching becomes uniform and guides other staff also to follow the systematic way. Improvement can be achieved as and when modern technology is introduced. It avoids the waste of time and labor of the instructional staff in case of change of syllabus or introduction of latest technology.

Why lesson plan is necessary? Because it performs some specific functions as described here:

a. It forces consideration of:
   - Goals and objectives,
   - Selection of subject matter,
   - Selection of procedure,
   - The planning of activities, and
   - The preparation of test of progress.
b. It keeps the teacher on the track, ensures steady progress and a definite outcome of teaching and learning procedure.
c. It is essential to effective teaching. It requires to look ahead and planning a series of such activities as will progressively modify learner's attitudes, habits, information and abilities in desirable direction.

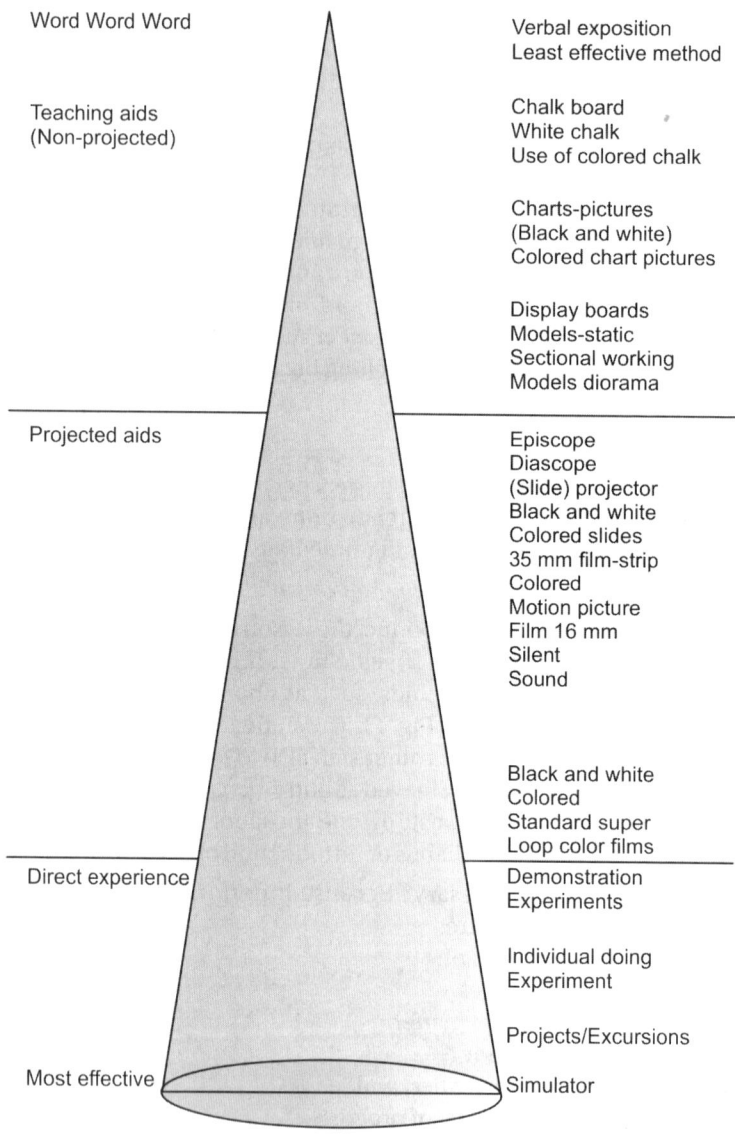

Fig. 1: Relative effectiveness of audiovisual (AV) aids (cone experience).

d. It prevents wastage of time and labor. It helps the teachers to be systematic and orderly. It encourages good organization of the subject matter and activity. It prevents haphazard teaching. It goes a long way toward eliminating disorder and other ills of thoughtless teaching.

e. It helps the teacher to limit the field in which he is teaching. It gives him immediate impetus to realize the aims and objectives set.
f. It encourages proper consideration of the learning process and the choice of appropriate learning procedure. The teacher gains confidence. He employs the best technique to judge the outcome of instructions.
g. It serves as a check on unplanned curriculum. It provides a sensible framework to help the work directing along the lines of the syllabus at a suitable rate. Continuity is achieved in the education process. Needless repetition is avoided.
h. It gives the teacher greater confidence and therefore greater freedom in teaching. It can assure that the teacher does not "dry up" or forget a vital point. It can remind him of the telling phrases, apt quotation or the effective illustrations, at the right moment from the lesson. A specimen lesson plan is appended in **Box 1**.

Box 1: Format of a lesson plan.

Subject: Psychology
Course: Basic BSc (Nursing) I Year
Topic: Emotions
Unit : I
Method of teaching: Lecture cum discussion/role play
Group No:
Audiovisual aids: Blackboard
                     OHP Charts,
                     Slides
Duration : I Hour   Teacher
Date: Designation

Central Objective
The students will be able to understand the different aspects of emotions, appreciate the knowledge, and able to practice the knowledge whenever necessary.

Specific Objectives
1. Define emotions
2. Explain the origin of emotions
3. List down the major types of emotions
4. Illustrate the types of emotions
5. Physiological changes in emotion
6. Give the different theories of emotion
7. Describe the significance of emotions in our life

Contd...

Contd...

Subject: Psychology
Course: Basic BSc (Nursing) I Year
Topic: Emotions
Unit : I
Method of teaching: Lecture cum discussion/role play
Group No:
Audiovisual aids: Blackboard
                    OHP Charts,
                    Slides
Duration : I Hour   Teacher
Date: Designation

Central Objective
The students will be able to understand the different aspects of emotions, appreciate the knowledge, and able to practice the knowledge whenever necessary.

Specific Objectives
1. Define emotions
2. Explain the origin of emotions
3. List down the major types of emotions
4. Illustrate the types of emotions
5. Physiological changes in emotion
6. Give the different theories of emotion
7. Describe the significance of emotions in our life

References
1.
2.
3.

Specific objective	Duration	Content	Teachers activity	Student activity	Evaluation
a. Defines the term emotion	3 minutes	Lesson coverage points in chronological order (must know points underlined)	Show transparency on definition	Observes and writes	How do you define emotions
		Definition of Emotions			
		1.			
		2.			
		3.			
b. Explain the origin of emotions	5 minutes	Origin of Emotion			

Contd...

Contd...

		Historical Background	Chart Presentations	Observer Understands		
c. List down the major types of emotions	4 minutes					
d. Illustrate the types of emotions	10 minutes		Arrangement for role play and introduction	Role play	Ask question	
e.	5 minutes	Physiological changes in emotion	Slides, OHP	Observes and writes	Questions to the class	
f.	10 minutes	Theories of emotions	Slides, charts	Observes and writes		
g.	5 minutes	Emotion and the nurse	Slides, charts	Observes and writes		
h.	5 minutes	How to control emotion	Slides, charts	Observes and understands		
	3 minutes	Recapitulation (summary)		Ask questions to clear doubts		
	3 minutes	Question by the class		Questions		
	2 minutes	Question to the class		Answers		
	2 minutes	Conclusion (Importance of emotions in the lives of patients, their families and nurses and how nurses should control their emotions and lead a balanced life)				
	2 minutes	Home assignments				

Lesson Plan Approved by:

FOR EFFECTIVE HEALTH TEACHING

1. Establish a good relationship with the learner.
2. Select "must know", "should know", and "could know" points. Plan the lesson.
3. Motivate the learner.
4. Teach a little at each time, in phases.
5. Know the learners, their aspirations and needs. Come down to their level. Have empathy with the learners.
6. Communicate clearly and in simple language.
7. Repeat important points to reinforce and reduce forgetting.
8. Use audiovisual aids.
9. Demonstrate and give chance to learner to practice.
10. Check assimilation.

Key Points ● ● ●

+ Motive, matter, and method are three ingredients of communication.
+ The curriculum is the sum total of all the experiences which the student undergoes in a school or college.
+ A lesson plan is a plan of action of the teacher for his students/learners.

STUDY QUESTIONS

Short Essays

1. Ingredients of education process.
2. Curriculum appraisal.
3. Lesson plan.

Short Answers

1. Education process.
2. Needs of learner.
3. Teacher qualities.

Multiple Choice Questions

1. How would an effective teacher help students take on another person's perspective?
    a. They would use role playing
    b. They bring in a guest speaker
    c. They use detailed case studies
    d. They get to know their students

2. Which of the following is the key teaching behaviour to make a teacher effective?
   a. Teacher comments made for the purpose of organising the upcoming teaching process
   b. Use of content or process questions by teacher
   c. Engagement of students in learning process
   d. Using students ideas and contributions

3. Assertion (A): All teaching should aim at ensuring learning.
   Reason (R): All learning results from teaching.
   Choose the correct answer from the following code:
   a. Both (A) and (R) are true, and (R) is the correct explanation of (A).
   b. Both (A) and (R) are true, but (R) is not the correct explanation of (A).
   c. (A) is true, but (R) is false.
   d. (A) is false, but (R) is true.

4. Which of the following learner characteristics is highly related to effectiveness of teaching?
   a. Prior experience of the learner
   b. Educational status of the parents of the learner
   c. Peer groups of the learner
   d. Family size from which the learner comes

5. The best method of teaching is to:
   a. Impart information
   b. Ask students to read books
   c. Suggest good reference material
   d. Initiate a discussion and participate in it

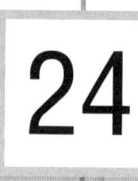

24. Role and Functions of a Teacher

Chapter Outline
- Teacher
- Planning
- Instructions
- Subject Matter
- Teaching Quality
- Student Counselor

Learning Objective

Students will be oriented to roles, functions, and qualities of a good teacher.

INTRODUCTION

Role refers to the behaviors expected of an individual in a given position. Role can also be referred to as a pattern of activity, i.e., what a person has to do (or thinks he has to do) in order to validate the position he holds. A teacher has three different roles:
1. Instructional role,
2. Faculty role, and
3. Individual role.

INSTRUCTIONAL ROLE

Instructional role is the central role or function of a teacher. It involves:
1. Planning and organizing courses
2. Creating and maintaining a desirable group climate which will encourage learning
3. Preparing instructional material of varying interests, needs and abilities of the students
4. Motivating and challenging students to pursue and sustain learning activities

5. Teaching, which consists of:
   - Supplying information needed or telling them where they can be formed
   - Explaining clarifying and interpreting
   - Demonstrating or explaining a procedure
   - Serving as a resource person for individual groups
   - Surprising performance in the classroom, laboratory, and hospitals wards
   - Evaluating the course outcome

FACULTY ROLE

Faculty is the staff of a college or the university. As a member of faculty of college of nursing, the duties of a teacher will include as a:
- Chairman, secretary, or member of one or more committees such on curriculum committee
- Student counselor
- Researcher as and when needed
- Resource person for outside institutions, health agencies
- College representative to professional nursing organizations
- A public relation agent of his institution

INDIVIDUAL ROLE

As a member of the family, community and a citizen, a teacher brings his/her basic dignity and distinct personality into every area where he/she functions.

To assume all the three roles above, he/she needs the necessary educational and professional qualifications and experience in his/her specialty and adequate related experience in other nursing specialties. With his/her experience, he/she should be able to be aware of the different situations the student nurses are likely to meet. He/she should also have excellent communication skills and interpersonal relationships.

QUALITIES OF A GOOD TEACHER

Those who can, do; those who cannot, teach.
—**George Bernard Shaw**

- **A well balanced person:** He knows when to laugh and when to be serious which makes teaching effective.

- **Professionally well groomed:** He has poise, self-confidence, neat, clean and attractive in personal appearance.
- **Kind and patient:** Sincere person, has intense love for old and young people alike. He is never too busy to give a word of encouragement.
- **Tolerant and fair:** No partiality. Always seems to have time to listen whether the class is large or small.
- **Preparation:** Presents lecture outlines to the students which contain objectives and main points of the lesson. Good knowledge of subject matter.
- **Clear exposition of subject matter:** Well-presented lecture so that students can understand the matter fully.
- Good quality voice, clear, distinct, pleasant, and well-modulated.
- **Teaching quality:** Teaches at the level of the students. Students are treated as intelligent and mature. Discussion and questions are encouraged.
- Assignments are given with references to books in the library.
- **Leadership quality:** Personality coupled with a deep interest in each individual student.
- Evaluation of the student for the entire course with reference to class discussion, midterm, and final examinations.
- Direct personal contact with each individual student.
- Helps the student how to think, plan, and act. Teacher plays the role model—friend, philosopher, and guide.
- Helps the students to develop their own personal philosophy of life and interest in nursing.

CHARACTERISTICS OF EFFECTIVE TEACHING

- The teacher must be clear about the objectives of the lesson being taught.
- In general, the teacher must be knowledgeable.
- He must have made a thorough preparation by studying the matter available in textbooks and periodicals. The additional background knowledge will come handy for answering unexpected questions from the students.
- He must have shifted the matter and prepared the relevant lesson plan with "must know" and "should know" points, underlined.
- Students must be informed what they are going to learn and why. Motivation charts will be very useful.
- Students should be provided with a handout containing the outline of the lesson and important teaching points. Students can fill in the details as the lesson progresses.

- The lesson should be properly "tied in" with the previous lesson. References should be included in the lesson plan.
- A particular lesson may be taught by different methods. The method selected must match the intellectual capacity and motivational needs of the students.
- The method must suit the teacher personally and should provide ample scope for using the special talents and assets of the teacher. The method must be used creatively by the teacher.
- Lesson should be conducted strictly as per the lesson plan. As many training aids should be used as planned in the lesson plan.
- Lesson should be summarized after each phase.
- Question technique must be perfect. Question first to the entire class and then to individual. Students should be encouraged to ask questions and clear their doubts. In general, the teacher has to be knowledgeable with clear voice, vocabulary and communication skills.
- He must be impartial without any prejudices.
- Homework and assignments should be given after the final summary.

Key Points

+ Teacher has different roles to play.
+ Teacher must be clear about the objectives of the lesson being taught.

STUDY QUESTIONS

Short Essays

1. Roles of a teacher.
2. Qualities of a teacher.
3. Characteristics of effective teaching.

Multiple Choice Questions

1. What kind of lessons must a teacher create to be effective in the role of educator?
    a. Lessons that are easy
    b. Lessons that are fast
    c. Lessons that are accessible to all students
    d. Lessons that are fun

2. Which of these roles is important for a teacher?
   a. Educator
   b. Caregiver
   c. Colleague
   d. All of these are important roles for a teacher
3. Why is teacher training necessary?
   a. Increase teaching skills
   b. Understand methods of school organization
   c. Upgrade knowledge of content
   d. All of the above
4. The most important quality of a good teacher is:
   a. Sound knowledge of subject matter
   b. Good communication skills
   c. Concern of student welfares
   d. Effective leadership qualities
5. An effective teacher will ensure
   a. Cooperation among students
   b. Laissez-faire role
   c. Competition among students
   d. Competition or cooperation as situation demands

25

Evaluation

Chapter Outline

- Evaluation
- Essay Type Questions
- Objective Type
- Longitudinal Assessment
- Formative Assessment
- Summative Assessment

Learning Objectives

♦ Students will be oriented to functions and principles of evaluation.
♦ Students will be introduced to objective and essay type questions with their pros and cons.

INTRODUCTION

Evaluation is an essential element of teaching learning process. It is a process of describing some quality-character of an individual, a program of an institution as a basis for judgment of that individual, program or institution. It is a systematic process of determining the extent to which the educational objectives of the institution are achieved by the learners. Evaluation includes both qualitative and quantitative measurements.

GENERAL FUNCTIONS OF EVALUATION

❖ To determine the level of knowledge and understanding of the student,
❖ To determine the level of knowledge and understanding of the students' clinical performance,
❖ To find out the weakness and strength of students in different areas,
❖ To locate specific difficulties,

- To improve self-directed knowledge,
- To select students for higher courses and jobs,
- To check the effectiveness of teaching,
- To improve teaching methods,
- To check the program in any institution,
- To gather information needed by any institution, and
- To provide financial security (audit) to the students, staff, parents and the institution (college).

PRINCIPLES OF EVALUATION

1. Anything that exists in some amount can be measured.
2. Judging human activities cannot be done satisfactorily and accurately.
3. The chief goal of evaluation is change and improvement.
4. For development, student needs approval and recognition.
5. Judgment of individual's potentialities is complex. Always there is a chance of error which cannot be avoided but can be reduced.
6. Evaluation by a group is better than by a single individual.
7. Approval methods should be reliable, valid, objective, and related to the subject.
8. Evaluation is an ongoing and continuous process.
9. Evaluation should be done continuously, systematically, and scientifically.
10. Tools used for evaluation should be appropriate and the teacher should have skill in using these tools. Use of tools should be based on the educational objectives.
11. Evaluation should be done at the appropriate time.
12. Purpose of evaluation should be told to the staff and students. Areas of evaluation also should be indicated.
13. Evaluation is an integral part of the education process.
14. Accountability for effectiveness should be established.
15. Evaluation should facilitate individual growth.
16. Evaluation of teaching and learning methods should be carried out.
17. Evaluation of student's process should be done by the teacher by student's performance, student's response and responses by others.
18. Evaluation of the outcome should also be carried out.

METHODS OF EVALUATION

Evaluation should be based on three domains:
1. Formative,
2. Summative, and
3. Longitudinal.

Formative

Concurrent evaluation/continous evaluation at regular intervals daily/weekly/monthly. It is done by using rating scales, checklists.

Summative/Terminal

Evaluation done at the end of the course, e.g., semester examinations.

Longitudinal

Evaluation done at the end of the entire program, e.g., at the end of the 4 years in the case of B.Sc. (Nursing).

EVALUATION OF INSTRUCTION

Competency based evaluation methods are used. It is done to determine students' progress. It helps to assess effectiveness of teaching. Teaching environment must be evaluated. Community involvement and involvement of other professionals should be evaluated. Senior tutors, HODs, examiners and teacher herself can evaluate the effectiveness of classroom instruction. Outsiders also can be requested to help in evaluation. Departmental seniors and experts from outside can be requested to evaluate. They evaluate the intelligence of the teacher, her subject knowledge, educational background, and attitude toward teaching. Availability of nursing care, health services, interest of the agency in giving care, location of the agency, availability of finance, resources personnel and their intellectual capacity should be considered while evaluating the teacher.

Students can be tested by giving oral/written tests and assignments (called programmed instruction).

For higher level students, precourse test can be conducted to assess what they already know.

Self-evaluation by teacher and students is important to keep themselves up to date. Evaluation in clinicals will improve their clinical skills.

BENEFITS OF EVALUATION

Evaluation is an ongoing process. Institutional learning and teaching is a cooperative effort, usually strengthened by frequent stock taking. Evaluation means the measurement plus quality judgment of one's ability.

Examinations are for evaluation and feedback. Terminal examination alone cannot be used for checking the adequacy of learning of the students. Although examination indirectly force students to take up their studies seriously, they are not able to ensure regular study habits. The gaps in any student's learning go unnoticed and unrectified. This limitation in the present day system can be overcome by substituting the end exams by tests of shorter duration held at regular and close intervals.

For students, a test can—
1. Provide a goal to be reached and promote a sense of achievement.
2. Confirm what has been learned and therefore assimilation.
3. Motivate the class by competition as each student wants to do well and excel.

For the instructor, a test can—
1. Make clear what the class knows at the start, if the test was conducted at the beginning of the course.
2. Grade the class by ability.
3. Measure progress and assimilations. This will also reveal the weakness in instruction.
4. Show how much revision is needed and when.

QUALITIES OF A GOOD TEST

To be fair and effective, a test must be:
1. Valid,
2. Reliable,
3. Predictable,
4. Comprehensive in scope, and
5. Discriminating.

Criteria for Selecting Question Papers

1. Sampling of objectives,
2. Sampling of syllabus contents,
3. Validity—accuracy, the degree to which it is measured,
4. Reliability, i.e., repeatability, and
5. Test of usefulness.

TYPES OF TESTS (FLOWCHART 1)

Essay Type

It reveals the higher mental processes of the students, such as organizing, and concising.

Advantages of Essay Type
1. Early to prepare the question paper.
2. Increases the ability to recall by the student.
3. Gives a deeper knowledge in that subject.
4. Students get an opportunity to answer questions without any binding or restriction.
5. The students get a good opportunity to express their individual ideas and talents. The answers are actually a clue to the student's personality.

Disadvantages of Essay Type
1. Takes a long time for correction.
2. Decreases sampling.
3. Lack of ability to organize; even if the student knows, they may find difficulty to organize.

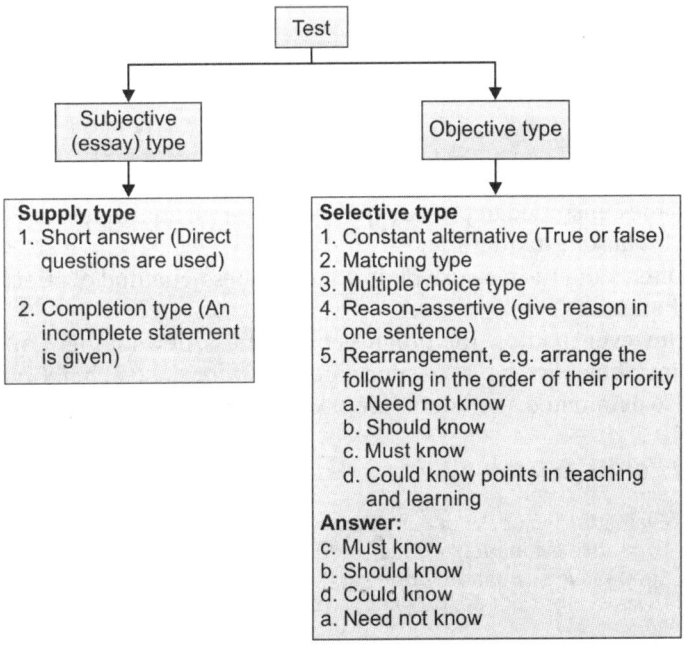

Flowchart 1: Types of tests.

4. They are unreliable.
5. They stress only on intellectual attainment.
6. The real evaluation of the ability of the student is not possible. Generally, teachers award marks on the basis of good handwriting or length of answers.

Preparation of Essay Type Question Paper

1. Question should be structured properly and marks allotted as per the content of each topic.
2. Questions must be worded properly avoiding grammar mistakes.
3. Questions should be specific and not vague and confusing.
4. Predetermined criteria for solution must be set before valuation starts.
5. To improve reliability of awarding marks, the teacher may read the answers of all the students and then only award marks.

Objective Type

Advantages of Objective Type

1. More reliable as the answers are predetermined.
2. More sampling; since objective types call for short answers, a large number of questions can be included, covering the entire syllabus.
3. Writing is reduced (minimized).
4. Easy to correct.
5. Scoring is easy; anybody including a computer can do it.
6. Free from biased correction.

Disadvantages

1. No chance for students to develop skills of essay writing.
2. Time consumed to prepare question paper in enormous.
3. May lack in standard.
4. Often students may use blind chance (guess) method of selecting the answer.

However to know the progress of the class/development of the subject, objective type questions are handy for the teacher. Choice is also eliminated as students are asked to answer all the questions.

Key Points ● ● ●

- ✦ Evaluation includes both qualitative and quantitative measurements.
- ✦ Formative evaluation is done at regular intervals.
- ✦ Summative evaluation is done at the end of the course.

STUDY QUESTIONS

Short Essays

1. Functions of evaluation.
2. Principles of evaluation.

Short Answers

1. Formative assessment.
2. Summative assessment.
3. Essay and objective type questions.

Multiple Choice Questions

1. Mr X always gives a test on the first day of class to help him plan for future instruction. These tests are not for a grade, but they give Mr X a good idea of what he needs to cover in his class. Mr X is using what form of evaluation?
    a. Diagnostic
    b. Final
    c. Formative
    d. Summative
2. When summative evaluation takes place:
    a. Anytime during the academic year
    b. At the beginning of the academic year
    c. At the end of the academic year
    d. After completion of the school
3. What are summative assessments used to determine?
    a. Instructional methods and student feedback
    b. If students have mastered specific competencies and to identify instructional areas that need additional attention
    c. Valid instruction
    d. Ongoing assignments, reviews, and observations
4. A classroom assessment used by students to self-assess and set goals is _____.
    a. Summative
    b. Neither
    c. Formative
    d. Longitudinal
5. Which is the characteristic of formative assessment?
    a. Evaluation occurs at the end
    b. Evaluation is done before the concept is introduced
    c. Evaluation relates to indicating learning outcome of teaching
    d. Evaluation is conducted during teaching

26

Our Social World

Chapter Outline

- Social Psychology
- Social Behavior
- Social Relations
- Groups
- Intergroup Conflict
- Stereotypes
- Prejudice
- Antisocial Behavior
- Group Morale
- Group Therapy
- Self-Help Groups
- Leadership

Learning Objectives

- Students will be introduced to social psychology.
- Students will be oriented to groups, its types and group morale.
- Students will be familiarized with the types of leadership.

SCOPE OF SOCIAL PSYCHOLOGY

Social psychology is the study of social behavior. Social behavior takes into account any of the four basic reactions.

1. When two individuals come into contact with one another, there will be mutual interaction between them.
2. When a person meets a group of individuals, his behavior is affected by that group.
3. The group which affects the individual, may itself get affected by the latter. The types of relationship in second and third reactions refer to person and group.
4. Finally, there is the interaction between individuals of two different groups or more than two groups. This type of relationships is between group and group. Social psychology studies the individual in relation to his fellow members in the group. The task of sociology

is to study the characteristics of group behavior along with scientific lines.

The world is beset with many social problems, such as racial prejudice, caste prejudice, crime and delinquency, industrial unrest, poverty, begging, divorce, alcoholism and so on. Many of these social ills may be due to difficulties in interpersonal relationships. It is the task of social psychology to have a thorough understanding of how these problems emerge, and how they can be predicted and controlled.

GROUP—THE UNIT OF STUDY

The basic unit of study in social psychology is the group which is made up of two or more persons who regularly relate with each other. Members of a group are united by social relations.

Groups may be primary or secondary. People in a primary group know each other well and have close emotional ties. They rarely leave the group. People enter a secondary group to accomplish some goal. They leave the group easily. Any group will last if relationships among its members are balanced.

The largest social groups are races, societies, and cultures. A race is a group with the same biological features. A society is an independent and self-sufficient group. A culture means the overall pattern of living which is passed from generation to generation.

The most important parts of culture are values, norms, and roles. Our behavior is molded on our society and culture. Roles, especially, are useful to help people know what kind of behavior to expect from each other.

A person may become a member of a new group through either assimilation or accommodation. Those who are assimilated become like all others in the group. Those who accommodate change some things but keep some cultural differences.

Two important sources of intergroup conflict are (a) Stereotypes, and (b) Prejudices. Stereotypes are images given to others from just a few facts.

Prejudice is a negative attitude against members of a particular group of people.

Lasting and constructive activities are possible through cooperative activity rather than competition.

ANTISOCIAL BEHAVIOR

Delinquency or antisocial behavior is one when the individual's behavior does not conform to the goals of the group.

Factors associated with antisocial behavior (delinquency) are:
a. Environmental factors, and
b. Personality factors.

Environmental Factors

1. Low economic income,
2. Living in a transitional area, and
3. Family breakdown.

Delinquency is the highest in areas which are in a process of transition from house to business (migrant). When a family disintegrates the child is deprived of affection, feelings of security, and social opportunities. If such a child comes in contact with a delinquent gang that can satisfy some of his needs, the child may follow that gang and become delinquent. Among mothers, it has been found that those who had been divorced or separated exhibit more anger and nonconformity.

Personality Factors

Delinquents find difficulty in correctly interpreting and evaluating both their own behavior and the behavior of others. They are morally blind. Once a person has committed a crime, the chances of committing another crime are very high.

Criminologists believe that an adult who is a habitual criminal cannot be rehabilitated. Prevention must start early if it is to be effective. Community planning (social institutions, social workers, etc.) and judicial action are the two methods commonly employed for prevention of crimes.

For the youth offender, the camp program must include education, trade training and recreation facilities like radio and television.

Delinquents should not be treated as hardened criminals. It is better to place them in the custody of trained psychologists and social workers.

STAFF GROUPS IN HOSPITALS

In hospitals, the nursing staff forms a separate group from the medical staff or maintenance staff. Nurses may at the same time belong to a professional organization, such as TNAI. The hospital staff, however, also forms a group with interests and activities concerning all the staff.

Unlike in industry, the main problems and conflicts among hospital staff are not those of policy or value systems. The disagreement arises over the way in which each member of the staff evaluates his own or other member's contributions. While the ward sisters, for example, feel that the doctors do not pay enough attention to their advice, student nurses tend to feel that the ward sisters do not credit them with any ability to contribute. When the ward sister feels that the nursing superintendent would not listen to her or be interested in her problem, junior nurses feel the same way about the ward sister and the patients may feel that no-one will listen to them. Administration should make efforts to eliminate, such feelings.

Group Morale

Morale is a positive group feeling of general satisfaction and enthusiasm for a task. Workers are happy and work well when their morale is high. Within a group, there can be vigorous argument and violent disagreement without damage to groups feeling. The purpose of this is to effect change. If the group is criticized or attacked by an outsider, it reacts as a whole by closing its ranks and protecting itself.

In hospitals where the morale is good, there can be very outspoken criticism from within, because all the group members have the same purpose of improving the existing practice. As soon as an outsider criticizes, all the staff are united in their defense.

Groups can be more efficient in solving problems than the individual members.

When a decision has been made by a whole group, the members feel more bounded by the decision than if it had been imposed on the group by one person, e.g., decisions about nursing procedure are more likely to be carried out, if they are made by the ward sisters themselves.

When the group morale is high, the group tends to be active and productive.

When the group morale is low, discussion is often avoided. People feel uneasy with each other. They cannot safely reveal their feelings and consequently avoid all topics which might arouse strong emotions. The result is that the group is unable to deal with its business.

Learning in Groups

During her training the student nurse may become a member of a small discussion group or of a group working on some educational projects. Group work has certain advantages more than other forms of instruction. It is active learning and, therefore, helps her to learn faster and more permanently. One important condition for successful group work is that the student should be willing to learn from her colleagues', respect their views and feel free to offer her own contributions.

Group Therapy

Much importance has been attached in recent years to the powerful effect of group on the ability of members to cope with change.

Patients with psychiatric problems were the first to benefit from organized group therapy. In some groups patients experience support from each other, develop awareness of the reasons for their problems and learn new and successful patterns of adaptation.

Many patients benefit from self-help groups in which they join fellow sufferers for mutual benefit. Examples of such groups are alcoholics anonymous, multiple sclerosis society, epileptic society, and weight watcher's group.

LEADERSHIP

Most people want to belong to a group and enjoy doing so but all the individuals are not satisfied simply to belong to a group. For them, the need for dominance (leadership) is more than the need for acceptance.

There cannot be any leader without the existence of followers. The leader exercises authority over the group and such authority is willingly accepted by the followers. Leader understands the individual feelings and problems of his followers. He/she accepts responsibility for the actions of his followers and he is impartial. Leadership cannot be ordered. It has to be earned.

Functions of a Leader

1. *Structuring the situation:* He/she has to interpret the situation to other members, emphasizing certain aspects, clarifying their doubts and focusing on certain goals. When there is any conflict among the members the effective leader must be sensitive to such conflict, help evaluate them objectively and provide a satisfactory compromise program.
2. Controlling group behavior.
3. Speaking for the group.
4. *Helping the group achieve its potential:* The leader should create a social climate which encourages individual members to participate in group activities.

Types of Leadership

1. Autocratic leadership,
2. Democratic leadership, and
3. Laissez-Faire or Free reign leadership.

Autocratic Leadership

The autocratic leader holds most authority and closely controls group activities; centralizes all power and decision making and tolerates no deviations, gets results but the leadership is as good as the leader is. If the leader is weak and inefficient, the followers also will be weak and inefficient.

Democratic Leadership

A democratic leader is one who formulates his policies through group discussion. There is decentralization of authority and he encourages the followers to function as a social unit and makes full use of their talents and abilities. The democratic leader is like the conductor of an orchestra rather than a one-man band.

a. He/she formulates his policies in group discussions.
b. Issues orders only after consultation with the group.
c. Permits his/her subordinates to participate in decisions which affect them.
d. Permits his/her subordinates to make important decisions in the areas of their functioning.

Laissez-Faire Leadership

The Laissez-Faire leader works with poorly defined lines of authority and responsibility and often allows the subordinates to set their own goals and make their own decisions. The system can work only if the subordinates are highly intelligent and duty conscious.

The leadership in most of the groups of which you are a member will be appointed by those in authority. Some may be chosen by the group. The nursing superintendent, nursing supervisors, ward sisters, and tutors are all appointed leaders. The leaders of your class will be chosen by the members of the class. Although successful leadership depends on both personality and situational factors, leadership ability can be taught. Training will improve leadership qualities.

Key Points ● ● ●

- Social psychology studies the individual in relation to his fellow members in the group.
- The basic unit of social psychology is the group.
- People in a primary group know each other well and have close emotional ties.
- A secondary group is formed to accomplish some goal.

Contd...

Contd...

- Two important sources of intergroup conflict are stereotypes and prejudices.
- Delinquents should not be treated as hardened criminals rather be rehabilitated under trained psychologists and social workers.
- Group tends to be active and productive when the group morale is high.
- Leadership is the ability of an individual or a group of individuals to influence and guide followers or other members of an organization.

STUDY QUESTIONS

Short Essays

1. Scope of social psychology.
2. Causes for delinquent behavior.
3. Types of leaders.

Short Answers

1. Group morale.
2. Group therapy.
3. Prejudice and stereotypes.
4. Primary and secondary group.
5. Functions of a leader.

Multiple Choice Questions

1. Stereotypes are:
    a. Generalizations that a small number of people have about particular social groups.
    b. Social behaviors.
    c. Generalizations that a large number of people have about particular social groups.
    d. An example of a social psychology research method.
2. Which one of the following is a "secondary group"?
    a. Nuclear family
    b. Peer group
    c. Association
    d. Joint family
3. Group morale refers to_____.
    a. Cooperation in a group
    b. Coordination in a group
    c. Unity in a group
    d. Team spirit in a group

4. What is one characteristic of Laissez-Faire leadership style?
   a. A leader gives opinion only when asked
   b. A leader takes charge
   c. Everyone works together and participates together
   d. Nobody gives any suggestions or instructions
5. Which is *not* a characteristic of the democratic leadership style?
   a. Leader asks before doing anything
   b. Leader enforces and relies on discipline
   c. Leader works together with the members as a group
   d. There is a mutual synergy between the leader and the team
6. Which of the following is an autocratic style of leadership?
   a. Directing style of leadership
   b. Consultative style of leadership
   c. Participative style of leadership
   d. Delegating style of leadership
7. What do you call a style of leadership that takes account of others' views, opinions and ideas?
   a. Laissez- faire
   b. People oriented
   c. Democratic
   d. Autocratic

27. Soft Skills and Nursing Empowerment

Chapter Outline

- Soft Skills
- Team Work
- Critical Thinking
- Adaptability
- Empathy
- Professionalism
- Nursing Empowerment

Learning Objectives

- Students will be introduced to the soft skills required to be a nurse.
- Students will be oriented to the concept, factors and abilities required for nursing empowerment.

SOFT SKILLS

Soft skills are skills that are necessary in all professions. The importance of soft skills is not restricted to a specific field. These thinking dispositions consist of a group of abilities that can be used in every aspect of people's lives, without any need to readapt them based on the situation. Soft skills are also known as common skills or core skills. These include critical thinking, problem solving, public speaking, professional writing, teamwork, digital literacy, leadership, professional attitude, work ethics, career management, and intercultural fluency.

Soft skills are a crucial component in nursing because they foster a collaborative, respectful and efficient workforce. Nurses without soft skills may fail to properly interact with patients, coworkers and other healthcare professionals, which may jeopardize a patient's health by obstructing the flow of care. Some of the soft skills required for nurses are described in **Table 1**.

Table 1: Soft skills for nurses by Kathleen Curtis.

Soft skills	Descriptions
Communication	Nurse has to communicate diagnosis, treatment plans to patients, caretakers, and updates about patient conditions to doctors and ensure that family members are also clear about the diagnosis and instruct caretakers about proper care for patients after discharge. They should also develop trust, offer guidance and answer the queries clearly
Listening	Nurses must be able to focus on what others say, address concerns, and accommodate preferences. Active and careful listening constitutes important part of nursing job. If incorrect information about patients is taken down then the patient's life will be in danger
Teamwork	Nurse needs to work along with a team. Working as a team improves patient outcomes, additional opportunities to engage with fellow professionals and higher job satisfaction
Critical thinking and problem solving	Critical thinking is the ability to analyze and evaluate information in a way to gather knowledge used in making informed decisions. Critical thinking plays an important role in nursing as these professionals must observe patients, gather information about their condition, and troubleshoot problems such as react quickly before condition worsens
Professionalism	Professionalism refers to maintaining patient confidentiality, taking feedback gracefully, maintaining a positive attitude, and keeping an attitude of compassion even in difficult working environments. Maintaining professionalism helps avoid work conflict, improve skills and have positive attitude at workplace
Empathy	Empathy is feeling with others. A nurse lacking empathy will be difficult to trust and has difficulty building rapport with the patients
Conflict resolution	This is an important skill required while dealing patients and coworkers. It is required while dealing with interpersonal conflicts, issue based conflicts, ego based conflicts, and ethics based conflicts
Leadership	In order to reach the peak of career, leadership skills are necessary. Leadership is not telling what others should do, it includes taking initiative, quality care, collaborative work and change management

Contd...

Contd...

Soft skills	Descriptions
Adaptability	More quick and flexible the nurse, adaptability is easier. Adjusting to shift work, working with variety of patients, adapting to new protocols, etc.
Time management	Managing time helps reduce stress. Nursing is a busy profession taking medical history, managing medications, intake of new patients, being organized and managing time helps a nurse to be successful

Source: EDUMED. Soft Skills Every Nursing Student Needs to Develop. [online] Available from: https://www.edumed.org/online-schools/nursing-rn-programs/soft-skill-development/. [Last Accessed April, 2022].

NURSING EMPOWERMENT

Nursing empowerment means the ability to effectively motivate and mobilize self and others to accomplish positive outcomes in nursing practice and work environment.

Factors Contributing to Empowerment

1. Decision making,
2. Autonomy,
3. Reward and recognition, and
4. Managing workload.

Abilities Required to be an Empowered Professional

1. Enhance leadership skills,
2. Be appositive change event,
3. Get certified, and
4. Being an evidence-based practice (EBP) cheerleader.

Key Points ● ● ●

- Soft skills, also known as common skills or core skills.
- Soft skills are a crucial component in nursing, because they foster a collaborative, respectful and efficient workforce.
- Empowerment helps nurses increase their job satisfaction.

STUDY QUESTIONS

Short Essay
1. Soft skills of a nurse.

Short Answer
1. Nursing empowerment.

Multiple Choice Questions
1. Empathy means:
    a. Ability to understand and share the feelings of another
    b. Talking to friends
    c. Asking for a favor
    d. Seeking therapy
2. Which among the following is a soft skill?
    a. Updating
    b. Analyzing
    c. Monitoring
    d. Counseling
3. Critical thinking concerns:
    a. Determining the cause of our beliefs
    b. Pinpointing the psychological basis of our beliefs
    c. Determining the quality of our beliefs
    d. Assessing the practical impact of our beliefs
4. Which of the following hinder nursing empowerment?
    a. Taking action to address system issues
    b. Eliminating divergent and conflicting views
    c. Collaborating and sharing in decision making
    d. Participating in institutional policies
5. Which of the following is not a barrier to effective communication?
    a. Poor listening skills
    b. Language
    c. Stereotyping
    d. Asking questions

Answer Keys

Chapter 1: Psychology and its Relation to Nursing
1. B 2. A 3. A 4. A 5. D

Chapter 2: Body-Mind Relationship
1. A 2. C 3. B 4. B 5. A

Chapter 3: Biology of Behavior
1. A 2. C 3. D 4. B 5. A

Chapter 4: Nature and Nurture: Individual Differences
1. A 2. C 3. D 4. B 5. B

Chapter 5: Observation: Attention, Sensation, and Perception
1. A 2. B 3. B 4. B 5. D

Chapter 6: The Learning Process
1. A 2. B 3. A 4. B 5. A 6. B 7. C 8. B 9. C 10. B

Chapter 7: Memory: Remembering and Forgetting
1. C 2. B 3. C 4. B 5. A

Chapter 8: Thinking and Reasoning: Concept and Language
1. A 2. B 3. D 4. B 5. A

Chapter 9: Intelligence and its Measurement
1. D 2. D 3. D 4. B 5. D 6. B 7. D 8. C 9. A 10. C

Chapter 10: Aptitude (Capacity or Innate Potential)
1. A 2. C 3. B 4. D

Chapter 11: Motivation
1. A 2. C 3. B 4. D 5. A

Chapter 12: Frustration and Conflicts
1. A 2. A 3. D 4. C 5. D

Chapter 13: Stress and its Management
1. A 2. B 3. B 4. D 5. A

Chapter 14: Defense Mechanisms
1. B 2. A 3. B 4. B 5. B

Chapter 15: Emotions in Health and Disease
1. A 2. C 3. A 4. C 5. B

Chapter 16: Attitude: The Way We See Things
1. C 2. D 3. B 4. C 5. C

Chapter 17: Personality (Is What the Man is)
1. C 2. C 3. B 4. C 5. C

Chapter 18: Developmental Psychology
1. B 2. A 3. C 4. A 5. C 6. A 7. A 8. B 9. D 10. C

Chapter 19: Mental Health and Mental Illness
1. B 2. A 3. D 4. D 5. D

Chapter 20: Psychological Tests: Measurement of Individual Differences
1. A 2. B 3. B 4. D 5. C

Chapter 21: Attribution: Our Explanations of Behavior
1. B 2. D 3. A 4. C 5. C

Chapter 22: Educational Psychology: Scope and Methods
1. D 2. D 3. B 4. C 5. B

Chapter 23: Effective Teaching
1. A 2. C 3. C 4. A 5. D

Chapter 24: Role and Functions of a Teacher
1. C 2. D 3. D 4. A 5. D

Chapter 25: Evaluation
1. C 2. C 3. B 4. C 5. D

Chapter 26: Our Social World
1. C 2. C 3. D 4. A 5. B 6. A 7. C

Chapter 27: Soft Skills and Nursing Empowerment
1. A 2. D 3. C 4. B 5. D

Index

Page numbers followed by *b* refer to box, *f* refer to figure, *fc* refer to flowchart, and *t* refer to table

A

Abraham Maslow hierarchy of needs theory 154, 154f
Abstract intelligence 118
Academic achievement 131
Acceptance 257
Achievement tests 280
Adaptability 338
Adaptation theory 175
Adjustment mechanism 167, 182
Administration 144
Adrenal glands 239
Adrenaline 196
Affection 150
Affective component 212
Affective disorders 267
Affective learning 62
Affiliation motives 150
Aggression motives 150
Aggressiveness 161
Agreeableness 233
Alarm reaction fight 175
Alcoholism 239
Alexander's pass along test 130
Alzheimer's disease 96
Amnesia 96
Anesthesia 54
Anger 172, 175, 206, 257
Anterograde amnesia 96
Antisocial behavior 329
Anxiety 172, 175, 181, 182
 disorders 267
 levels of 77
Applied psychology, branches of 10, 10t
Approach-approach conflict 162, 162f
Approach-avoidance conflict 163, 164f
Aptitude 141, 144, 280
 tests 142, 280
 uses of 143
Arousal theory 151, 153
Aspiration, levels of 236
Atmosphere 301
Attack 166
Attention 44, 45, 303
 degree of 48
 division of 48
 external determinants of 46
 internal determinants of 46
 span of 46
 types of 46
 varieties of 46
Attitudes 210, 212, 217, 237
 change of 216
 characteristics of 211
 components of 211
 development 213
  classification of 214f
 functions of 211
 general features of 211
 measurement of 215
 toward class 305
Attributional analysis 289
Attributions 285, 289
Audiovisual aids, relative effectiveness of 310f
Audition 45
Autocratic leadership 333
Autonomic nervous system 28
Autonomy 251
Aversion therapy 67

Avoidance-avoidance conflict 162, 163f
Axon 24

B

Backaches 171
Bad throat 20
Balance theory 215
Bandura's social cognitive theory 72, 231
Bargaining 257
Basal ganglia 28
Behavior 285
  biology of 24
  classifications of 3t
  glandular control of 31
  muscular control of 29
Behavioral component 212
Behaviorism 5
Behaviorist approach 245
Bell adjustment inventory 280
Big blooming buzzing confusion 201
Binocular cues 53
Biological amnesias 96
Biological theories 151, 152
Birth, complications of 172
Blood
  glucose level 239
  pressure 19
Bluffing 306
Body
  language 198
  mind relationship 18
  movement 121
  upon mind, action of 19
Boredom 206
Brain 26
  damage 97
  functioning of 49
Bruner's theory 125
Business management 11

C

Calcarine fissure 28
Cannon-Bard theory 204, 204f
Cardiac death 172
Carl Roger's self-theory 225, 230
Case history method 296
Cat cry syndrome 39
Catastrophic events 172
Cattell's theory 127, 232
Central fissure 28
Central nervous system 24, 26, 30f
Cerebellum 26
Cerebral
  cortex 27
  hemispheres 27
  palsy 135
Childhood amnesia 97
Children's apperception test 236
Chromosomal abnormalities 38, 135
Chromosomes 37
Citric acid 98
Classical conditioning 68t
  applications of 67
Clinical psychology 9, 10
Cloud, patch of 236
Cognition 120
Cognitive 212
  appraisal theory 204
  approach 246
  component 212
  development 123t, 238
    Piaget's theory of 122, 123, 247t
  learning 62
  personal factors 231
  symptoms 171
Colds 171
Common fate 52, 52f
Communication 112, 337
  barriers of 301
  basic elements of 113
  process of 300
Community 270
  psychology 10
Compensation 183
Compensatory education 297
Compromise 165, 166, 177
Concentration 20
  difficulty in 171

Concept formation, Bruner's theory of 125
Cone experience 310f
Conflicts 159, 161, 166
   types of 162
Confrontation 177
Conscientiousness 233
Conscious 227
Consciousness
   altered state of 20
   levels of 20, 21, 227
Consensus 288
Conservation principle 124f
Consistency 288
Consolidation theory 92
Constipation 19
Continuous reinforcement schedule 70
Control, locus of 231
Conversion 187
Corpus callosum 28
Counseling 274, 276
   psychology 10
Counselor, characteristics of 275
Creative thinking 104
Creativity 122
Cretinism 135
Crisis intervention 176
Cube construction test 130
Curriculum 308
   appraisal 308

D

Day-dreaming 188, 301
Defense mechanisms 178, 181, 182, 190-192
   characteristics of 182
   types of 183t
Defense-oriented reaction pattern 166
Delinquency 329
Delivery 305
Democratic leadership 333
Dendrites 24
Depression 171, 175, 257

Deprivation effects 247
Depth perception 53
Development 244, 245
   domains of 237
   Mahler's theory of 257
   Piaget's cognitive theory of 112
   process of 238
   stages of 257
Developmental method 9
Developmental psychology 10, 244
Developmental task 248, 249
   model 248b
Diabetes 172
Diet 239
Differential aptitude test 142, 280, 297
Discrimination 65
Dissociative disorders 267
Distinctiveness 288
Distress 172
Dominance, law of 37
Double approach-avoidance conflict 164f
Down's syndrome 38, 135
Dream amnesia 97
Drive reduction theory 151, 152, 153f
Drugs 239
Dyspepsia 19

E

Early childhood 251
Echoic memory 85
Education 213, 292, 300
   field of 11
   process, ingredients in 301
Educational psychology 10, 292, 294
   methods of 295
   objectives of 294
   scope of 294
   significance of 298
Effective health teaching 314
Effective learning, law of 63
Effective teaching 300
   characteristics of 318

Ego 225
    integrity 256
Emergency theory 198
Emotional conflicts 237
Emotional development 201, 246
    psychosocial theory of 228
Emotional intelligence 202
Emotional quotient 202
Emotional reactions 175
Emotional state 47
Emotional symptoms 171
Emotions 194, 195, 200
    characteristics of 195
    control of 206, 207
    development of 201
    effect of 197f
    external changes in 197
    importance of 200
    internal changes in 196
    measurement of 198
    parts of 195
    quotient test 199
    states of 205
    subjective experience of 204
    theories of 202, 203f
Empathy 337
Encoding 84, 95
Endocrine
    glands 27, 239
    system 31
Environment 39, 134, 213
Environmental factors 160, 239, 330
Epinephrine 196
Episodic memory 86
Erik H Erikson psychosocial theory 225
Erikson's eight psychosocial stages 250, 258, 258t
Ethological approach 246
Eustress 172
Evaluation 108, 120, 211, 321, 323
    benefits of 324
    general function of 321
    methods of 323
    principles of 322

Exercise, law of 63
Exhaustion, stage of 176
Experiences 213
Experiment 63
Experimental method 7, 296
Experimental psychology 10
Experimentation 7
Exposure, frequency of 49
External aggression 165
Extrasensory perception 57, 58f
Extraversion 233, 280
Extrinsic factors 90
Extrinsic motivation 147
Extroverts 222
Eysenck's personality
    inventory 240, 241t
    questionnaires 280

F

Facial expressions, observations of 198
Factors influencing
    attributions 288
    learning 76
    memory 87
    personality development 239
Factors theories 118
Failure, fear of 171
Family
    relationships 236
    triangle, period of 252
Fantasy 188
Fatigue 76, 171
    retards intellectual activity 19
Faulty memory process 92
Favoritism 306
Fear 171, 172, 175, 181, 206
Fetal alcohol syndrome 39
Figure-ground relationship 50
Flight syndrome 198
Forebrain 26
Forgetfulness 171
Forgetting 83
    curve of 87f
    processes of 95
    theories of 92
Formal operations 125

Fragile X syndrome 39
Freud analytical theory, stages of 258*t*
Freud's psycho-sexual stages 258
Freud's theory 227
    stresses 224
Frustration 159, 160, 166, 174, 237
    results of 160*f*
    sources of 160
Functionalism 4
Functioning, levels of 20

G

G factor theory 119
Galactosemia 135
Galvanic skin response 199
Gender identity 247
General adaptation syndrome 175
General aptitude test battery 297
General intelligence, Cattell's theory of 127
General psychology 10
Genes 37
Genetic
    abnormalities 135
    endowment 36
    method 9
Gestalt psychology 5, 73
Gestures 305
Glands 32
Goddard form board test 130
Gonads 32
Good teacher, qualities of 317
Good test, qualities of 324
Gratification, delay of 232
Gratitude, develop attitude of 216
Gregariousness 150
Group 329
    learning in 331
    morale 331
    test 280
    therapy 332
Growth 29, 229, 238
Guidance 143, 276
    characteristics of 275
    field of 11

Guilford's model 120*f*, 121*f*
Guilt 206
Gustation 45

H

Halo effect 281
Havighurst's developmental tasks model 248
Headaches 171
Healey's picture completion test 130
Health
    determinants of 171*fc*
    emotions in 194
    for-all 272
Heart
    disease 174
    pounding of 171
Heredity 36, 134, 269
Heterogeneity 303
High blood pressure 171
Hindbrain 26
Homeostasis 148
Homo sapiens 103
Homogeneity 303
Hormones 196
Hospitalization, stress of 174
Human body 31
Humanism 6
Humanistic theory 225, 229
Humor 306
Humpty Dumpty 89
Hunger drive 148
Hyperthesia 54
Hyperthyroidism 20
Hypnosis 20
Hypothesis
    evaluation of 108
    formulation of 108
Hypothyroidism 20

I

Iconic memory 84
Id 225
Imitation, principle of 72

Immediate memory 84
   test for 129
Impressions, strengthening of 302
Incentive theory 152, 154
Indigestion 19, 171
Individual test 280
Industrial psychology 10
Information processing 84
Inheritance, Mendel's laws of 37
Inner fantasies 236
Instinct theory 151, 152
Integrating mechanism 27
Intellect, Guilford's model of 120f, 121f
Intellectualization 184
Intelligence 117, 133, 134, 136
   assessment of 127
   Bhatia's battery of performance tests of 280
   cubical model of 121f
   individual differences in 36, 132
   information processing theories of 126
   measurement 117
   process oriented theories of 122
   quotient 128, 202
   tests 137, 280
      types of 118, 130
      uses of 130
   theories of 118
Interference
   theory 93
   types of 94
Internal aggression 165
Internal growth 224
Interpersonal intelligence 121
Interviews 234, 280
Intonation 114
Intrapersonal intelligence 122
Intrinsic motivation 147
Inventory method 8
IQ
   current status of 131
   limitations of concept of 131
Irritability 171, 175

J
James-Lange theory 202, 203f, 204
Job performance 131

K
Klinefelter's syndrome 38, 135
Kohlberg's moral level 257, 258, 258t
Kohs block design test 129, 130
Krebs' cycle 98

L
Laboratory method 7
Laissez-Faire leadership 333
Language 111-113
   ability 307
   development 112
Lateral fissure 28
Law, field of 12
Leader, functions of 332
Leadership 332, 337
   quality 318
   types of 332
Learner
   nature of 76
   needs of 302
Learning 62, 64, 73, 79, 239
   characteristics of 74
   curves 77, 78f
   method, nature of 77
   modes of 63
   process 61, 295
      evaluation of 295
      steps in 76
   transfer of 78
   types of 62
Legal psychology 10
Lesson plan 309
   format of 311b
Lethargy 20
Lie detector 199
Life changing unit points 172
Life cycle, development in 248
Life's little hassles 172
Limbic system 28

Linguistic intelligence 120
Listening 337
Local adaptation syndrome 175
Loci, method of 89, 98
Logical learning 77
Longitudinal fissure 28

M

Mahler's theory 260*t*
Major developmental tasks 260, 261
Major endocrine glands 31, 31*t*
Major fissure 28
Major life stressors 172
Major personality theories 225*b*
Mannerisms 305
Maslow's hierarchy of needs 152, 155
Mathematical intelligence 121
Matrices test 130
Maturation 201, 238
Mature adulthood 255
McClelland theories 151
Mechanical intelligence 118
Medicine, field of 11
Meditation 21, 178
   six steps in 21
Memory 83, 97
   disorders 96
   long-term 84, 85
   network theory 87
   process of 91
   short-term 84, 85, 91
   system 84
   three stages of 84
   trace decay theory 92
Mental
   age 128
   factors 239
   health 265, 267, 268, 271
      foundations of 269
   hygiene 267
      movement 266
   illness 265
      medical classification of 267
   imagery 303
   imbalance 19
   mechanisms 182
   retardation 131
      causes of 134
   stroll method 89
Mentally healthy individual, characteristics of 268
Message 113
Metabolic disorders 135
Midbrain 26
Mid-career crisis 255
Middle age
   crisis 255
   slump 255
Military psychology 10
Mind
   division of 227
   structure of 227
   upon body, action of 19
Minnesota multiple personality inventory 235, 280
Mixed emotions 196, 196*f*
Monocular cues 53
Monozygotic twins 134
Mood swings 172
Moral development, Kohlberg's stages of 257, 261*t*
Motivated forgetting 95
Motivation 49, 146, 155, 159, 194, 236
   theories of 151, 152
   types of 147
Motivational cycle 147*f*
Motives 147, 301
   types of 147
Motor development sequence 250*t*
Motor learning 62
Movement 46
Multifactor theories 119
Multiphasic questionnaire 235
Multiple approach-avoidance conflicts 164
Multiple sclerosis 172
Muscle 27
   control 30
   tension 171
Musical intelligence 121

N

National Mental Health Program for India 273
Natural intelligence 122
Nature 34
Nature-nurture
   controversy 41
   debate 244, 245
Negative attitudes 215
Negative emotions 206
Negative punishment 71
Nerve 24
   cell 24
Nervous system 24, 25f, 27
Neuron 24
Neuroticism 233, 280
Nonverbal communication 198
Nonverbal group intelligence tests 130
Nonverbal individual intelligence test 130
Nonverbal tests 137
Noradrenaline 196
Norepinephrine 196
Nurse 21, 136, 144, 155, 156, 217, 239, 251, 254, 256, 289
   education 73
   patient relationship 271
   personality traits of 223
   role of 250, 271, 273
Nursing 12
   care 13
   empowerment 336, 338
Nurture 34, 35
   view 245

O

Observation 44, 49, 56, 296
   method 7, 234
Obsessive compulsive disorder 227
Olfaction 45
Openness 233
Operant conditioning 68, 68t
   applications of 71
   basic concepts in 69
Optimism 206
Organic defects 76
Organic mental disorders 267
Organism, behavior of 49
Organization 87, 95
   tree 88f
Organizational psychology 10
Overcompensation 189
Overlearning 88, 89f, 99
Oxidation 98

P

Paired comparison method 215
Pan Posthema's case 286
Pancreas 31
Paper-pencil test 280
Parapsychology 10, 57
Parasympathetic nervous system 29
Paresthesia 55
Partial reinforcement schedule 70
Pass along test 129
Pattern drawing test 129
Pavlov's experiment 64
Peplau's interpersonal theory 257, 261t
Perception 44, 49, 76
Perceptual organization 50
Performance
   Bhatia's battery of 129, 280
   tests 130, 280
Peripheral nervous system 24, 28
Peripheral theories 202
Personal adjustment 268
Personal frustrations 161
Personal inadequacies 160
Personality 220, 239
   anatomy of 225
   assessment 234, 240
      techniques of 233
   classifications of 221
   development 237
      theories of 224
   disorders 267
   dynamics 227
   Eysenck's theory 225
   factors of 223, 280, 330
   humanistic theory of 225

inventories 234
structure of 225, 226f
subsystems of 225
tests 223, 280
types 174
Phallic stage 252
Phenylketonuria 135
Physical
   change 254
   development 238
   discomfort 301
   factors 270
   symptoms 171
Physiological changes 196
   measurement of 199
Physiological motives 148
Physiological psychology 10
Piaget's intellectual stages 257, 258, 258t
Piaget's scheme 246
Piaget's system 123
Piaget's theory, criticism of 125
Picture arrangement test 130
Picture construction test 129
Political psychology 10
Polygraph-lie detector 199
Positive attitudes 215
Positive emotions 205
Positive punishment 70
Posture sense 45
Power
   motives 150
   test 279
Practical experiment 137, 142, 240
Practice periods, distribution of 77
Pregnancy, complications of 172
Pressure 166, 174
Primary emotions 196, 196f
Primary motives 148
Proactive inhibition 94, 94t
Professionalism 337
Projection, phenomenon of 236
Projective techniques 234
Projective tests 235, 236, 280

Promote positive feelings 207
Proper learning method 98
Proximity 50, 51t
Psyche, topographical description of 227
Psychoactive drugs 21
Psychoanalysis 4
Psychoanalytic approach 245
Psychoanalytical theory 224
Psychokinesis 57
Psychological amnesia 97
Psychological development 238
Psychological feedback 77
Psychological tests 279
   kinds of 279
   purpose of 279
Psychological theories 152, 154
Psychology 1-3, 11, 12, 14, 15, 29, 146, 293
   abnormal 10
   beginnings of 1
   father of 3, 16
   importance of 11
   methods of 6
   schools of 4
   scope of 9
   subfields of 9
   systems of 4
Psychosexual disorders 267
Psychosexual stages 226
Psychosocial development theory, relevance of 229
Psychosomatic diseases 177
Psychosomatic illness 208
Psychotherapy 271
   use in 66
Psychotic disorders 267
Psychoticism 280
Puberty 254
Public opinion polling 215
Pull theories 154
Punishment 70
Pure psychology, branches of 10, 10t

Q

Questionnaires 234, 280
    method 296

R

Rank order method 215
Rapid breathing 171
Rating scale 280, 281
Raven's progressive matrices 280
RB Cattell's 16 personal factors test 280
Reaction formation 189
Readiness, law of 64
Recall, process of 91
Referent confusion 301
Regression 189
Reinforcement 69
    schedules of 70
Reinforcers, types of 69
Repression theory 93
Respiratory drive 149
Retention curve 87f
Retrieval 84
    problems 95
Retroactive inhibition 93, 93t
Rhyming system 99
Rorschach's ink blot test 236, 280
Rote plus reasoning 306
RPM test booklet 137

S

Sadness 206
Sarcasm 305
Schachter-Singer theory 204, 205f
Scholastic aptitude test 142, 297
    scores 133f
Segregation, law of 37
Self, development of 246
Self-confidence 206
Self-criticism 171
Self-development, field of 12
Self-efficacy 232
Self-image, growth of 229
Self-observation method 6
Self-sufficiency 20
Semantic memory 86
Semantotonic 222
Senile dementia 96
Sensation 44, 45
    plus interpretation 49
    psychology of 29
Sense organs 27, 29, 45, 45t
    functioning of 49
Sensorimotor 123
Sensorimotor stage 123
Sensory experience 45, 45t
Sensory memory 84, 86f, 91
    functions of 85
    types of 84
Sensory perception, abnormalities in 54
Sensory process 45
Sentence completion test 236, 237, 280
Sentiments 210
Septic tonsils 20
Sex drive 149
Sex glands 239
Sex urge, functioning of 237
Sexual behaviour, abnormal 267
Sheldon's classification 224
Shooting line 306
Sigmund Freud psychosexual theory 225
Sign learning, Tolman's theory of 75
Simple reactions 165
Situational tests 280
Skeletal muscles 30
Skill learning 62
Sleep drive 149
Sleeping, difficulty in 171
Smell 45
Social cognitive theory 230, 231f
Social distance scales 215
Social factors 239, 270
Social intelligence 72, 118
Social learning theory, applications of 73

Social psychology 10
   scope of 328
Social readjustment rating scale 173*t*
Social relationships 236
Socialization 246
Sociometry 297
Soft skills 336, 337
Somatic nervous system 28
Somatoform disorders 267
Space binocular depth cues, perception of 53
Spatial intelligence 121
Spearman's two factor theory 119
Speech, manner of 305
Speed test 279
Spinal cord 26
Stanford-Binet test 127, 280
State dependent memory 95
Stereoscopic vision 53
Stimuli, grouping of 50
Stimulus
   intensity of 46
   location of 46
   material, perception of 91
   nature of 46
Stop clock 137, 142
Stress 170, 174, 177, 182
   chronic societal sources of 174
   management 170
   reaction 178
   sources of 172
   symptoms of 171
   types of 172
Strong's vocational interest blank 297
Structural theories 118
Structuralism 4
Student nurse, personality description of 280
Study, unit of 329
Studying psychology, relevance of 13
Subject, motivation of 236
Sublimation 186
Submissiveness 165
Substance use disorders 267
Sudden emotion 19
Sulci 28
Summated rating scales, Likert's method of 215
Superego 226
Suppression 190
Survey method 8
Sweet lemon 185
Symmetry 51
Sympathetic division 196
Sympathetic nervous system 29
Systematic desensitization 67
Systematic observation 7

T

Task-oriented reaction pattern 165
Taste 45
Teacher
   functions of 316
   personal qualities 305
   problems 302
   role of 316
Teaching quality 318
Teamwork 337
Tegmentum 26
Telencephalon 26
Telepathy 57
Terri's case 212
Terri's negative attitude 212
Tests, types of 325, 325*fc*
Thematic apperception test 236, 280
Theoretical perspectives 245
Theories adopting
   developmental approach 225
   trait approaches 225
Thinking
   four stages of development of 123
   kinds of 104
Thirst drive 148
Three memory process 84
Thurston's scale 215
Thyroid 31
   glands 239
Tolman's theory 75

Tongue, tip of 86
Training aids, value of 307
Trait approach 223
Trait theories 232
Transmission
    manner of 305
    methods of 304
Tuberculosis 172
Turner's syndrome 38
Two factor theory 204

U
Ulcers 171
Unconscious 227

V
Verbal communication 113
Verbal group intelligence tests 130
Verbal individual intelligence test 130
Verbal learning 62
Verbal test 280
Verbalism 301
Verification 108
Violent reactions 165
Vision 45
Visual monocular cues 53
Voice 305

W
Wastes, elimination of 149
Wechsler scales 129
Wechsler tests 129
Word association test 236, 237, 280
Working memory 85
Writing materials 137, 142, 240

Y
Yerkes-Dodson law 153, 153f
Yoga 178
Young adulthood 254